RHEUMATOLOGY & ORTHOPAEDICS

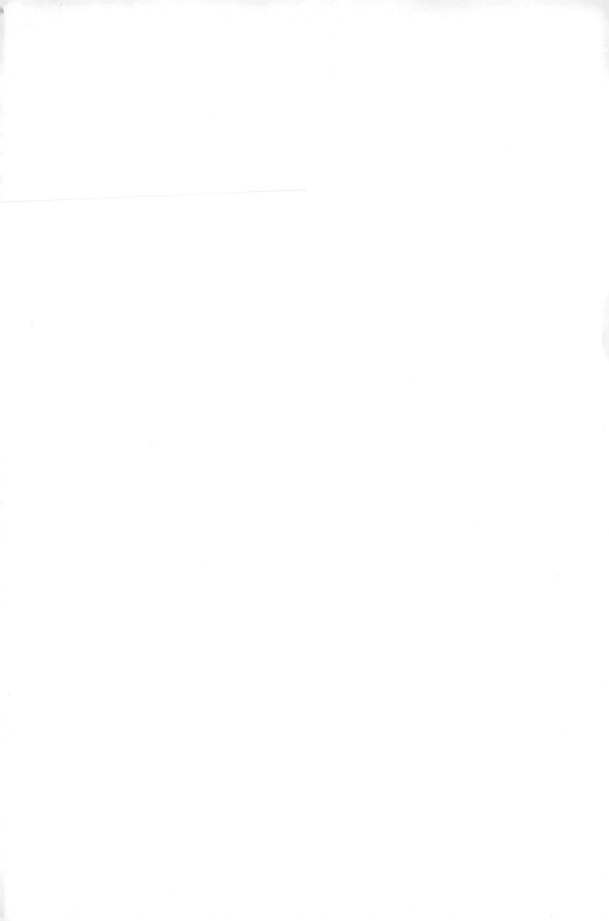

RHEUMATOLOGY & ORTHOPAEDICS

Andrew Brown MBChB MRCP PhD
Senior Lecturer in Medical Education and Rheumatology, Hull York Medical School, University of York
Consultant Rheumatologist, York Teaching Hospital NHS Foundation Trust

Maria Slade BSc (Hons) MBChB (Hons) MRCP MSc
Specialist Registrar in Rheumatology
Health Education England Yorkshire and the Humber

Helen Ingoe MBBS MRCSEd MD MSc PGCert
Specialist Registrar in Trauma and Orthopaedics
Health Education England North East, Newcastle Hospitals Foundation NHS Trust

Alan Middleton MBChB FRCSEd (Tr & Orth)
Consultant Trauma and Orthopaedic Surgeon
North Tees and Hartlepool NHS Foundation Trust

Scion

© **Scion Publishing Ltd, 2021**

ISBN 9781911510673

First published 2021

A CIP catalogue record for this book is available from the British Library.

Scion Publishing Limited

The Old Hayloft, Vantage Business Park, Bloxham Road, Banbury OX16 9UX, UK
www.scionpublishing.com

Important Note from the Publisher

The information contained within this book was obtained by Scion Publishing Ltd from sources believed by us to be reliable. However, while every effort has been made to ensure its accuracy, no responsibility for loss or injury whatsoever occasioned to any person acting or refraining from action as a result of information contained herein can be accepted by the authors or publishers.

Readers are reminded that medicine is a constantly evolving science and while the authors and publishers have ensured that all dosages, applications and practices are based on current indications, there may be specific practices which differ between communities. You should always follow the guidelines laid down by the manufacturers of specific products and the relevant authorities in the country in which you are practising.

Although every effort has been made to ensure that all owners of copyright material have been acknowledged in this publication, we would be pleased to acknowledge in subsequent reprints or editions any omissions brought to our attention.

Registered names, trademarks, etc. used in this book, even when not marked as such, are not to be considered unprotected by law.

Line artwork by Matthew McClements at Blink Studio Ltd (www.blink.biz)
Cartoons by James Pollitt (www.jamespollitt-graphicnarratives.co.uk)
Cover design by Andrew Magee Design Ltd
Typeset by Evolution Design & Digital Ltd, Kent, UK
Printed in the UK
Last digit is the print number: 10 9 8 7 6 5 4 3 2 1

Contents

Preface

Musculoskeletal conditions are common and a leading cause of disability and chronic pain worldwide. Rheumatology and Orthopaedics are specialties that manage a spectrum of emergency, acute and chronic conditions, affecting patients of all ages.

This book will help you to navigate these varied presentations, whether you are seeing a patient in primary care, an outpatient clinic or the emergency department.

The first chapter guides you through basic musculoskeletal anatomy and physiology. The second chapter introduces the essential clinical tools you need to assess the musculoskeletal patient.

Armed with this foundation, the clinical chapters go on to discuss important musculoskeletal conditions. A clinical case at the start of each chapter describes a typical presentation of a selected condition and guides you through important clinical reasoning steps, explaining the pertinent investigations and outlining the appropriate management. We also use 'starter questions' to test your existing knowledge, inspire interest and direct you towards the key points in each chapter. Colourful figures and photographs of clinical signs make the information more memorable and easy to digest, and we have highlighted key clinical learning points in yellow 'tips' boxes. Cartoons bring cases to life and introduce some of the wider issues that you need to be aware of in order to offer the best possible care for your patient.

The final chapter offers you some single best answer questions to test your knowledge and prepare for your exams.

We hope this book gives you the confidence to assess an individual presenting with a musculoskeletal problem, the knowledge to recognise an emergency and the awareness of appropriate initial management and onward referral.

Andrew Brown
Maria Slade
Helen Ingoe
Alan Middleton

Acknowledgements

We wish to thank patients and colleagues at York Teaching Hospital, Royal Victoria Infirmary Newcastle upon Tyne, Harrogate District Hospital and Leeds Teaching Hospitals.

Special thanks go to:

Dr David King, Consultant Radiologist at York Teaching Hospital, for providing images.

Dr Neal Larkman, Consultant Radiologist at Harrogate Hospital, for providing images and annotations.

Alison Styles, Physiotherapist at Harrogate Hospital, for the use and explanation of equipment for photographs in *Chapter 2*.

Kirstie Neat, Occupational Therapist at Chapel Allerton Hospital, for assisting with photographs of occupational therapy aids in *Chapter 2*.

Dr Lorraine Green at Chapel Allerton Hospital, for providing nail capillaroscopy images (Figure 4.9) with detailed explanations, for *Chapter 4*.

Dr Andrew Grainger of Cambridge University Hospitals (previously Leeds Teaching Hospitals), for providing the plain radiograph of rickets (Figure 5.4) in *Chapter 5*.

Dr Alvin Karsandas, Consultant Radiologist at Newcastle Hospitals, for providing radiographic images.

And finally, very warm thanks to the patients who have allowed their photographs to be published in the interests of medical education.

We also would like to thank our families, friends and colleagues for their support during the writing of this book.

Abbreviations

ACE	angiotensin-converting enzyme		**CMCJ**	carpometacarpal joint
ACh	acetylcholine		**CNS**	central nervous system
ACL	anterior cruciate ligament		**COX**	cyclooxygenase
ACPA	anti-citrullinated protein antibody		**CPA**	citrullinated protein antibody
ADL	activities of daily living		**CPK**	creatine phosphokinase
ADP	adenosine diphosphate		**CPPD**	calcium pyrophosphate dihydrate
ALP	alkaline phosphatase		**CRP**	C-reactive protein
ALT	alanine aminotransferase		**CSF**	cerebrospinal fluid
ANA	antinuclear antibody		**CT**	computed tomography
ANS	autonomic nervous system		**CTS**	carpal tunnel syndrome
AOSD	adult onset Still's disease		**DAS**	Disease Activity Score
AP	anterior–posterior		**DDH**	developmental dysplasia of the hip
APLS	antiphospholipid syndrome		**DEXA**	dual energy X-ray absorptiometry
aSpA	axial spondyloarthritis		**DIC**	disseminated intravascular coagulation
AST	aspartate aminotransferase		**DIP**	distal interphalangeal
ATP	adenosine triphosphate		**DIPJ**	distal interphalangeal joint
AVN	avascular necrosis		**DMARD**	disease-modifying antirheumatic drug
bDMARD	biologic DMARD			
BMD	bone mineral density		**dsDNA**	double-stranded DNA
BMI	body mass index		**DVT**	deep vein thrombosis
bpm	beats per minute		**ECM**	extracellular matrix
CASPAR	ClASsification criteria for Psoriatic ARthritis		**ECRB**	extensor carpi radialis brevis
			EDS	Ehlers–Danlos syndrome
CCP	cyclic citrullinated peptide		**eGFR**	estimated GFR
CK	creatine kinase		**EGPA**	eosinophilic granulomatosis with polyangiitis
CKD	chronic kidney disease			
CKD–MBD	chronic kidney disease – mineral and bone disorder		**EMG**	electromyography
			ENA	extractable nuclear antigen
CMC	carpometacarpal		**ENT**	ear, nose and throat

ESR	erythrocyte sedimentation rate		**NAI**	non-accidental injury
FBC	full blood count		**nbDMARD**	non-biologic DMARD
FDG	fludeoxyglucose		**NCS**	nerve conduction studies
FPL	flexor pollicis longus		**Nr-aSpA**	non-radiographic aSpA
GABA	gamma-aminobutyric acid		**NSAID**	non-steroidal, anti-inflammatory drug
GALS	gait, arms, legs, spine		**OA**	osteoarthritis
GCA	giant cell arteritis		**OI**	osteogenesis imperfecta
GCT	giant cell tumour		**PAN**	polyarteritis nodosa
GFR	glomerular filtration rate		**PCL**	posterior cruciate ligament
GGT	gamma glutamyl transferase		**PET**	positron emission tomography
GI	gastrointestinal		**PIP**	proximal interphalangeal
GPA	granulomatosis with polyangiitis		**PIPJ**	proximal interphalangeal joint
HIV	human immunodeficiency virus		**PMR**	polymyalgia rheumatica
HLA	human leucocyte antigen		**PNS**	peripheral nervous system
HRCT	high resolution CT		**POP**	plaster of Paris
IBD	inflammatory bowel disease		**PPI**	proton pump inhibitor
ICE	ideas, concerns, expectations		**PsA**	psoriatic arthritis
IL	interleukin		**pSpA**	peripheral SpA
IMRT	intensity-modulated radiation therapy		**PTH**	parathyroid hormone
INR	international normalised ratio		**PV**	plasma viscosity
IPJ	interphalangeal joint		**RA**	rheumatoid arthritis
IV	intravenous		**RANK**	receptor activator of nuclear factor kappa-B
JAK	Janus kinase		**RF**	rheumatoid factor
LCL	lateral collateral ligament		**SCFE**	slipped capital femoral epiphysis
LFT	liver function test		**SIJ**	sacroiliac joint
MCH	mean cell haemoglobin		**SIRS**	systemic inflammatory response syndrome
MCL	medial collateral ligament		**SLE**	systemic lupus erythematosus
MCP	metacarpophalangeal		**SpA**	spondyloarthritis
MCPJ	MCP joint		**STI**	sexually transmitted infection
MCV	mean corpuscular volume		**TB**	tuberculosis
MDT	multidisciplinary team		**TENS**	transcutaneous electrical nerve stimulation
MPA	microscopic polyangiitis		**TNF**	tumour necrosis factor
MPO	myeloperoxidase		**TPMT**	thiopurine methyltransferase
MRI	magnetic resonance imaging		**TSH**	thyroid-stimulating hormone
MSC	mesenchymal stem cell		**U&Es**	urea and electrolytes
MSU	monosodium urate		**UTI**	urinary tract infection
MTP	metatarsophalangeal		**WCC**	white cell count
MTX	methotrexate			
NAC	*N*-acetylcysteine			

Chapter 1
First principles

Answers to questions are to be found in *Section 1.17*.

Starter questions

Overview of the musculoskeletal system

1. Where would you take a bone marrow biopsy? i.e. what type of bones store the reddest marrow?

Development of the musculoskeletal system

2. What are the secondary ossification centres of the distal humerus and when do they appear?

3. How are fingers and toes formed?

4. Why are growth plates radiolucent on radiographs?

The immune system in musculoskeletal disease

5. Why are women more predisposed to autoimmune disease than men?

6. Why are people with rheumatoid arthritis more prone to having heart attacks?

7. Why are people more at risk of autoimmune disease in temperate climates?

Bone anatomy and physiology

8. Does increasing dietary calcium make bones strong?

9. What are the consequences of reaming (removing the bone with a drill) the canal of the long bones to insert an intramedullary nail on fracture healing?

10. What effect does reduced weight bearing have on bones?

The nervous system

11. At what vertebral level would you undertake a lumbar puncture?

12. What clinical signs and symptoms would be present if only the right side of the spinal cord at L1 is transected?

13. How does Botox work?

Muscles and soft tissues

14. What is a muscle strain?

15. What is rhabdomyolysis?

Locomotion

16. What are static and dynamic joint stabilisers?

17. How is gait assessed?

18. How does a prosthetic limb affect gait?

1.1 Overview of the musculoskeletal system

The musculoskeletal system comprises the bony skeleton and other supporting connective tissues such as ligaments, cartilage, tendons and joints. Its function is to provide support and protection for the internal organs and to allow movement, both of which are important for survival. The bony skeleton is also the biggest store of calcium and produces almost all blood cells.

1.1.1 Skeleton

The skeleton has four principal roles:
- locomotion (movement)
- protection of organs
- calcium metabolism
- production of blood cells (haematopoiesis).

Protection
Vital organs such as the heart and lungs are protected by the ribcage; the brain and spinal cord by the skull and vertebrae; and pelvic organs by the bony pelvis. The abdomen is unprotected by the skeleton and damage to internal organs can be catastrophic. Fractures to the bones protecting the organs, although painful, often readily heal within weeks.

Calcium metabolism
Calcium and phosphate levels are maintained in the bloodstream by regulating how much is stored within the skeleton. The mechanism of fine tuning the mineral levels in the blood is one of the many homeostatic mechanisms maintaining balances within the body.

Production of blood cells
All bones contain marrow in their core, an area of the bone which is highly vascular and where all blood cells are made in the body. It is also where lymphocytes – the body's immune cells – are made and stored. In the adult human, the most active haematopoietic bones are the flat bones (pelvis and sternum); in children the long bones, thymus, spleen and lymph nodes also produce blood cells.

1.1.2 Connective tissue
Connective tissues facilitate movement of the skeleton and include:
- muscle
- ligament
- cartilage
- tendon.

Each muscle is attached to the bone at an origin and insertion on either side of a joint. By contracting and relaxing they produce movement at the joints.
- The **origin** of a muscle is its direct attachment to the bone proximally (towards the centre of the body).
- The **insertion** is its indirect attachment distally (further away from the body), usually via a tendon.

Ligaments directly attach bone to bone. They do not produce active movement but provide a check rein to joints, allowing some gliding but preventing dislocation.

Cartilage is the smooth, hard covering of an area on the surface of a bone where it forms a joint with another bone. Cartilage allows smooth gliding of the two bone surfaces with respect to each other and prevents wear of the bones at the joints. An alternative name for a joint is an articulation; the cartilaginous surface is referred to as the articular surface.

1.2 Embryology

The formation of the musculoskeletal system *in utero* derives from two primary germ layers: the ectoderm – which forms the rudimentary spinal cord and brain – and the mesoderm, forming most of the muscles, bones and cartilage (**Table 1.1**).

Table 1.1 *Embryological cells involved in the formation of the musculoskeletal system*

Primary germ layer	Somites	Precursor cells	Adult tissue
Ectoderm	Neural crests	Neuroblasts	Dorsal root ganglia Sensory nerves
			Anterior root ganglia Motor nerves
Mesoderm	Dermomyotome	Dermoblasts	Skin
		Myoblasts	Muscle
	Sclerotome	Chondroblasts	Cartilage
		Osteoblasts	Bone
		Fibroblasts	Tendon/ligament

1.2.1 Ectoderm

Neural tube

Ectoderm is the outermost layer of the developing embryo (**Figure 1.1a**). During the first few weeks it thickens and folds in towards itself to make the neural tube – the precursor of the central nervous system and the spinal cord (**Figure 1.1b**). The 'in' folding of the neural plate is influenced by chemical factors secreted from the notochord – mesoderm that eventually forms the vertebral discs. These factors help the closure of the neural tube and form the neural crests that spread outwards and lie on either side of the tube (**Figure 1.1c**).

> **Folate is a key nutrient in the diet that helps closure of the neural tube.** Failure of the neural tube to close can lead to a birth defect in which the spinal cord and its coverings are exposed, known as spina bifida.

Neural crests

The crests are able to differentiate into several cell types but in general form the peripheral nervous system by expanding into the newly formed limb buds. Sensory nerves are formed at the back of the embryo (dorsal root ganglia) and motor nerves are formed at the front (anterior root ganglia). The formation of a nerve plexus (a group of closely related nerves) enters the premuscle tissue that has surrounded the skeletal core of the limb. Even at this early stage the muscles are arranged in groups and intermuscular septa (thin dividing layers) are seen.

1.2.2 Mesoderm

The mesoderm is the middle layer of the developing embryo, appearing early at week 3. It has three distinct components: the paraxial (nearest the centre), intermediate and lateral (furthest from the centre) plate mesoderm.

Early development

Somites

The paraxial mesoderm forms paired buds called somites which are the precursors of the developed muscles, cartilage, bone and skin (**Figure 1.1d**). The intermediate mesoderm forms the kidneys, bladder and gonads and the lateral plate mesoderm forms the limbs and circulatory systems. The precursor of the axial skeleton starts to form at week 3 with the paired somites derived from para-axial mesoderm. By week 5 there are paired somites for each of the vertebrae: 4 occipital, 7 cervical, 12 thoracic, 5 lumbar, 5 sacral and 3–5 coccygeal vertebrae.

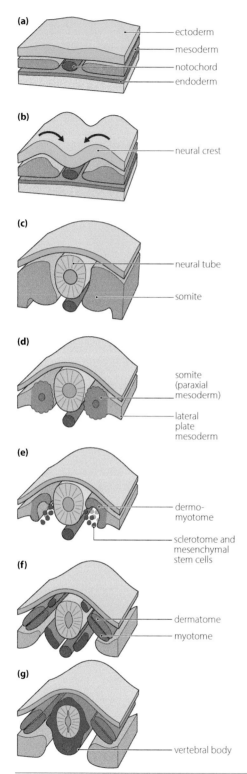

(a)
— ectoderm
— mesoderm
— notochord
— endoderm

(b)
— neural crest

(c)
— neural tube
— somite

(d)
— somite (paraxial mesoderm)
— lateral plate mesoderm

(e)
— dermo-myotome
— sclerotome and mesenchymal stem cells

(f)
— dermatome
— myotome

(g)
— vertebral body

Figure 1.1 The neural tube and vertebral column are formed from the mesoderm, endoderm and ectoderm.

Sclerotome and dermomyotome

Each somite divides into two parts – the **sclerotome** (**Figure 1.1e**), which appears closest to the neural tube and specifically goes on to form cartilage, bone or ligaments; and the **dermomyotome**, which forms furthest away from the neural tube and produces either a **myotome**, which is a muscle precursor, or a **dermatome** – a skin precursor (**Figures 1.1f** and **g**).

Mesenchymal stem cells

The mesodermal cells of the sclerotomes form a jelly-like substance known as mesenchyme. The mesenchymal stem cells (MSCs) are able to differentiate into three different cell types. Fibroblasts produce ligaments and tendons, osteoblasts produce bone and chondroblasts produce cartilage (**Table 1.2**).

Formation of the axial skeleton

The vertebral bones are formed when the paired sclerotomes come together. The cranial part (towards the head) of one sclerotome and the caudal part (tail end) of the sclerotome above fuse, forming a column around the notochord which is a rod-like structure of mesoderm. The mesenchymal cells go on to form the intervertebral disc between the vertebral bodies. The notochord enlarges in and around the intervertebral disc, forming the central spongy nucleus pulposus. The vertebral bodies, the weight-bearing part of the spine, form in between each segment as the notochord regresses.

Formation of the limbs

Limb buds form at week 4 as an outgrowth of the lateral mesoderm plate covered with ectoderm (**Figure 1.2**). The advancing ectodermal cells form the apical ridge, which thickens as the limb bud grows. The limb extends longitudinally and by week 5 a limb paddle is formed distally. The limbs rotate through 90° so that the thumbs turn outwards and the big toes turn inwards. The apical ridge then starts a process of programmed cell death within the web spaces to form digits.

Table 1.2 *Cells involved in the formation and remodelling of musculoskeletal tissues*

Description	Cell	Function
Forming cells (-*blast*)	Osteoblast	Forms extracellular matrix and collagen in bone
	Chondroblast	Forms extracellular matrix and collagen in cartilage
	Fibroblast	Forms extracellular matrix and collagen in connective tissue
	Myoblast	Muscle-forming cell
Mature cell (-*cyte*)	Osteocyte	Mature bone cell
	Chondrocyte	Mature cartilage cell
	Fibrocyte	Mature connective tissue cell
	Myocyte	Mature muscle cell
Resorbing cell (-*clast*)	Osteoclast	Resorbs bone cells
	Chondroclast	Resorbs calcified cartilage

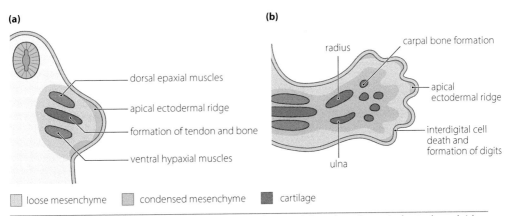

(a)

- dorsal epaxial muscles
- apical ectodermal ridge
- formation of tendon and bone
- ventral hypaxial muscles

(b)

- radius
- carpal bone formation
- apical ectodermal ridge
- interdigital cell death and formation of digits
- ulna

☐ loose mesenchyme   ☐ condensed mesenchyme   ■ cartilage

Figure 1.2 The limb buds are formed from the mesoderm and the advancing apical ectodermal ridge: (a) week 4; (b) week 5–6.

Cartilage and joints

The MSCs condense and differentiate into chondrocytes, firstly in the shaft or centre of the newly forming long bones. Joints are formed in a process of resorption and cavitation of the newly formed primitive cartilage, known as segmentation. The process of developing bone is known as ossification and starts when the embryo is 8 weeks old.

Children with limb defects often have other congenital abnormalities and several syndromes are well known. **VACTERL** is a syndrome in which there are abnormalities in the structures derived from mesoderm. It is associated with **V**ertebral anomalies, **A**nal atresia, **C**ardiac malformations, **T**racheo-o**E**sophageal fistula, **R**enal anomalies/**R**adial aplasia and **L**imb anomalies.

Muscles

Skeletal muscle is derived from the myotomes of the paraxial mesoderm. It follows the lateral plate mesoderm to form the limb buds. The myotome is split into a large anterior hypaxial division forming all the limb muscles and the flexor muscles of the trunk, and a smaller posterior epaxial division forming the extensor muscles of the back. Myoblasts are mesenchymal cells that produce skeletal muscle and are seen at 3 months' gestation, producing myofibrils which are components of adult muscle (see *Section 1.14.6*).

1.3 Skeletal development in childhood

Ossification or osteogenesis is the formation of bone and describes both the formation of bone in the embryo as well as the process of forming new bone after a fracture. There are two types of bone formation.

- **Intramembranous** ossification forms the flat bones (clavicles, sternum and facial bones) and is formed directly from MSCs and not from cartilage.
- **Endochondral** ossification forms the long bones and has a cartilage precursor.

1.3.1 Intramembranous ossification

Intramembranous ossification is a four-step process by which new bone forms without having to first make cartilage (**Figure 1.3**). Within the mesenchyme, MSCs replicate and group together tightly to form the ossification site. The MSCs turn into osteoblasts, the cells that form bone (**Figure 1.3a**). The central osteoblasts begin to directly make osteoid which is an uncalcified matrix. A ring of osteoblasts is formed and the central osteoid calcifies and hardens within a few days. As more osteoblasts are made, they get stuck in the osteoid that they produce. These osteoblasts then transform to become osteocytes, which are mature bone cells (**Figure 1.3b**). New capillaries are formed and osteoid is deposited around it, forming the trabecular matrix of woven bone (**Figure 1.3c**) (see *Section 1.8.2*). Periosteum is a thick covering of connective tissue that forms on the outer surface of the bone and is formed from the mesenchyme (**Figure 1.3d**). Underneath the periosteal layer compact bone forms.

1.3.2 Endochondral ossification

Endochondral ossification is the process in which long bones and some short bones are formed from cartilage at the primary and secondary ossification sites (**Figure 1.4**). These ossification

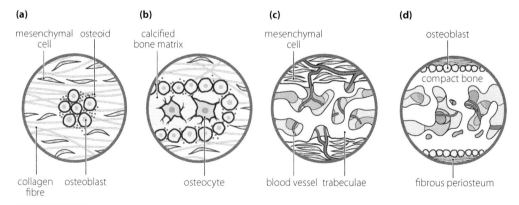

(a) mesenchymal cell   osteoid   collagen fibre   osteoblast

(b) calcified bone matrix   osteocyte

(c) mesenchymal cell   blood vessel   trabeculae

(d) osteoblast   compact bone   fibrous periosteum

Figure 1.3 Bone is formed directly from mesenchymal stem cells without the formation of a cartilage precursor: (a) development of ossification centre; (b) calcification; (c) formation of trabeculae; (d) formation of periosteum.

(a) IN EMBRYO   **(b)** IN FOETUS   **(c)** IN CHILD

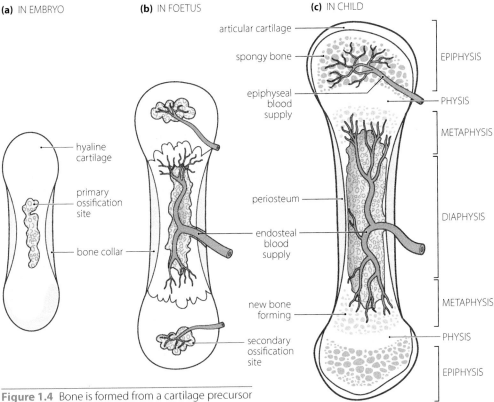

Figure 1.4 Bone is formed from a cartilage precursor by the process of endochondral ossification.

sites are responsible for the length of the bone. The periosteum on long bones covers the diaphysis but not the joint surfaces at the epiphysis; it is responsible for increasing the circumference and strength.

Primary ossification site

Chondrocytes are cells that produce cartilage. During foetal development they condense into a small area, forming a primitive cartilage matrix where the centre of the bone will form (**Figure 1.4a**). A perichondral layer surrounds the primitive cartilage matrix, formed at 6–8 weeks after conception. It then calcifies. Nutrients required to form new chondrocytes are disrupted when the matrix becomes calcified, causing the chondrocytes to fail and disintegrate. Spaces are left when the chondrocytes disintegrate and are then replaced by blood vessels that deliver bone-forming cells (**Figure 1.4b**).

A periosteal collar is formed encircling the cartilage matrix and provides a support for osteocytes to start laying down bone. The perichondral layer transforms into bone, forming the periosteum (**Figure 1.4c**). In children the periosteum is thick, as it is also full of osteoblasts producing calcified bone which increases the circumference (appositional growth).

The primary ossification site replaces the cartilage matrix in the middle of the bone. It is from this primary ossification site that the bone grows longitudinally to form the length. Soft cartilage is laid down by the chondrocytes and it elongates; however, it is progressively resorbed by osteoclasts (bone-resorbing cells). After the osteoclasts resorb the bone, osteoid (mature bone) is laid down by osteoblasts and it is then calcified. A vascular supply is formed from within the bone, known as the nutrient artery. It transports the bone-forming osteoblasts away from the primary ossification centre and towards the growing ends of the bone. The primary ossification centre forms the diaphysis of the bone.

Secondary ossification site

Secondary ossification centres form dense cartilage at each end of each bone after birth (except the distal femur, in which they are already present from 36 weeks' gestation). The secondary ossification centre has its own blood supply that enters into the ends of the bone, delivering firstly the osteoclasts that break down the cartilage, followed by osteoblasts that lay down osteoid. This secondary ossification centre forms the epiphysis.

1.3.3 The growth plate

The growth plate (**Figure 1.5**), also known as the physis, is the area between the metaphysis and the epiphysis. In the growing child the physis is where most of the length of the bone is formed by endochondral ossification, i.e. from cartilage. The physis is a layered structure in which the chondrocyte cells graduate and become larger as they travel from the epiphysis towards the metaphysis. The cartilaginous matrix that is formed is invaded by the metaphyseal blood supply that feeds osteoblasts and osteoclasts that replace the cartilage with osteoid, the mature bone.

> **Achondroplasia** is a congenital deformity in which patients are short in stature due to a failure to produce chondrocytes at the physis. As intramembranous ossification and periosteal ossification are normal, the long bones have a normal circumference but are short and the flat bones form normally.

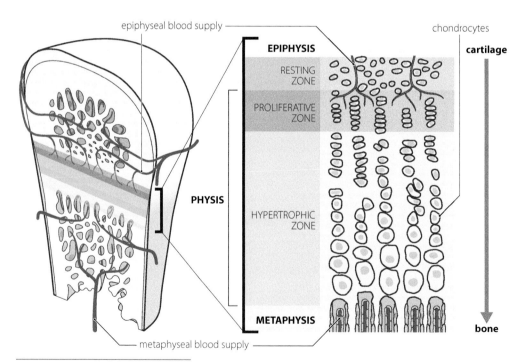

Figure 1.5 The physis (growth plate).

The elbow is a common site for injury in children and fractures can often be mistaken for normal secondary ossification sites (**Figure 1.6**). The secondary ossification sites form and ossify at different times during maturation and can be remembered by the mnemonic **'CRITOL'** (**Table 1.3**).

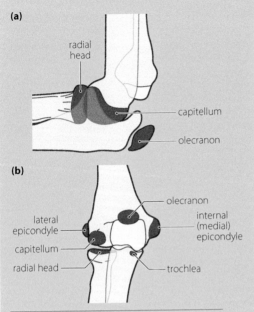

(a)

radial head

capitellum

olecranon

(b)

olecranon

lateral epicondyle

internal (medial) epicondyle

capitellum

radial head

trochlea

Figure 1.6 Ossification centres of the elbow: (a) lateral; (b) posterior view.

Table 1.3 *Formation of the ossification centres around the elbow; females usually ossify one year before males*

Ossification centre	Age at formation (years)	Age at fusion (years)
Capitellum	2	12
Radial head	4	15
Internal epicondyle	6	17
Trochlea	8	12
Olecranon	10	15
Lateral epicondyle	12	12

1.4 The immune system in musculoskeletal disease

The immune system is vital in the defence against infection and in organising repair of tissues following insult. When it becomes deregulated, immune deficiency or autoimmune disease occur. Elements of the musculoskeletal system, particularly joints and connective tissue, are affected by several such deficiencies and diseases. Knowledge of normal pathways, the immune cells and chemical messengers of the immune system will help you understand the effects of autoimmune disease and the immunological targets for new and emerging treatments.

1.4.1 Innate and adaptive immunity

When a 'non-self' material is present, the immune system detects the abnormality and responds with a complex set of interactions between different cell types and communicator molecules. These types of immunity are often distinguished by the terms *innate* (rapid non-specific response) and *adaptive* (slow specific response), but this is arbitrary as usually both processes are complementary and begin at the same time. Inflammation inevitably occurs before the cells and chemicals act to dampen down the response, allowing healing of the host tissue. Examples of 'non-self' are a bacterium or virus, or a cancer cell where mutations occur to the point where a cell no longer resembles its host tissue.

1.4.2 Innate immunity

Innate immunity is the rapid response to a foreign object or tissue. It is non-specific and comprises both physical defence and cellular response. In the musculoskeletal system, skin acts as a primary barrier to infection or injury, whilst the joint capsule provides an internal barrier. Cells of the innate immune system are myelocytes, e.g. macrophages and dendritic cells. They circulate continuously and are primed to identify foreign particles and mount an attack.

Complement

Part of the innate immune response, the complement system comprises a large number of proteins. In their activated form (following stimulation from foreign materials) these proteins act firstly to stimulate the adaptive immune response; they then coat foreign particles and attract macrophages. The proteins C3 and C4 play a major role in the complement cascade and are of clinical relevance in monitoring disease activity in autoimmune disease, e.g. systemic lupus erythematosus (SLE) (see *Sections 2.6.11* and *4.4*).

1.4.3 Adaptive immunity

Adaptive immunity is a targeted response built up over time, although it can be initiated rapidly. Adaptive immune responses are characterised by their ability to bring about a specific, tailored response and provide the immune system with memory. It is the adaptive system that is the main driver in the development of autoimmunity. Cells of adaptive immunity are lymphocytes. **Table 1.4** shows some of the different cells involved in both the adaptive and the innate immune responses.

1.5 Chemical messengers of the immune system

Chemical messengers control the immune response and inflammation in a number of rheumatological diseases. It is these chemical messengers that are targets for specific immunological therapies (see *Section 2.8.5*).

1.5.1 Cytokines

Cytokines are the major chemical mediators of the immune response, helping to up- or down-regulate the cascade of inflammation at a given site. They are communicator molecules, which bind to receptors on the surface of cells, causing the cells to respond in a specific way:

■ pro-inflammatory cytokines such as tumour necrosis factor alpha (TNF-α), interleukin 1 (IL-1), IL-2 and IL-6. TNF-α is produced by many cells but predominantly by macrophages. It exerts its pro-inflammatory effects through changes in immune cell function; its role in inflammation is shown in **Figure 1.7**.

■ suppressants of inflammation when resolution of inflammation is required (the threat or antigen has been dealt with); e.g. IL-10.

Whilst acting locally, cytokines are responsible for the systemic effects of the acute phase response, including appetite suppression, pyrexia and lethargy.

1.5.2 Other messengers

Other compounds are also important in the interplay between cells (**Figure 1.8**), in particular:

■ prostaglandins and leukotrienes, molecules derived from arachidonic acid, act like hormones within a local area, regulating inflammation through vasodilatation and cell maturation

■ calcineurin is a protein phosphatase which activates T cells.

Table 1.4 *Cells involved in the innate and adaptive immune systems*

	Cell	Role	Relevance in disease
Innate (myelocytes)	Macrophage	Rapid phagocytosis of pathogen Development of inflammatory response by release of cytokines	Front-line cell for detecting and rapidly killing pathogens, initiating inflammatory cascade, recruiting other cells to area of damage Present in all immune responses
	Dendritic cell	Antigen presentation	Initiates the adaptive response, e.g. in infected joints and also in autoimmune disease
	Neutrophil	Killing of pathogens	Responsible for purulence, e.g. in infected joint Can cause significant collateral tissue damage
	Mast cell	Release of pro-inflammatory mediators and proteases	Present in acute inflammation (e.g. septic arthritis) but also chronic conditions
	Eosinophil	Degranulate to release toxic granules, killing pathogens, particularly parasites	Implicated in allergic reactions and vasculitis
Adaptive (lymphocytes)	B cells	Antibody production (plasma cells), cytokine secretion	Responsible for autoantibody formation in autoimmune disease
	T cells	T helper cells (CD4) boost inflammatory responses T killer cells/CD8 T cells kill infected cells and tumour cells T regulatory cells are anti-inflammatory	T helper cells enhance antibody production T regulatory cells act to balance response (may be important in the development of autoimmunity)

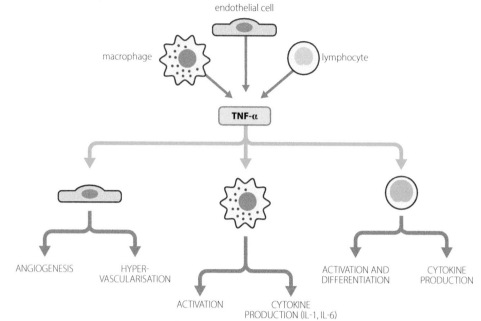

Figure 1.7 The role of TNF-α in inflammation.

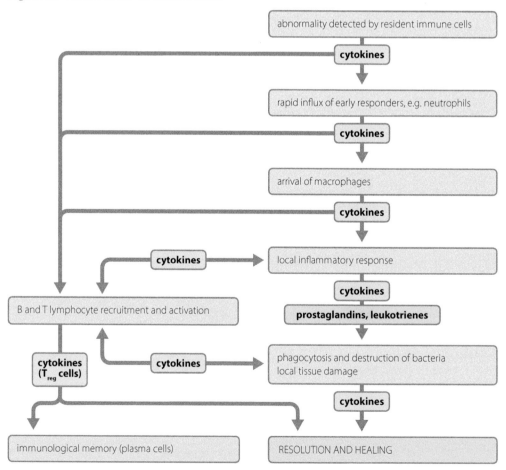

Figure 1.8 The role of cytokines in the immune response.

1.6 The role of the immune system in healing and infection

The immune system must act rapidly and efficiently to protect against infection and trauma. *Sections 1.6.1–1.6.3* describe three examples of its role and the consequences of its dysregulation within the musculoskeletal system: wound healing, infection and sepsis.

1.6.1 Wound healing

Following damage to host tissue, the immune system plays a role in coordinating the healing process. The stages of wound healing are shown in **Figure 1.9** and begin with clot formation. Platelets are cells in the blood that clump together to form a plug and release cytokines which attract immune cells to the site. Neutrophils and macrophages act to debride the wound area, phagocytosing foreign bodies and bacteria.

Macrophages also release reactive radicals, cytokines and growth factors (e.g. fibroblast growth factor and vascular endothelial growth factor). Fibroblasts are recruited to the area where there is active endothelial cell proliferation, angiogenesis and collagen synthesis.

People who are immunosuppressed experience difficulties with wound healing. For example, glucocorticosteroid drugs delay wound healing through effects such as reduced fibroblast proliferation, reduced collagen synthesis and de-amplification of chemical messengers in the inflammatory response.

An elevated white blood cell count is common after trauma and surgery. This can trigger concerns that there is an infection but often it simply represents a normal physiological response.

HAEMOSTASIS

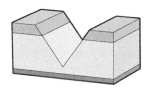
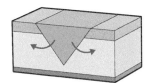

Platelets aggregate
Vasoconstriction
Cytokine release to attract leucocytes

INFLAMMATION

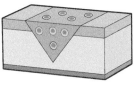

Leucocytes drive inflammatory response, attracting fibroblasts and activating endothelial cells

PROLIFERATION

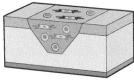

Fibroblasts proliferate
Epithelialisation occurs

MATURATION

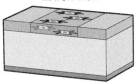

Fibroblasts remain for weeks or years
Remodelling of site

Figure 1.9 The stages of wound healing.

1.6.2 Infection

A joint or muscle is very different from the environment of the gut or skin, where organisms are found in high numbers, often contributing to a healthy microbiome. Joints in particular are aseptic spaces, and any microorganism in synovial fluid or muscle compartments is considered abnormal, and infection here can be difficult to manage.

In the immunosuppressed patient (**Table 1.5**), a failure to contain the initial infection can lead to systemic infection, e.g. bacteraemia and significant tissue damage as the episode becomes chronic. In other patients, an over-exuberant immune response leads to overwhelming inflammation and organ damage. Whilst a pathogen can cause significant harm, it is often an overwhelming immune response that leads to the most damage.

Immunosuppression can be due to genetic or environmental factors. Drugs used to treat autoimmune disease induce a degree of immunosuppression. If a patient has several causes for immunosuppression, care is taken on initiating drugs that will amplify this effect.

Patients presenting with an infection should be considered as being at high risk of serious sequelae if they are immunosuppressed and action needs to be taken to minimise their immunosuppression, where possible.

Systemic inflammatory response syndrome (SIRS)

- Tachycardia (heart rate >90 beats per minute (bpm))
- Tachypnoea (respiratory rate >20 breaths per minute)
- Abnormal body temperature (fever >38°C or hypothermia <36°C)
- Abnormal white blood cell count (leucocytosis >1200mm^3 or leucopenia <4000mm^3).

Patients with two or more of these criteria are deemed to have SIRS. However, it does not differentiate what is the cause of the response.

1.6.3 Sepsis

A diagnosed infection with a SIRS response is termed sepsis. There are degrees of sepsis which help to identify patients who need the most support.

Table 1.5 *Risk factors for immunosuppression*

Risk factor	Mechanism
Drugs, e.g.:	
■ corticosteroids	Reduced cytokine expression, effects on both innate and adaptive immune cell types
■ methotrexate (MTX)	Reduction of rapid immune cell turnover
■ adalimumab	Blocks TNF-α
Age	Reduction in number and differentiation of antigen-presenting cells, T and B lymphocytes
Malnutrition	Poorly developed lymphoid tissue in children
	Increased stress hormones can impair the immune response
Smoking	Impairs immune response to infection and increases general inflammatory response
Asplenia, e.g. post splenectomy	Loss of spleen's role as blood filter, antigen-presenting site, etc.
Genetic predisposition	e.g. complement deficiency, lymphocyte deficiencies
Infection	e.g. HIV-led depletion of T lymphocytes

■ **Severe sepsis** signifies that there is sepsis with organ dysfunction, e.g. renal failure.
■ **Septic shock** signifies sepsis-induced hypotension which persists despite adequate fluid resuscitation.

A significant immune system reaction can also trigger the coagulation system to become affected. Disseminated intravascular coagulation (DIC) occurs when the usual clotting factors are used up very quickly, to the point where there is both inappropriate clot formation and bleeding.

1.7 Autoimmune disease

In autoimmune disease, the immune system is misdirected and attacks host tissue directly. When this happens in rheumatoid arthritis, immune cells are recruited and attack a joint. A pannus, a layer of abnormal and immunologically active tissue, is formed and turns the normally protective synovium into an invasive and destructive growth (**Figure 1.10**).

1.7.1 The mechanism of autoimmunity

Because the immune system is constantly producing large numbers of immune cells, it occasionally produces autoreactive cells that mistakenly recognise host cells as foreign (**Figure 1.11**). To prevent them attacking bodily tissue, these cells are normally killed or quiesced. This process is called self-tolerance.

Self-tolerance is broken if this process fails (**Figure 1.12**). Both genetic and environmental factors play a role. It is likely that there are several genes (polygenic) that need to be switched on or off for a vulnerability to be exposed. Environmental factors further drive the progression towards autoimmunity. Environmental factors include drugs, diet and infections.

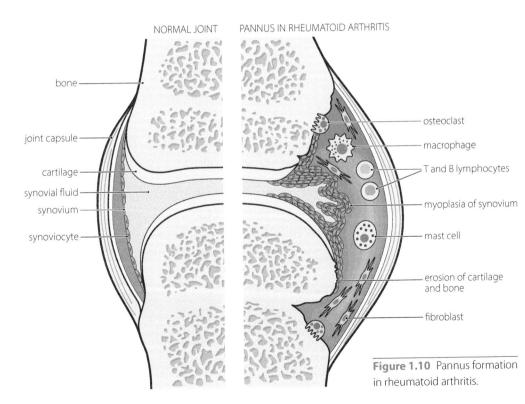

NORMAL JOINT PANNUS IN RHEUMATOID ARTHRITIS

bone
joint capsule
cartilage
synovial fluid
synovium
synoviocyte

osteoclast
macrophage
T and B lymphocytes
myoplasia of synovium
mast cell
erosion of cartilage and bone
fibroblast

Figure 1.10 Pannus formation in rheumatoid arthritis.

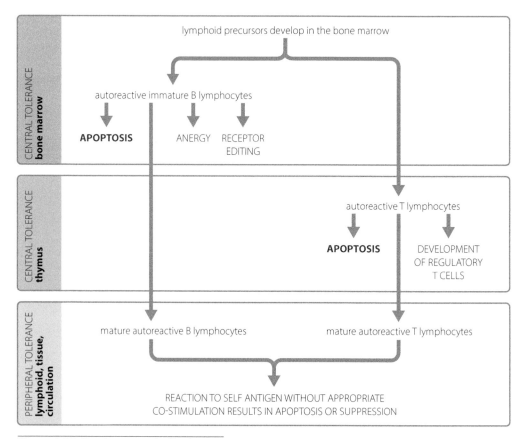

Figure 1.11 Development of self-tolerance.

Autoantibodies

Mature B cells (plasma cells) produce antibodies (also known as immunoglobulins). These Y-shaped proteins have unique molecular shapes, allowing them to bind to a variety of different antigens. They are termed 'autoantibodies' when the antigen recognised is a host protein (see **Figure 1.12**). They are specific or non-specific in their clinical context. For example, rheumatoid factor, whilst a sensitive predictor for rheumatoid arthritis, can be increased in several different autoimmune conditions and infections, whereas anti-double-stranded DNA is more specific for SLE. Therefore, it is always necessary to interpret autoantibodies in the context of an individual patient's clinical symptoms and signs. Autoantibodies initiate and aggravate the immune response by binding to a host antigen and activating an inflammatory response, e.g. complement cascade. They also bind to cell receptors to induce a phenotypic change within that cell, e.g. production of a different cytokine. Autoantibodies with a role in rheumatological disease are discussed in *Sections 2.6.11, 3.2* and *4.5–4.12*.

Human leucocyte antigens

Human leucocyte antigens (HLAs) are the human version of the major histocompatibility complex. They are proteins expressed on the surface of many cells where they act as self-recognition molecules and, by binding to and displaying antigens, play a role in the presentation of antigen to the immune system.

The genes for HLAs are grouped closely together on chromosome 6 and comprise a haplotype (a group of genes that are so closely linked that they are inherited together from a single parent). Some HLA haplotypes confer a genetic predisposition to autoimmune disease, e.g. HLA-B27 is associated with axial spondyloarthritis, inflammatory bowel disease, uveitis, psoriatic arthritis and reactive arthritis.

Drugs affecting the immune system

The treatment of autoimmune disease aims to reduce the immune response to self, whilst preserving an adequate response to infection. Modern drugs target specific mediators of inflammation such as cytokines and immune cell receptors. These therapies are discussed further in *Section 2.8.5*.

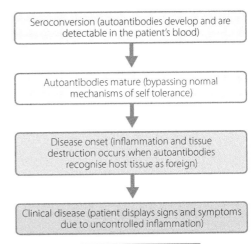

Figure 1.12 Phases of development of seropositive autoimmune disease.

1.8 Bone anatomy and physiology

There are three main functions of bones:
- They provide a mechanical support for the body's soft tissue and provide protection to the internal organs.
- The bone marrow is central to blood cell production, generating millions of red blood cells, platelets and white blood cells.
- Bones store most of the calcium within the body and, in conjunction with the body's regulatory systems, keep the calcium levels within normal levels by either releasing or storing more calcium within the bone.

1.8.1 Macrostructure of bone

There are five types of bone, all with different functions: long bones are mostly used for locomotion, while the irregular bones are specially shaped for their function (**Table 1.6**; **Figure 1.13**).

Most of the skeleton comprises long bones. These are formed by endochondral ossification. They have three distinct anatomical zones (**Figure 1.14**):
- diaphysis (shaft)
- epiphysis (the end of the bone)
- metaphysis (the region between diaphysis and epiphysis).

1.8.2 Bone microstructure

Bone has two components:
- a matrix of collagen fibres in which hard inorganic mineral salts (e.g. calcium hydroxyapatite and phosphates) are deposited
- organic cells, e.g. osteoblasts, osteoclasts and osteocytes.

The various types of bone contain differing amounts of these components and differ in how they are structured (**Table 1.7**).

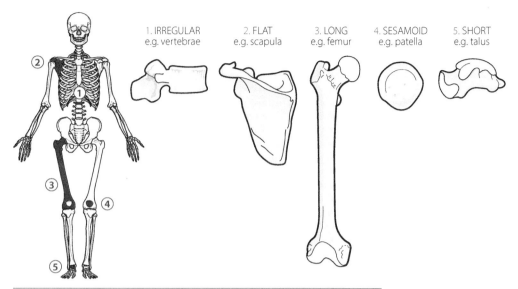

Figure 1.13 Types of bone: (1) irregular; (2) flat; (3) long; (4) sesamoid; (5) short.

Table 1.6 *Five types of bone and examples*		
Bone	**Description**	**Examples**
Irregular	Irregular bones have specific roles in the body	Vertebrae, sacrum and facial bones
Flat	Protection of the vital organs Formed by intramembranous ossification	Pelvis, ribcage and skull
Long	Longer than they are wide Numerous muscle attachments Joints at each end to allow movement	Femur, tibia, humerus, metacarpal, metatarsal and phalanges
Sesamoid	Present within a tendon Reduce the forces placed on the tendons while being stretched over a joint	Biggest sesamoid bone is the patella (kneecap)
Short	Wider than they are long Covered in thick layers of ligaments Individually not very mobile	Bones of the wrist (carpal) and midfoot (tarsal)

Table 1.7 *Properties of immature and mature bone*				
Bone	**Matrix**	**Calcification**	**Timing**	**Function**
Woven (immature)	Soft disorganised collagen	Not calcified	Made quickly (days to weeks)	Childhood growth Initial stability of fractures
Lamellar (mature)	Organised collagen fibres	Calcified hydroxyapatite	Forms slowly (months to years)	Mature adult bone Remodelled bone after fracture

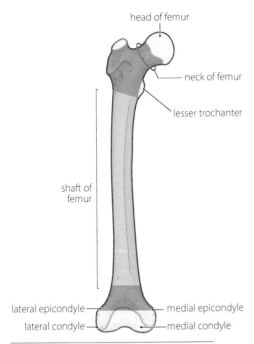

Figure 1.14 The diaphysis (shown in blue), epiphysis (yellow) and metaphysis (red).

1.8.3 Woven bone

Immature (woven) bone is a mass of collagen fibres that are not mineralised but are randomly and quickly made by osteoblasts. This bone is mechanically weak but, as it can be made quickly, it is seen in the growing child and in early fracture healing.

1.8.4 Lamellar bone

Mature (lamellar) bone is a composite material that has a soft collagen matrix that is hardened by deposited mineral salts. The hard scaffold made of calcium hydroxyapatite as well as other mineral salts makes the bones strong but brittle, while the soft collagen makes the bone more elastic and therefore more resistant to fracture. Osteocytes are the bone cells that are formed as a result of osteoblasts being trapped in this hardened matrix.

There are two different types of lamellar bone that are structurally different:

- **Cortical bone** is the hard outer part of the bone.
- **Trabecular bone** is the soft core of the bone (found in the epiphysis and metaphysis).

This arrangement allows bones to be strong yet light in weight (**Figure 1.15**).

Cortical (Haversian) bone

The hard outer cortical bone is structured into multiple long columns called osteons. The osteons contain concentric rings (lamellae) of osteoblasts and osteoclasts and are supplied by a central vascular channel called the Haversian canal (**Figure 1.16**).

Trabecular (cancellous) bone

Trabecular bone is structurally similar to cortical bone, but is less dense. The collagen fibres form thin rod-like trabeculae and they orientate their position in line with the greatest mechanical stress on the bone.

> Looking for mal-aligned or disrupted trabeculae on radiographs can help diagnose minimally displaced or angulated fractures (see *hip fracture, Case 6.1* and *Section 6.5*).

The trabecular bone is found in the epiphyseal and metaphyseal parts of the long bones and in the central part of other bones such as the vertebrae. It is highly vascular and metabolically active.

1.8.5 Bone marrow

Bone marrow is the substance found within the cancellous bone of mostly long, vertebral and flat bones and is the primary site of blood cell formation (haematopoiesis). Haematopoietic stem cells within the bone marrow can differentiate into red blood cells (erythrocytes), white blood cells (lymphocytes) and myelocytes (see **Table 1.4**).

Haematopoiesis

Erythrocytes are small red cells that do not have a nucleus. Billions of red blood cells are made every day and circulate round the vascular system, transporting oxygen and carbon dioxide. It takes around seven days for the immature erythropoietic stem cells to form into erythrocytes. They are then released into the circulation and last around 120 days.

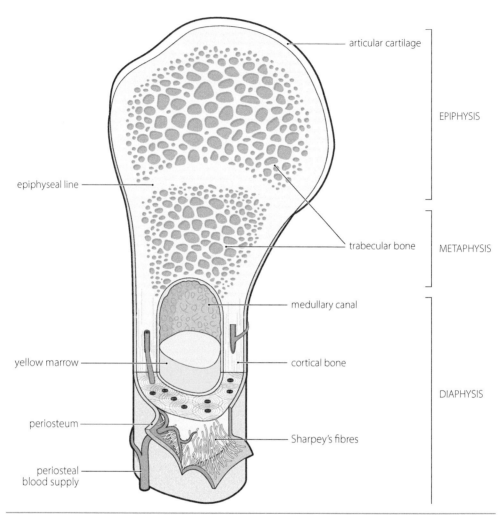

Figure 1.15 The structure of a long bone, showing the soft central cancellous bone, hard compact bone and periosteal covering.

Although white blood cells differ from red blood cells in that they contain a nucleus, they are derived in much the same way from haematopoietic stem cells in the marrow.

1.8.6 Vascular supply

Blood is supplied to bones by three routes (**Figures 1.4**, **1.5**, **1.15** and **1.16**):

■ endosteal, from inside the bone
■ periosteal, from outside the bone
■ metaphyseal–epiphyseal, around the joints.

Endosteal blood supply

The internal endosteal supply comes from the nutrient artery that enters in the centre of the diaphysis (**Figure 1.4**). Once inside the medulla, the blood is distributed through the shaft towards the metaphysis via the Haversian systems (**Figure 1.16**).

The endosteal blood supply is compromised when reaming and inserting intramedullary nails for fracture fixation. This can cause problems with bone healing (see *Section 2.9*).

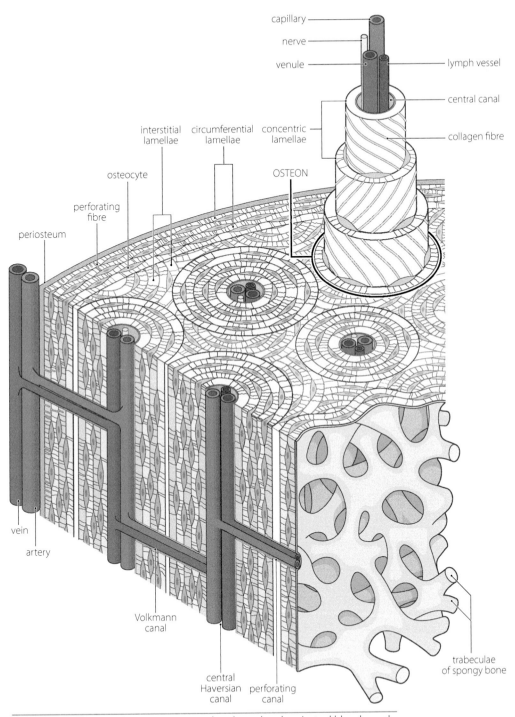

capillary
nerve
venule
lymph vessel
central canal
collagen fibre
interstitial lamellae
circumferential lamellae
concentric lamellae
osteocyte
OSTEON
perforating fibre
periosteum
vein
artery
Volkmann canal
central Haversian canal
perforating canal
trabeculae of spongy bone

Figure 1.16 Haversian bone structure and endosteal and periosteal blood supply.

Periosteal blood supply

Blood supply to the external periosteal layer comes from blood capillaries that enter along the length of the diaphysis but which are particularly numerous at muscle attachment sites (**Figure 1.15**). This external blood supply is important in children as the periosteum is where appositional (layered, increasing diameter) bone growth occurs.

The endosteal and periosteal blood supply are connected via the Volkmann canals and distribute the blood through the cortex layers.

Metaphyseal–epiphyseal blood supply

After growth plate fusion, the original separate blood supplies to both metaphysis and epiphysis still remain but they begin to anastomose and form a plexus (network between the two systems) around the joints (**Figure 1.5**).

> **The anastomosis of blood supply to the head of the femur in adults is important.** If the capillaries that enter through the capsule are disrupted in an intracapsular neck of femur fracture, then the blood supply is disrupted, meaning the fracture is unlikely to heal and/or the head becomes avascular and dies (avascular necrosis). Conversely, if the fracture is extracapsular then the blood supply is likely to be intact (see *Section 6.5*).

1.9 Mineral exchange and bone turnover

Bone is metabolically active, storing most of the body's minerals within its structure.

1.9.1 Bone metabolism

The amount of calcium and phosphate within bone is regulated by parathyroid hormone (PTH) and vitamin D, so the levels within the blood serum are maintained within tight limits. Mineral levels are maintained by excretion or resorption by the kidneys, or by resorption and deposition of bone by osteoclasts and osteoblasts (see **Table 1.8**).

Table 1.8 *The effect of hormones on bone metabolism*

	Osteoblasts	Osteoclasts	Calcium	Phosphate
PTH effect	Inhibits	Increases	Increases serum calcium	Increases serum phosphate
Calcitonin effect	Increases	Inhibits	Lowers serum calcium	Lowers serum phosphate
Vitamin D effect	No effect	Reduced activity in response to high serum calcium absorbed from the gut	Increases intestinal absorption and serum calcium	Increases intestinal absorption and serum phosphate
Oestrogen effect	Increases	Decreases	Lowers serum calcium	Lowers serum phosphate
Steroid effect	Inhibits	Increases	Lowers serum calcium	Lowers serum phosphate

Calcium

Calcium is used in many processes including muscle contraction, nerve conduction and blood clotting. Calcium is absorbed from the gut into the serum, promoted by vitamin D, and it is also resorbed by the kidneys in response to PTH (**Figure 1.17**). Over 98% of the body's calcium is stored in the bones as hydroxyapatite crystals.

Phosphorus

Phosphorus is used in active metabolic processes as adenosine triphosphate (ATP). Around 85% of the body's phosphorus is stored within the bone, together with calcium as hydroxyapatite crystals. Phosphorus is absorbed as phosphate from the gut in response to vitamin D but is excreted by the kidney in response to PTH (**Figure 1.17**).

Vitamin D

Vitamin D is absorbed from the diet and by action of sunlight on the skin. Vitamin D3 (cholecalciferol) is synthesised from the skin or absorbed from the gut, along with vitamin D2 (ergocalciferol).

Vitamin D3 and D2 undergo hydroxylation in the liver to produce 25-hydroxyvitamin D. The final hydroxylation and activation occur in the kidneys (catalysed by PTH), resulting in the formation of 1,25-hydroxyvitamin D (**Figure 1.18**).

Parathyroid hormone

PTH is secreted from the parathyroid glands in the neck in response to low levels of calcium in the serum. In the kidney, PTH is responsible for activating the inactive vitamin D by hydroxylation (**Figure 1.17**).

1.9.2 Bone remodelling

Bone remodelling is a continuous active process by which bone is resorbed and replaced; it is influenced by many factors including exercise, age and medications. In this process osteoclasts first excavate a cavity within the bone. After a few weeks, osteoblasts begin to produce osteoid and the osteoclasts enter programmed cell death.

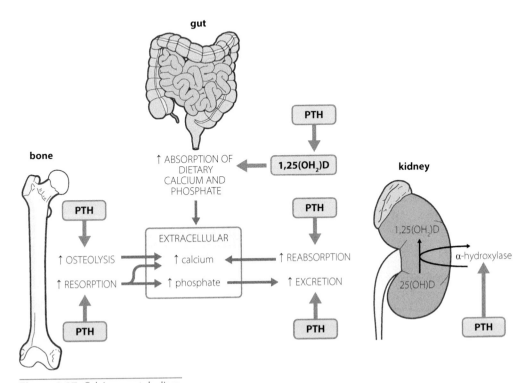

Figure 1.17 Calcium metabolism.

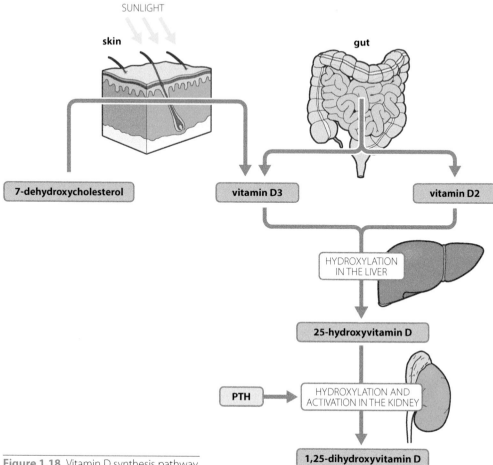

Figure 1.18 Vitamin D synthesis pathway.

Within three months the newly formed osteoid is then mineralised, forming new bone.

Age-related bone changes

Bone mass increases rapidly in childhood until around 30 years of age, as the intratrabecular spaces are filled in and the bone cortices become thicker. After the age of 30 there is a slow but steady loss of bone mass as the trabeculae become thinner and the bone becomes more porous. Women rapidly lose bone mass during the menopause in response to a reduction in oestrogen that decreases osteoblast and increases osteoclast activity (**Figure 1.19**).

> **Hormone replacement therapy** with oestrogen in menopausal women can help maintain peak bone mass.

1.9.3 Fracture healing

A fracture is a break in the cortex of the bone and it can heal by two separate mechanisms:
- primary bone healing (intramembranous ossification – forms without callus)
- secondary bone healing (endochondral ossification – forms from a cartilage precursor).

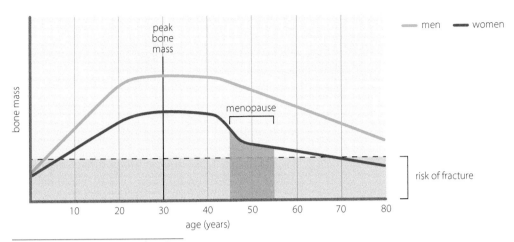

Figure 1.19 Bone mass and ageing.

Primary bone healing requires bone ends to be aligned with no gaps and no movement at the fracture site. Osteoclasts create cutting cones (a tunnel) which reaches across the fracture and is directly followed by capillaries and osteoblasts that lay down new bone.

Secondary bone healing has four stages (**Table 1.9**). Fracture healing can be influenced by the amount of mechanical strain placed on the fracture. In a high strain environment when bone ends are mobile, granulation tissue is formed; when bone ends become less mobile (low strain), bone is formed.

Table 1.9 *Fracture healing is a four-step process lasting up to 5 years (this process is quicker in children)*

	Timing	Stability	Description
Inflammation	1–7 days	Unstable	Exposed blood vessels bleed and form a clot, neutrophils and other inflammatory cells are transported to the clot and a fibrin network is made and gradually replaced by granulation tissue
Soft callus	2–3 weeks	Bone ends stop moving	Granulation tissue is replaced by disorganised fibrous tissue and cartilage (extracellular matrix)
Hard callus	3–4 months	Firmly united	The extracellular matrix becomes calcified (woven bone)
Remodelling	Up to 5 years	Firmly united	Woven bone is replaced by lamellar bone

1.10 Bone and joint anatomy

Joints are articulations between bones that allow for movement. There are three types of joint:
- synovial
- cartilaginous
- fibrous.

They are structurally different to facilitate different functional demands.

1.10.1 Synovial joints

Synovial joints (e.g. the hip and shoulder joints) give the most freedom of movement and are designed to absorb loads during exercise. All synovial joints contain a joint capsule, hyaline cartilage and synovial fluid. However, the shape of these joints varies depending on what functional movement is required.

Joint capsule

Synovial joints have a strong capsule which holds fluid inside the joint for lubrication. The capsule is made from a strong fibrous material, with the outer portion of the capsule being a strong ligament-type structure, while the inside of the capsule secretes the synovial fluid. The joint capsule is avascular and gains most of its nourishment required to keep supple and strong from surrounding tissues. This diffusive process happens more readily during exercise as compression and moving of fluid within the joint adds a convectional property to transfer nourishment more quickly.

Articular (hyaline) cartilage

Inside the capsule the ends of the bone are covered in articular hyaline cartilage which is smooth like glass and has almost no friction. Hyaline cartilage is composed of a complex inorganic matrix and the organic chondrocyte cells (**Figure 1.20**). The inorganic or extracellular matrix is a criss-cross of fibres of collagen and elastin that acts as a scaffolding to resist tensile stretching forces. Proteoglycans (aggrecan) and its side chains of glycosaminoglycans make up the rest of the matrix and are attached to a hyaluronic acid backbone to form the larger proteoglycan aggregate called aggrecan aggregate. These aggregate proteins are large and negatively charged molecules that attract large amounts of water into the matrix. Articular cartilage can be thought of as reinforced concrete. The collagen and elastin are like the steel rods resisting tension forces and the glycosaminoglycans, proteoglycans and water are a jelly-like concrete resisting compressive forces (**Table 1.10**).

Synovial fluid

Synovial fluid is a protective lubricant to the joints, allowing them to slip past each other with little

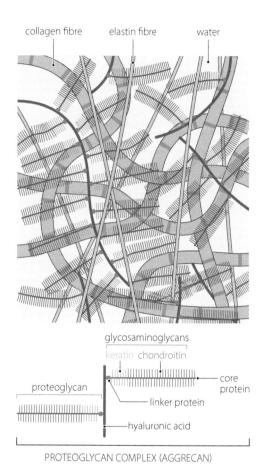

PROTEOGLYCAN COMPLEX (AGGRECAN)

Figure 1.20 Hyaline cartilage.

frictional resistance. Synovial fluid is the same basic fluid as blood plasma; however, it has no blood cells or clotting factors, making it a clear viscous yellowish fluid. Its four base components are:

- lubricin
- hyaluronate
- proteinase
- collagenase.

Synovial joint types

The synovial joints of the body are specifically designed for their purpose, with each small ridge and notch being present to create or limit movement. Joints come in different sizes, shapes and with different ranges of movement (**Table 1.11**).

Table 1.10 *Zones of articular cartilage*

Zone	Collagen	Proteoglycans	Cells	Calcification	Vascularity
Superficial	Type II parallel to the joint	Sparse	Flattened chondrocytes	None	Avascular
Intermediate	Type II random organisation	Abundant	Round chondrocytes	None	Avascular
Deep	Type II perpendicular to the joint	Highest concentration	Round chondrocytes in columns	None	Avascular
Tidemark	Division between non-calcified avascular cartilage and calcified vascular cartilage				
Calcified cartilage	Type II perpendicular to the joint	Sparse	Small	Calcified	Vascular

Table 1.11 *Types and examples of synovial joints*

Synovial joint	Description	Movement	Example
Hinge joints	Hinge joints allow movement in only one plane	Flexion/extension	Knee joint
Pivot joints	Pivot joints allow a rotational movement around only one axis	Internal/external rotation	Proximal and distal radio-ulnar joints Atlanto-axial joint
Ball and socket	Ball and socket joints allow movement in all planes around a common centre	Flexion/extension Abduction/adduction Internal/external rotation	Hip joint between femoral head and the pelvic acetabulum
Saddle Joint	A saddle joint has one concave surface and an opposite convex surface and is saddle-shaped	Flexion/extension Abduction/adduction Opposition	First carpometacarpal joint (thumb)
Condylar joint	Oval-shaped surface	Flexion/extension Abduction/adduction	Metacarpophalangeal joint

Hinge – knee joint

The knee joint is a hinge joint, articulating the distal femur with the proximal tibia. The patella-femoral articulation is not part of the hinge joint but is important for reducing forces within the knee. The bony elements of the knee provide only a small amount of stability within the joint. The knee is stabilised further by the static ligaments, menisci and dynamic muscles (**Figure 1.21**). The ACL and PCL are important internal stabilisers of the knee, resisting rotational and anterior/posterior translational forces. The medial and lateral collateral ligaments resist lateral/medial movement.

Osteology

The distal femur has two smooth condyles that are convex and a central depression called the intercondylar notch that is not covered in articular cartilage. The medial femoral condyle is larger than the lateral which, when flexing, causes a slight internal rotation of the tibia on the femur or, conversely, external rotation when the knee is extended. The tibia surface also has two condyles split by the intercondylar eminence which projects upwards to fit in the intercondylar notch of the femur when the leg is extended. The medial tibial condyle is larger and concave and the lateral is convex; the lateral compartment's meniscus is a lot more mobile than the medial. Both these aspects allow a greater translational movement over the top of the tibia. This greater mobility of the lateral side contributes to the rotational element of the knee when it flexes and extends.

Menisci

The menisci are two discs of fibrocartilage which sit between the femur and tibia and help increase shock absorption and gliding.

Knee ligaments

As the bone shape only allows flexion and extension with a small amount of rotation, ligaments provide extra restraints to prevent abnormal movements. The cruciate ligaments are inside the knee joint and are so called as they cross over each other. The anterior cruciate ligament (ACL) is important to resist anterior translation of the tibia on the femur, but also resists some internal rotation. The insertion of the ACL is anterior-medial on the tibial spine and it extends backwards and laterally to insert on the femur.

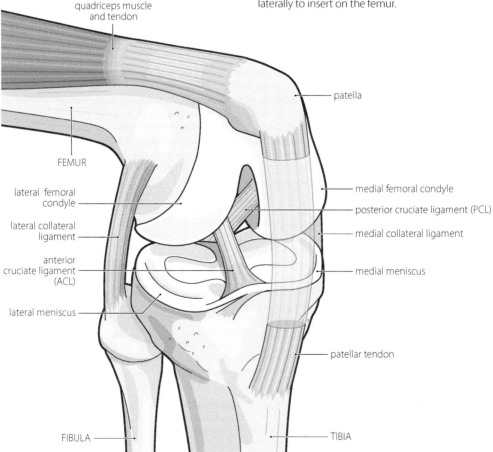

Figure 1.21 The knee joint is an example of a hinge joint with multiple ligaments.

The ACL is often injured when the foot is connected with the floor and a valgus stress or internal rotation of the knee occurs. It is a common injury after a side tackle in football.

The posterior cruciate ligament (PCL) is stronger than the ACL; it stretches from its insertion on the posterior lateral part of the tibial eminence to the medial femoral insertion. The PCL restrains posterior translation of the tibia on the femur and is injured when the knee is flexed and the tibia is forced backwards, e.g. knee hitting the dashboard in a car accident.

Medial and lateral collateral ligaments (MCL and LCL, respectively) are outside the knee joint. On each side of the knee they extend from the femoral condyles to insert at the tibia on the medial side and head of the fibula on the lateral side. The main function of these ligaments is to resist valgus and varus stresses on the knee joint.

Pivot – atlanto-axial joint

The atlanto-axial joint is the articulation of the first cervical vertebra on the second and is a pivot joint (**Figure 1.22**). The tight transverse ligament holds the odontoid peg of C2 within the ring of C1, allowing up to 100° of lateral rotation. Combined with the rest of the C spine movements, up to 180° of lateral rotation is normal.

Atlas is the C1 vertebra and it sits on top of the **axis**, the C2 vertebra. Think of the earth sitting on its axis.

The axis bone (C2), like all vertebrae, has a ring structure but also has a projection upwards that inserts through the wide spinal canal of the atlas bone (C1). This projection allows rotation of the head to 90° on each side. There is an incredible amount of movement in this joint; however, this is limited by the strong ligaments connecting the two bones. This part of the skeleton, although highly mobile, also protects the brainstem which if damaged almost certainly leads to death.

Radio-ulnar joints of the forearm

Another example of a pivot joint is the radio-ulnar joints of the forearm. The pronation and supination movement in the forearm occurs due to the shape of the forearm bones. The ulna is the fixed bone and the radial bone moves around it due to the cup shape of the proximal radial head. The radial head articulates with the capitellum of the distal humerus and it rotates around this axis with 85° of supination and 75° of pronation. The proximal ulnar articulation with the humerus only allows flexion and extension. At the distal end of the forearm the radius and ulna articulate again and this time the radius has to roll around the ulna and has a full arc of 130° (**Figure 1.23**).

Ball and socket – hip joint

The hip joint is a ball and socket joint. It has a significant range of movement and it is able to flex/extend, aBduct/aDduct, rotate internally/externally, and has a large arc of circumduction. The femoral head is round and fits into the socket known as the acetabulum. The proximal femur has two trochanters which are projections just distal to the neck and are the attachment of the muscles around the hip (**Figure 1.24**). The pelvis is made up of three bones: the ischium, pubis and ilium, plus the sacrum; these are held in place by strong fibrous ligaments. The hip capsule and labrum are important to stabilising the hip joint and allowing circumduction of the hip.

The head and acetabulum are covered by a strong joint capsule that attaches to the neck

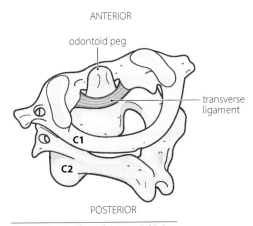

ANTERIOR

odontoid peg

transverse ligament

C1

C2

POSTERIOR

Figure 1.22 The atlanto-axial joint.

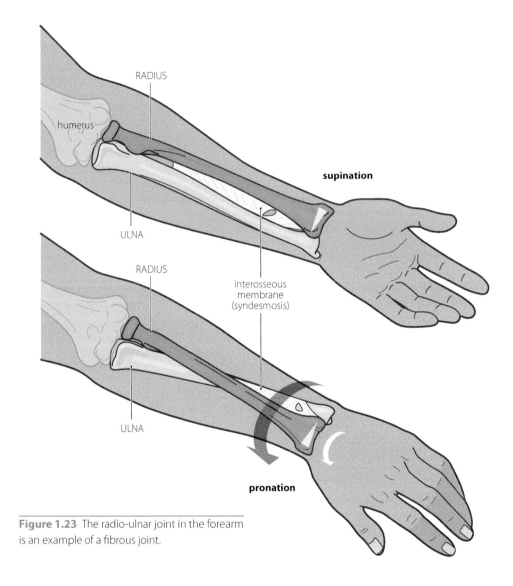

RADIUS

humerus

supination

ULNA

RADIUS

interosseous
membrane
(syndesmosis)

ULNA

pronation

Figure 1.23 The radio-ulnar joint in the forearm
is an example of a fibrous joint.

of the femur in between the two trochanters.
This is very important anatomically as almost all
the blood supply to the neck and head of the
femur enters within this capsule (see hip fracture
Case 6.1 and *Section 6.5*). The acetabular labrum is
a fibrocartilage lip that surrounds the acetabulum
beneath the capsule. It aids with joint stability as
well as sealing in the synovial fluid.

Saddle – carpometacarpal joint

The first carpometacarpal joint is a saddle joint
and is the articulation of the trapezium (carpal
bone) and the metacarpal bone. It is shaped like a
saddle and permits all movements except rotation

(**Figure 1.25**). The movements of this joint can be
difficult to distinguish and are often the opposite
of what you might think. These are explained in
Table 1.19. Oppositional movement is unique
to the saddle joint of the thumb; this movement
of the thumb crosses the palm to touch the
little finger. The interossei muscles attach the
metacarpals to the proximal phalanges to abduct
and adduct the MCP joints. The extensor tendons
insert to the distal phalanges and control DIPJ
extension. A wrap-around expansion of the same
tendon, called the hood, attaches to the middle
and proximal phalanges, controlling extension of
the MCP and PIP joints.

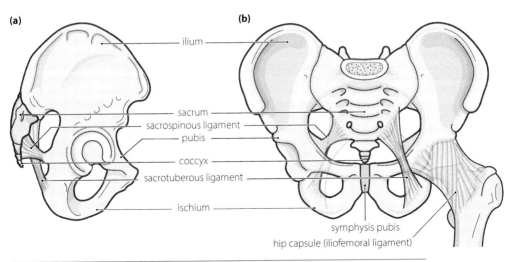

(a)   **(b)**

ilium

sacrum

sacrospinous ligament

pubis

coccyx

sacrotuberous ligament

ischium

symphysis pubis

hip capsule (iliofemoral ligament)

Figure 1.24 The pelvic bones, ligaments and hip joints: (a) lateral view; (b) anterior view.

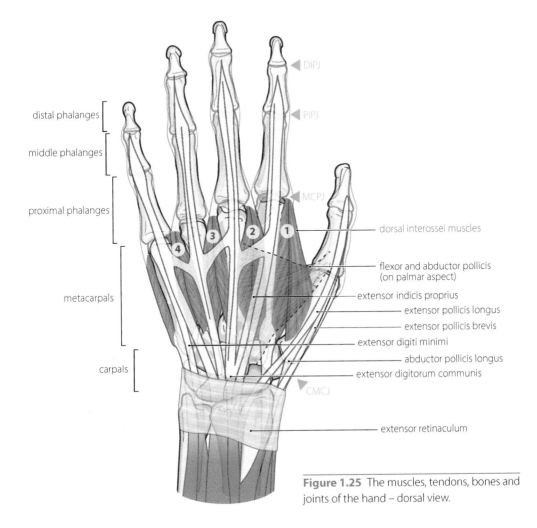

DIPJ

PIPJ

distal phalanges

middle phalanges

proximal phalanges

MCPJ

dorsal interossei muscles

flexor and abductor pollicis
(on palmar aspect)

extensor indicis proprius

extensor pollicis longus

extensor pollicis brevis

metacarpals

extensor digiti minimi

abductor pollicis longus

extensor digitorum communis

carpals

CMCJ

extensor retinaculum

Figure 1.25 The muscles, tendons, bones and joints of the hand – dorsal view.

Condyloid – metacarpophalangeal joints

The small joints of the fingers and toes are condyloid joints. The joints between the metacarpals and the phalanges are called the metacarpophalangeal joints (MCPJ); they are oval in shape and movements include circumduction as well as flexion and extension. The proximal and distal interphalangeal joints (PIPJ and DIPJ, respectively) are between the proximal, middle and distal phalanges. These are bicondylar hinge joints as they have two condyles but only permit flexion and extension of these joints.

Plane joints

Plane (arthrodial/gliding) joints are surrounded by a tight joint capsule and only permit a small amount of gliding motion. These joints are often very flat. Plane joints include those of the intertarsal and intercarpal joints of the feet (**Figure 1.26a**) and hands (**Figure 1.26b**), respectively. In the foot, the tarsal bones form longitudinal and transverse arches, maintained by the plantar ligaments. In the hand, the carpal bones also form an arch towards the palm, which is covered by the transverse carpal ligament; this is where the median nerve enters the wrist. The ulnar nerve enters between the pisiform and hamate bones.

1.10.2 Cartilaginous joints

Cartilaginous joints are covered in articular hyaline cartilage and have a fibrocartilage pad in between; examples include the sternal joints and the intervertebral joints of the spine. One of the strongest cartilaginous joints is the symphysis pubis (see **Figure 1.24**) which holds the two pubic bones of the pelvis together at the front.

The vertebral column and intervertebral joints

The vertebrae are the bones of the spine that are specifically designed to protect the spinal cord, hold the body upright and allow movement. There are 7 cervical, 12 thoracic, 5 lumbar and 5 fused sacral vertebral bones and the coccyx (**Figure 1.27**). Each of these types of vertebra has a different shape:

■ cervical and lumbar vertebrae are lordotic, i.e. curved in the sagittal plane with the apex anterior

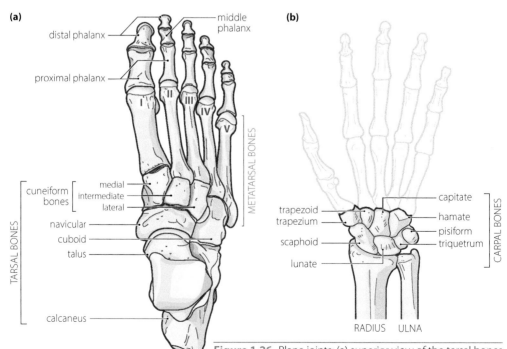

Figure 1.26 Plane joints: (a) superior view of the tarsal bones of the foot; (b) palmar view of the carpal bones of the wrist.

■ thoracic vertebrae and the sacrum are kyphotic (apex posterior), giving an overall straight alignment of the mechanical axis.

Strong ligaments hold the vertebral column together while the intervertebral and facet joints allow movements within the spine.

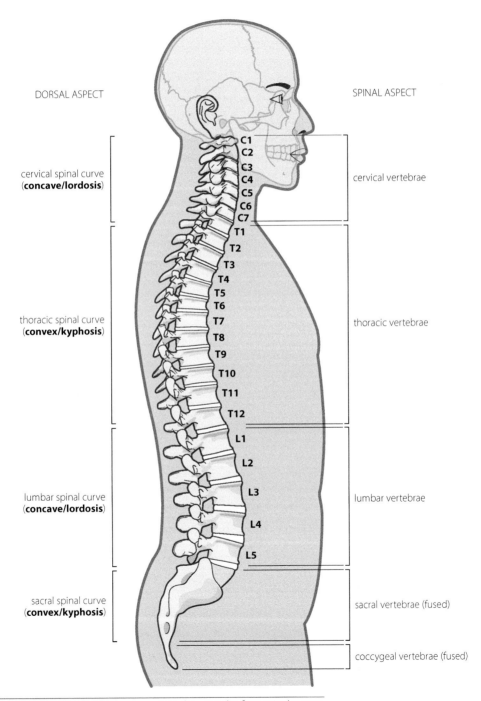

DORSAL ASPECT

SPINAL ASPECT

cervical spinal curve
(**concave/lordosis**)

C1
C2
C3
C4
C5
C6
C7

cervical vertebrae

T1
T2
T3
T4
T5
T6
thoracic spinal curve
(**convex/kyphosis**)
T7
T8
T9
T10
T11
T12

thoracic vertebrae

L1
L2
lumbar spinal curve
(**concave/lordosis**)
L3
L4
L5

lumbar vertebrae

sacral spinal curve
(**convex/kyphosis**)

sacral vertebrae (fused)

coccygeal vertebrae (fused)

Figure 1.27 The vertebral column regions showing the four spinal curves.

The shapes of the vertebral bones are different for each spinal level as each has a different role. All consist of a weight-bearing body part that is interspersed by intervertebral discs. Attaching to the body and extending posteriorly are the paired pedicles, which form the anterior rim of the spinal canal. Connecting at the back are the two laminas, which form the posterior ring of the spinal canal (**Figure 1.28**).

Spreading laterally on each side where the pedicles and lamina meet are the transverse processes. Underneath the transverse processes, the pedicles form the intervertebral foramen where the spinal nerves exit. Sitting just on top of the transverse processes are the superior articular processes and below, the inferior articular processes. The area in between is called the pars interarticularis. These joints above and below articulate with the adjacent vertebra as a synovial facet joint. The shape of these joints dictates the movements allowed in the spinal column. The spinous processes extend backwards from the lamina, providing protection of the spinal cord from the back (**Table 1.12**).

The longest spinous process is at C7, making it an easy anatomical landmark to palpate.

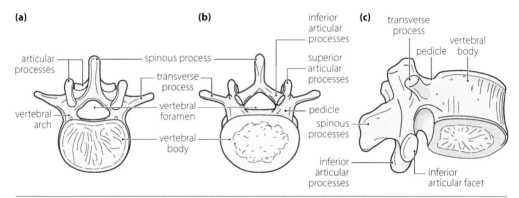

Figure 1.28 The structure of the vertebrae showing (a) a superior view; (b) an inferior view; (c) lateral and inferior views.

Table 1.12 *Characteristics of different vertebral levels and their respective movements*

	Cervical C3–C7	Thoracic T1–T12	Lumbar L1–L5
Body	Small and oval	Medium and heart-shaped	Large
Spinous process	Small and bifid (except C7)	Large and down-sloping	Short and more parallel
Facet joint slope	45°	60°	90°
Facet joint direction	Posteriorly	Lateral	Medial
Movements	Flexion and extension Lateral flexion	Rotation Limited flexion/extension	Flexion and extension No rotation
Distinguishing features	Transverse foramen	Costal facets	Large and no costal facets
Curve	Lordosis	Kyphosis	Lordosis

Intervertebral disc

The intervertebral discs (**Figure 1.29**) are responsible for the shock absorption of the spine, while permitting some movement. The specific arrangement of the fibrocartilage discs makes it ideal for resisting compressive forces. The discs have multiple outer rings of strong fibrous material called the annulus fibrosus. The layers of the rings are orientated at 90° to each other to resist forces in all directions. The nucleus pulposus is the centre part of the disc and is jelly-like, containing lots of collagen, proteoglycans and water.

> You are 1 cm taller in the morning than in the evening. This is due to the compression on the vertebral discs during normal daily activities causing water to be squeezed out of the discs.

1.10.3 Fibrous joints

Fibrous joints do not have any hyaline cartilage but connect two bones together with a strong band of fibrocartilage. One example is the sutures of the skull, which are narrow, linear joints between the skull bones and allow no movement. Two other examples are the joints between the tibia and fibula at the ankle and between the radius and ulna, both called the syndesmosis (see **Figure 1.23**).

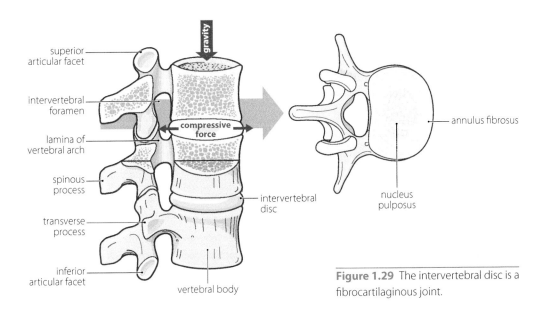

Figure 1.29 The intervertebral disc is a fibrocartilaginous joint.

1.11 The nervous system

There are three separate nervous systems that control different parts of the body.

- The central nervous system (CNS) includes the brain and spinal cord and is the conscious control centre for all processes.
- The autonomic nervous (ANS) system supplies the body's solid organs and is involuntary.
- The peripheral nervous system (PNS) relays messages to and from the CNS to control movement and sensory feedback; it also has its own unique reflex system.

1.12 Nerves

1.12.1 Axon

The most basic unit of a nerve is the neuron formed from a large cell body that has branching dendrites and a long thin tail-like axon (**Figure 1.30**). The axon's long thin body is surrounded by long lines of Schwann cells which are covered in a myelin sheath. The myelin sheath acts as an insulating cover to keep the chemical and electrical signals within the cells. Between the Schwann cells are the nodes of Ranvier which are not covered by myelin and are free to conduct outside the myelin sheath. Their existence is vital to the rapid transmission of signals along the axon.

1.12.2 Nerve structure

Nerve fibres are long multi-layered structures covered in connective tissue. Neurons are covered in the thin connective tissue called the endoneurium. Multiple neurons are bundled together into fascicles which are separated by perineurium. The whole nerve consisting of

multiple fascicles is then covered in supportive and protective epineurium (**Figure 1.31**).

1.12.3 Neuronal communications

Neurons communicate with each other by action potentials which are electrical signals that travel down each neuron. At the end of each neuron a synapse connects to another neuron or end organ such as muscle via the neuromuscular junction.

Resting membrane potential

This electric energy is created by the movement of ions from inside and outside the nerve cells. Charged ions cannot diffuse through the phospholipid bilayer as they are not water soluble and require an ion channel to bypass the hydrophobic part of the cell membrane (**Figure 1.32**). Ions move down the channels and through the cell membranes by diffusion from a high concentration to a low concentration to maintain a chemical equilibrium. Despite the maintenance of a concentration gradient, the electrical gradient

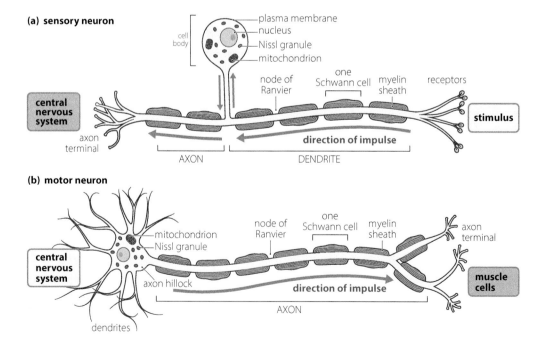

Figure 1.30 Myelination of axons: (a) sensory neuron; (b) motor neuron.

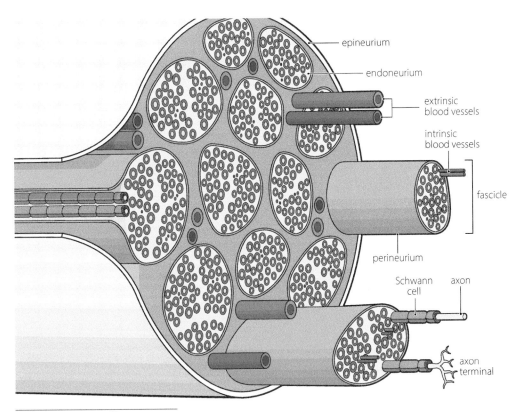

Figure 1.31 Nerve fibre structure.

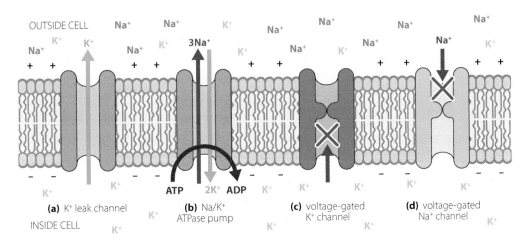

Figure 1.32 Ion channels and the resting membrane potential.

is disrupted. Inside the cell has the highest concentration of the positively charged potassium (K⁺) ions and large negatively charged proteins. Conversely, outside the cell there is a higher concentration of sodium (Na⁺) and chloride (Cl⁻) and relatively small amounts of K⁺. Nerve cells have a natural resting potential of energy which is −70mv. Three types of channel maintain the resting membrane potential (electrochemical gradient):

- leak channels
- Na⁺/K⁺ ATPase pump
- voltage-gated channels.

Leak channels

A steady flow of K⁺ leaks through the diffusion channels to try to maintain a chemical concentration equilibrium (**Figure 1.32a**). However, as the K⁺ leaves the cell the electrical gradient becomes more negative inside the cell and wants to attract the K⁺ back through the channels. K⁺ diffuses more readily outside the cell than Na⁺ diffuses into the cell, due to Na⁺ leak channels being tightly closed when the nerve cell is at rest.

Na⁺/K⁺ ATPase pump

At rest there is some movement of ions against the concentration and electrical gradient but this requires energy in the form of ATP, the universal unit of chemical energy (**Figure 1.32b**). The active Na⁺/K⁺ pump uses ATP to exchange three Na⁺ molecules out of the cell for two K⁺ going in. As K⁺ diffuses more readily out of the cell and less K⁺ is actively pumped back in, the resting potential is negative within the cell.

Voltage-gated Na⁺ and K⁺ channels

At rest the voltage-gated Na⁺ and K⁺ channels are inactive and closed; they are activated by an increase in the resting membrane potential. (**Figure 1.32c** and **d**)

1.12.4 Action potentials

Action potentials are the chemical and electrical messages that are transmitted down the axon to the synapse.

Depolarisation

A stimulus triggers a chemical wave of messages down the axon by opening the voltage-gated Na⁺ channels, causing a large influx of Na⁺ and a rise in the charge across the cell membrane (**Figure 1.33**).

Repolarisation

The Na⁺ channels then close and the ongoing leak of K⁺ through the diffusion and voltage-gated K⁺ channels begins to restore the membrane potential back to −70mv (repolarisation). There is a small dip below resting membrane potential before restoration to equilibrium, due to K⁺ channels taking longer to close and Na⁺ channels being in the inactive state rather than the resting phase. Na⁺ channels are unique, as once stimulated they open rapidly. However, once shut, they stay shut for a few milliseconds more.

Refractory period

Calcium (Ca²⁺) binds to the Na⁺ channel, preventing the Na⁺ channel being fired again too quickly; this is called the refractory period. So, no matter how many times the Na⁺ channels are stimulated within the refractory period, another action potential will not commence.

> Uncontrolled muscle spasms known as tetany occur secondary to low Ca²⁺ levels in the blood. Na⁺ channels lose the normal refractory period in the presence of low Ca²⁺ and continue to fire uncontrolledly.

Propagation

Propagation of the action potential down the axon is dictated by its size and whether or not the nerve is myelinated. Non-myelinated fibres propagate as a slow wave of conductance having to depolarise the whole length of the nerve. Myelinated fibres are covered in the non-conducting myelin sheath. This allows the wave of depolarisation to quickly 'bunny-hop' down each of the unmyelinated nodes of Ranvier to the synapse (known as saltatory conduction) (**Figure 1.34**). The depolarised region, showing the creation of local currents that enable the spreading of the depolarisation wave, is indicated in **Figure 1.34**.

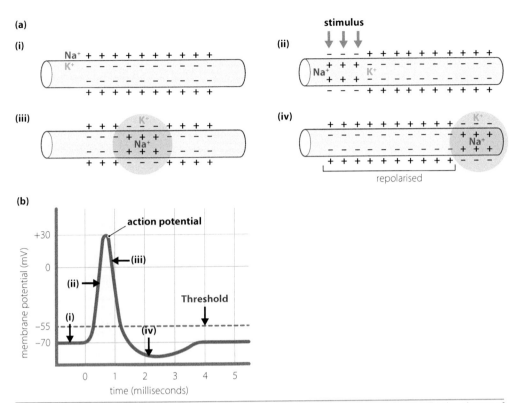

Figure 1.33 (a) Action potential and nerve conduction along an unmyelinated neuron; (b) the phases of action potential.

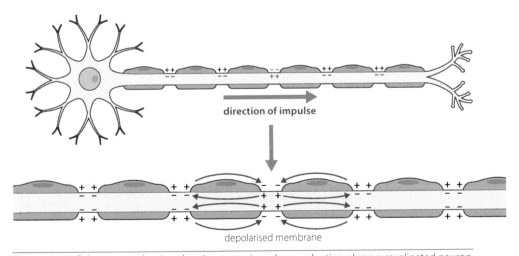

Figure 1.34 Saltatory conduction showing nerve impulse conduction along a myelinated neuron.

1.12.5 Synaptic transmission

The axons and dendrites connect to form synapses like a spider's web to transmit chemical or electrical signals down the interconnected pathways from the presynaptic neuron to the postsynaptic neuron.

Chemical synapse

When the depolarised wave hits the synapse, Ca^{2+} enters the presynaptic neuron from the synaptic cleft through voltage-dependent Ca^{2+} channels. This in turn releases neurotransmitters out of the nerve cell to diffuse across the synaptic cleft to the dendrites of the postsynaptic neuron, where they attach to receptors that modulate the action potential (**Figure 1.35**).

Neurotransmitters

The neurotransmitters are either excitatory (glutamatergic), that depolarise the cell, or inhibitory (gamma-aminobutyric acid; GABA) and hyperpolarise the cell or have a specialised role. The neuromuscular junction secretes acetyl choline (cholinergic) and some neurons can secrete hormones such as adrenaline (adrenergic). Receptors present on the postsynaptic membrane bind the neurotransmitters and activate the postsynaptic neuron. Leftover neurotransmitters in the synaptic cleft are reabsorbed by the presynaptic cleft or are broken down metabolically.

Summation

Both excitatory and inhibitory transmitters can be fired at the same time; the additive effect of multiple waves is called summation.

Spatial summation

The inhibitory GABA neurotransmitter acts to hyperpolarise (negatively charge) the cell. It does this by two methods: allowing K^+ to quickly leave the cell and the negative chloride ion to enter. The overall effect is to make the charge of the cell more negative. As the starting point for depolarisation is now more negative, the effect is that it requires a bigger excitatory stimulation to bring about a depolarisation.

Temporal summation

Similarly, small excitatory impulses on their own are not able to bring about a depolarisation but if several are fired together from a single neuron quickly enough, the threshold for depolarisation can be reached by this summation process (**Figure 1.36**). Temporal summation generates an action potential from one excitatory neuron which, when stimulated several times, will produce an action potential. Spatial summation generates an action potential from several presynaptic neurons.

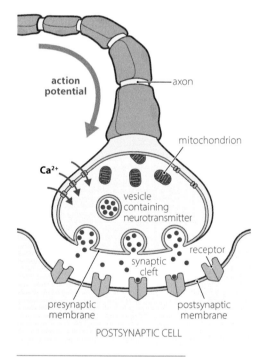

Figure 1.35 The chemical synapse.

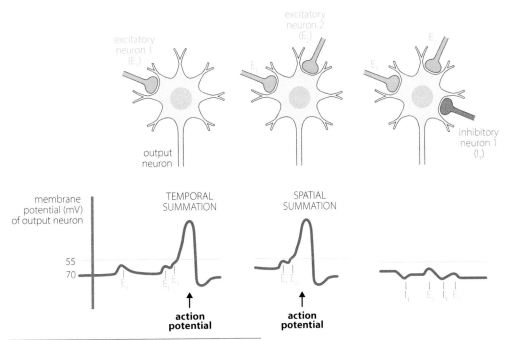

Figure 1.36 Summation and integration of synapses.

1.13 Central nervous system

The CNS processes sensory signals that are transmitted through the spinal cord up from the PNS and then coordinates a response before sending signals back down the spinal cord to the periphery.

1.13.1 Structure

The CNS contains the brain and spinal cord and it is bathed in a protective covering of meninges and cerebrospinal fluid (CSF).

White and grey matter

The brain and spinal cord consist of both white and grey matter due to their difference in cells. The innermost white matter consists of mostly long myelinated axons without many cell bodies. The outer grey matter holds mostly neuronal cell bodies and dendrites as well as the unmyelinated fibres.

Non-neuronal cells

Glial cells, of which there are several types, are the non-neuronal cell of the CNS, keeping the neuronal cells protected as well as regulating the environment around them.

- Oligodendrocytes produce the protective myelin sheath that also gives it a layer of electrical insulation to improve conduction down the nerves.
- Astrocytes are the most abundant glial cell and their star-shaped long projections help support the neurons as well as other multiple functions. They buffer the metabolic products of the neuron, so they are chemically balanced and also help maintain the blood supply and blood–brain barrier.

Meninges and CSF

The brain and spinal cord are covered in layers of protective tissue and fluid (**Table 1.13**). The innermost layer is called the pia mater. This is a very thin but impermeable fibrous sheath and it is closely related to the brain as it enters into all the small sulci. A spider-like arachnoid mater is the next covering. Underneath this layer is the subarachnoid space in which the CSF flows.

Table 1.13 *Layers and spaces surrounding the spinal cord*

Meninges	Description or contents
Epidural space	Spinal cord blood vessels
Dura mater	Tough protective layer
Subdural space	The dura and arachnoid mater are usually adherent, but this is a potential space for haematoma to collect
Arachnoid mater	Middle spider-like protective layer
Subarachnoid space	CSF
Pia mater	Thin innermost protective layer
Cord	Long ascending and descending axons

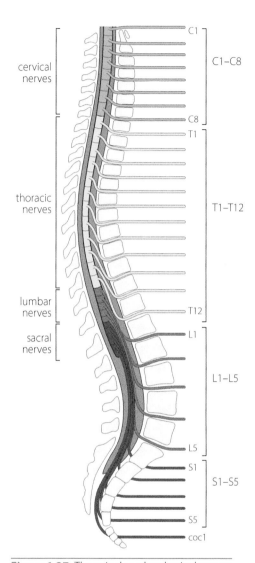

Figure 1.37 The spinal cord and spinal nerves.

Dura mater

The dura mater is the outermost covering and it is also the strongest. Small venous projections from the arachnoid mater enter the dura CSF and communicate with the venous cerebral blood flow that circulates within the subdural space. Outside the dura is the extradural space in which the lymphatics and arterial systems flow. The dural sac ends at the S2 level of the spinal column; however, the innermost pia mater continues down further to cover the final nerve roots and anchors itself to the coccyx as the filum terminale.

1.13.2 Spinal cord

The spinal column consists of 8 pairs of cervical nerves, 12 pairs of thoracic nerves, 5 pairs of lumbar nerves, 5 pairs of sacral nerves and one coccygeal nerve. The spinal nerves exit the spinal canal at the same level as their corresponding vertebral body. The spinal cord starts at the level of the medulla (respiratory centre of the brain that sits at the exit of the skull) and extends down to the L1–2 level in the adult (**Figure 1.37**).

After the L1–2 level the spinal cord splits into its terminal paired spinal nerves (also known as the cauda equina); they continue inside the spinal canal and exit at their corresponding vertebral levels, as before. There are multiple ascending and descending tracts within the spinal cord but four distinct areas are important in the musculoskeletal system (**Table 1.14**). The white matter in the outer part of the spinal cord groups together different sensory and motor tracts. The central grey matter consists of the crossing tracts, interneurons and the cell bodies.

Table 1.14 *The spinal cord is a highway for the electrochemical action potentials and is divided into separate ascending and descending tracts*

Type	Tract	Location	Decussations (crossing the midline)	Cell body	Action
Ascending sensory	Dorsal column	Posterior medial	Medulla	Dorsal root ganglion	Light touch Vibration Proprioception
	Spinothalamic tract	Anterior lateral	Spinal cord	Dorsal root ganglion	Crude touch, pain and temperature
Descending motor	Lateral corticospinal tract	Posterior lateral	Medulla	Anterior horn	Motor fine skills
	Anterior corticospinal tract	Anterior medial	Spinal cord	Anterior horn	Motor fine skills

Ascending sensory tracts

The ascending sensory tracts take sensory inputs from the periphery to the brain. Sensory tract cell bodies (where they synapse with the PNS) are outside the spinal column in the dorsal root ganglion (**Figure 1.38a**). Light touch and proprioception ascend in the dorsal columns which travel on the ipsilateral (same side) as it enters and then decussate (cross to the opposite side) at the level of the medulla in the brain. This is in contrast to the spinothalamic tract, which decussates at the same level as it enters the spinal cord.

Descending motor tracts

The descending motor tracts send information from the motor cortex in the brain to the muscles. The descending motor tract cell bodies are in the ventral horn inside the cord. The lateral corticospinal tract decussates high up in the medulla, whereas the anterior corticospinal tract decussates at the level it exits the spinal cord (**Figure 1.38b**). The lateral corticospinal tract is the main motor tract; the anterior corticospinal tract is only present to the mid-thoracic level.

Cauda equina

The spinal cord splits into its final nerve roots at the level of the L1–2 vertebrae and its terminus is called the conus. The fibres of L2–S5 fan out and, as paired nerves exit the spine, the density of the bundle becomes less. Overall the appearance resembles a horse's tail, giving these nerves the collective Latin name 'cauda equina'. The nerves of the cauda equina transmit sensation and motor signals to and from the legs, the anal and urethral sphincters and the sexual organs.

Blood supply

Along the whole length of the spinal cord three main arteries run within the arachnoid space. The anterior spinal artery supplies the ventral and lateral columns and two posterior spinal arteries supply the dorsal columns. The cord and the meninges are also supplemented with branches from the aorta and vertebral arteries. In the cervical region the vertebral artery branches, called the segmental medullary arteries, penetrate from outside at each level. In the thoracic and lumbar area posterior and anterior radicular arteries that arise from the aorta enter with the dorsal and ventral nerve roots to directly supply the spinal cord. Despite the spinal arteries and radicular arteries supplying the same area, they do not anastomose within the cord and their supply is independent of one another (**Figure 1.39**).

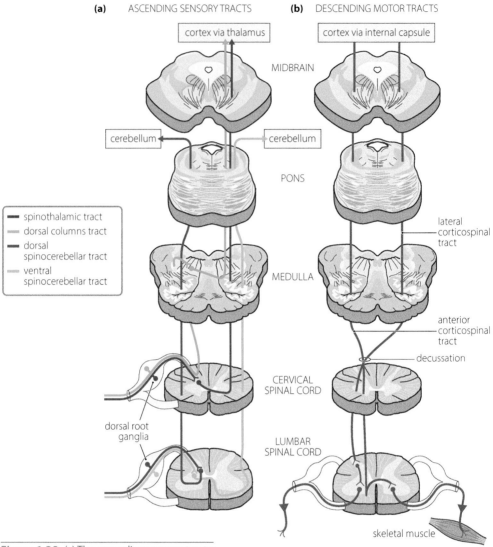

Figure 1.38 (a) The ascending sensory tracts;
(b) descending motor tracts.

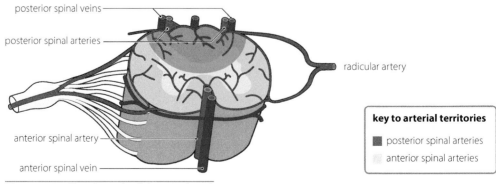

Figure 1.39 Blood supply of the spinal cord.

The blood supply below the level of the cervical vertebrae from the anterior and posterior spinal arteries is poor and relies very heavily on the radicular blood supply. During surgery on the aorta the large radicular branches are at risk of becoming damaged, which could result in paralysis below this level.

1.14 Peripheral nervous system

The PNS consists of both the sensory and motor nerves supplying the limbs, face and visceral organs. It connects the CNS to the end organs via the paired spinal and cranial nerves. The somatic nerves of the PNS are under conscious control and supply the limbs. The autonomic nervous system is part of the PNS but this supplies the visceral organs and is not under conscious control.

1.14.1 Spinal nerves

There are 31 pairs of spinal nerves: 8 cervical, 12 thoracic, 5 lumbar, 5 sciatic and one coccygeal. The paired spinal nerves consist of a sensory and motor component which originate and synapse with the spinal cord. Each paired spinal nerve has a corresponding sensory area on the skin, known as a dermatome, and a corresponding muscle group, known as a myotome.

Inside the spinal canal

The sensory part of the nerve synapses posteriorly with the dorsal root ganglion, while the motor synapses within the spinal cord at the ventral horn but exits via the ventral root ganglion. The separate parts of the nerve come together very close to the cord just before exiting through the intervertebral foramen of the bony spine. Once out of the spinal column they again split into the dorsal and ventral rami, which now contain both motor and sensory elements together (**Figure 1.40**). The dorsal ramus supplies the posterior skin and muscles (epaxial) and the ventral ramus the frontal muscles and skin (hypaxial).

Outside the spinal canal

The somatic peripheral nerves are long and only synapse once, making them quick to transfer messages. The downside to this is that they are vulnerable to noxious stimuli, due to their lack

of meningeal coverings, and also to penetrating injury as they are not protected by the bony skeleton. The outgoing motor messages from the spinal cord travel in the efferent (exiting) nerves and the incoming sensory messages travel in the afferent (inbound) nerves (**Figure 1.40**).

1.14.2 Peripheral sensors

The distal part of the sensory nerve starts with a specific type of nerve sensor (**Table 1.15**). Mechanoreceptors respond to mechanical stimulation; nociceptors are stimulated by noxious or painful stimuli and proprioceptors are for position sense. Once activated by the stimuli, the nerve sends messages through the afferent sensory nerves back towards the dorsal root ganglion to synapse with the CNS.

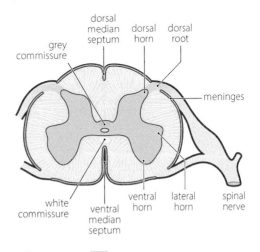

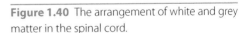

Figure 1.40 The arrangement of white and grey matter in the spinal cord.

Table 1.15 *Peripheral nerve sensors detect several sensations and trigger action potentials in the sensory nerves*

Sensor type	Sensation	Nerve type	Structure
Merkel	Pressure	Slowly adapting Myelinated	
Ruffini	Stretch	Slowly adapting Myelinated	
Pacinian	Vibration	Fast Myelinated	
Meissner	Light touch	Rapidly adapting Myelinated	

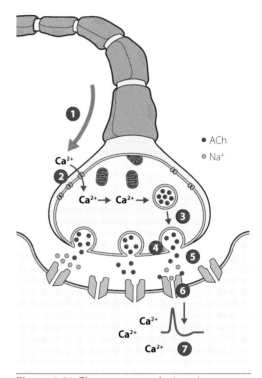

1.14.3 Neuromuscular junction

The distal part of the motor nerve ends with the neuromuscular junction. This is a special synapse that initiates muscle contraction by synapsing directly to a muscle fibre (**Figure 1.41**). Similar to other synapses, a Ca^{2+} influx stimulates the docking of synaptic vesicles full of neurotransmitters to the presynaptic membrane via SNARE proteins. As the vesicles are incorporated into the cell membrane, the neurotransmitter is emptied into the synaptic cleft.

Acetylcholine (ACh) is the neurotransmitter that binds at the motor end-plate, increasing the permeability to Na^+ and K^+ and causing a depolarisation wave. A little of the leftover ACh

Figure 1.41 The neuromuscular junction: ① action potential; ② Ca^{2+} enters plasma membrane; ③ the synaptic vesicle is activated by calcium and moves towards synaptic membrane; ④ vesicle fuses with presynaptic membrane and releases ACh into the synaptic cleft; ⑤ ACh diffuses across synaptic cleft and binds to Na^+ channel receptor; ⑥ Na channel is opened and Na flows into the motor end-plate, causing depolarisation; ⑦ depolarisation in the motor end-plate releases calcium that stimulates muscle contraction.

in the synaptic cleft is reabsorbed back into the presynaptic membrane but most is broken down by the enzyme acetylcholinesterase.

Myasthenia gravis is a disease in which the ACh receptors on the motor end-plate become blocked by antibodies. The muscles are unable to contract as the action of ACh is ineffective at generating an end-plate potential. Clinically muscles appear to work at first but rapidly tire as all the ACh is quickly used up.

Acetylcholinesterase inhibitors are a class of drugs used in myasthenia gravis to increase the amount of ACh in the synaptic cleft. As the enzyme is inhibited, less of the ACh is broken down and it keeps a higher concentration within the cleft. A higher concentration of ACh is able to compete with the antibodies for the binding site.

1.14.4 Nerve plexus

Both hypaxial and epaxial spinal nerves exit the spinal column and form multiple plexuses, i.e. intersections where nerves join and divide into branches. This allows crossover between nerves, so that areas of the body are innervated by multiple spinal nerves, rather than a single nerve. The grouping of nerves allows one larger nerve to disseminate the complex array of messages between the CNS and peripheral receptors. The three plexuses involved in movement are:

■ cervical plexus: cervical spinal nerves C1–4, which supply the neck
■ brachial plexus: cervical nerves C5–8 and the first thoracic nerve T1 supplying the arms

■ lumbosacral plexus: lumbar and sacral nerves L1–S4 supply the function of the legs and perianal area.

The brachial plexus

The spinal nerves C5–T1 supply all motor function to the arms and receive all sensory information from them. At the brachial plexus, they join together and diverge in a network (a 'plexus') (**Figure 1.42**). The 5 spinal nerve roots C5–8 and T1 come together to form three **trunks**: upper C5 and 6, middle C7 and the lower C8 and T1. At this point each **trunk** then divides into two, with one **trunk** going posterior and the others anterior before coming back to form the cords which are named in their relation to the axillary artery. The

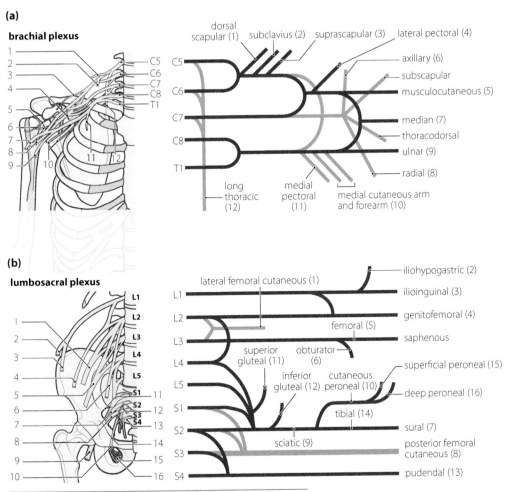

(a)

brachial plexus

(b)

lumbosacral plexus

Figure 1.42 (a) The brachial plexus; (b) the lumbosacral plexus.

posterior cord is formed from all of the posterior divisions, the lateral cord is formed from the anterior divisions of C5–6 and the medial cord is the anterior division of C8–T1. Finally, the **branches** form as the proper named nerves. The axillary and radial nerve are formed as a splitting of the posterior cord. The musculocutaneous nerve is a continuation of the lateral cord and the ulnar nerve is a continuation of the medial cord. The median nerve is formed by the joining of the lateral and medial cords.

> **The brachial plexus is injured following a stretching or crushing injury.** It is injured in childbirth if significant traction is placed on the arm, or if the arm is forced quickly above the head (e.g. when a person is thrown from a motorbike).

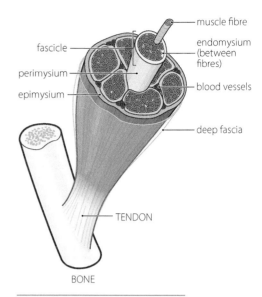

Figure 1.43 Muscle fibre structure.

1.14.5 Muscles and soft tissues

Muscles, tendons and ligaments are responsible for keeping the bones connected together, as well as for movement. Tendons attach muscle to the bones, while the muscles contract and relax and initiate movement. Ligaments attach bones to other bones around joints, allowing normal joint movement but preventing abnormal movement (instability).

1.14.6 Skeletal muscle

Muscle is made up of multiple groups of fibrils, fibres and layers of connective tissue (**Figure 1.43**). The smallest are the fibres which are surrounded by a connective tissue layer known as the endomysium. A group of around 100 muscle fibres form a fascicle which is separated from adjacent fascicles by perimysium. Groups of multiple long fascicles make up the larger muscle bulk and are surrounded by an overall covering of connective tissue called epimysium.

1.14.7 Skeletal muscle types and compartments

There are eight types of muscle shape (**Figure 1.44**; **Table 1.16**). The shape of a muscle

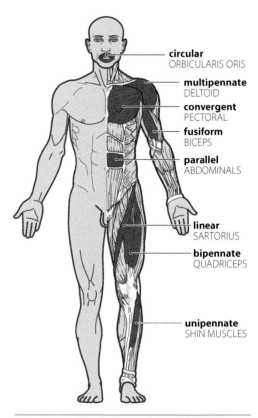

Figure 1.44 The function of a muscle is based on its shape and size.

Table 1.16 *Types of skeletal muscle, descriptions and examples*

Shape	Description	Example	Strength	Energy expenditure
Circular	Muscle fibres are circular	Orbicularis oris	Medium	Medium
Unipennate	Muscle fibres insert into tendon diagonally	Flexor pollicis longus	Strong	Tire quickly
Bipennate	Central tendon with muscle fibres that insert in two different diagonals	Rectus femoris	Very strong	Tire quickly
Multipennate	Multiple diagonal fibres inserting on several central tendons	Deltoid	Very strong	Tire quickly
Convergent	Triangular in shape. Wide proximal attachment but converges to insert onto a single tendon	Pectoralis major	Very strong	Tire quickly
Parallel (strap)	All fibres run in parallel	Sartorius, Rectus abdominus (tendinous intersections)	Weak	Good endurance
Fusiform	Fibres are parallel but the muscle belly is wider than the tendon it originates and inserts	Biceps brachii	Medium	Medium

depends on its functions and location. Many muscles are grouped into fascial compartments; each compartment is covered in a thick layer of fascia called a septum. There are fascial compartments in the lower leg, thigh, arm and forearm; small compartments are found in the hands and feet. A cross-section of the lower leg shows how its muscles are tightly encased within several compartments (**Figure 1.45**; **Table 1.17**).

A consequence of swelling in these compartments is compartment syndrome – see *Case 11.4*.

1.14.8 Sarcomere

Sarcomeres are the smallest building block structures within muscle and are only visible under the electron microscope (**Figure 1.46**). They contain two protein groups: the thinner actin filaments and the thicker myosin filaments.

These proteins interlock and slide relative to one another, causing muscle contraction (see *Section 1.14.10*). Areas in which they interlock have distinct names. The A (d**A**rk) bands represent where the **thick** myosin filaments are present, with or without the presence of the actin. The I (L**I**ght) bands are where the **thin** actin filaments

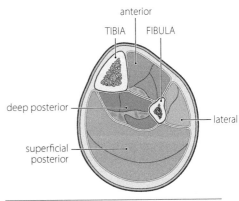

Figure 1.45 The four fascial compartments of the lower leg.

Table 1.17 *The four fascial compartments of the lower leg*		
Compartment	**Muscle group**	**Muscles**
Anterior	Ankle and toe extensors	Tibialis anterior Extensor hallucis longus Extensor digitorum longus Peroneus tertius
Lateral	Foot evertors	Peroneus/fibularis longus and brevis
Deep posterior	Ankle and foot flexors	Tibialis posterior Flexor hallucis longus Flexor digitorum
Superficial posterior	Ankle flexors	Gastrocnemius Soleus Plantaris

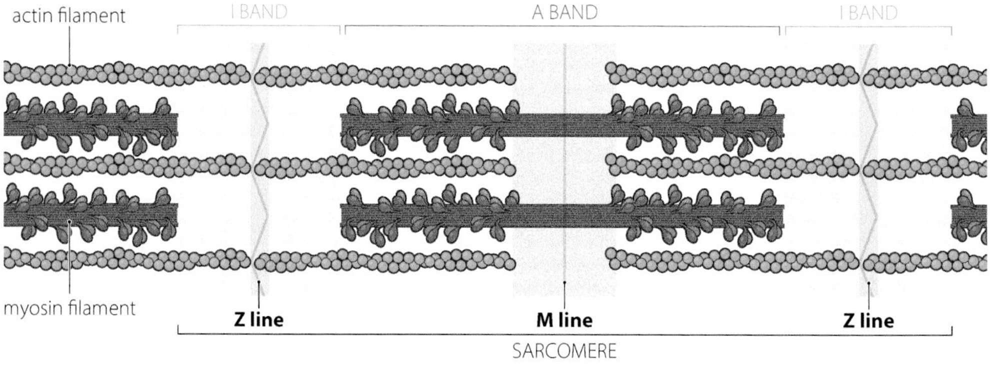

Figure 1.46 The structure of the sarcomere.

are on their own without any overlap with myosin. The M line is where myosin filaments join together and the Z line represents the attachment of one sarcomere to the next.

Actin

Actin is the main protein constituent of the thin filament but it also has little subunits, projections which either help bind to myosin (troponins) or block binding to myosin (tropomyosin).

Myosin

Myosin is a heavy protein formed into three distinct parts and shaped like a Y. The arms of the Y have globular heads which are the site in which actin binds. The neck has light protein chains that are flexible and move the head towards the actin to bind. The tail is a heavy chain helix.

1.14.9 Muscle fibres

The muscle fibres are covered in a plasma membrane called the sarcolemma (**Figure 1.47**). This has deep invaginations called T (transverse) tubules, which run transverse to the muscle fibres and between the I and A bands, so each sarcomere is encircled by two tubules. The sarcoplasmic reticulum is a membrane-like structure that is loosely networked over the surface of the muscle fibres. Its main purpose is calcium storage. The T tubules that overlie the sarcoplasmic reticulum are closely linked but have no direct contact. Little outpouchings of the sarcoplasmic reticulum where the T tubules cross over are called terminale cisternae (lateral sacs) and they are responsible for releasing calcium into

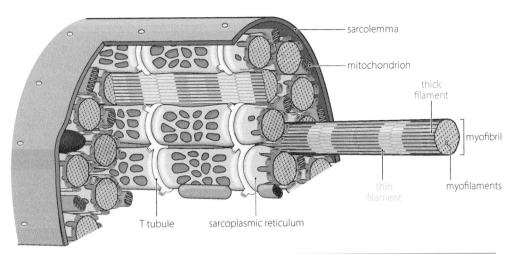

Figure 1.47 The sarcomere is covered in sarcoplasmic reticulum that stores calcium and is separated by T tubules.

the sarcomere to start a muscle contraction (see neuromuscular junction, *Section 1.14.3*).

1.14.10 Muscle contraction

Muscles take the electrical and chemical impulses from the central and peripheral nervous systems and turn them into contractions that move the joints of the body. The force of contraction depends on the cross-sectional area of the muscle, whereas the speed is dependent on the length of the muscle fibre.

Sliding filament theory

The structure of muscle with its thick myosin filaments and thin actin filaments allows movement over each other to either shorten (contract) or lengthen (relax) the sarcomere. To slide past each other, multiple chemical interactions need to take place to bind and release the myosin and actin filaments.

> It is important to note that although the overall muscle contracts and shortens, the actual length of the actin and myosin doesn't change; they merely slide past each other.

Motor end-plate

It all starts as the chemical signal arrives down the motor nerve to the neuromuscular junction.

The neurotransmitter ACh is released into the synapse and binds to the motor end-plate. The Na^+ channels open and the resulting depolarising wave travels from the motor end-plate through the T tubules that encircle each sarcomere. The T tubules are in very close proximity to the terminale cisternae of the sarcoplasmic reticulum and the depolarisation causes an interaction of the receptors on both their surfaces. This signal causes Ca^{2+} to be released from the sarcoplasmic reticulum into the sarcomere.

Cross-bridge cycling

Calcium is the main generator of muscle contraction, but it also requires energy in the form of ATP.

ATP binding

The binding of ATP to the myosin head causes a change in the myosin head shape and it detaches from the actin filament (**Figure 1.48a**). ATP is hydrolysed (splits) to adenosine diphosphate (ADP) and a single phosphate molecule (P_i). Again, this reaction causes a change in the shape of the myosin head into the 'cocked' position, allowing contact with actin as it weakly binds (**Figure 1.48b**).

Formation of the cross-bridge

To form a full cross-bridge between the actin and myosin, the actin binding site needs to be clear of

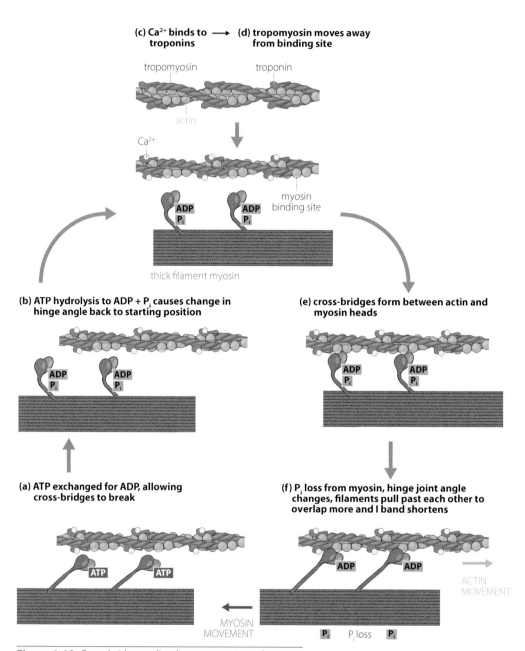

Figure 1.48 Cross-bridge cycling between actin and myosin.

the molecule tropomyosin, which in the resting state blocks the cross-bridge. The newly released Ca^{2+} binds to another molecule called troponin C that is present on actin (**Figure 1.48c**). This activated troponin C with the help of troponin T moves the tropomyosin away from the actin

binding site to allow both myosin heads to strongly bind to the actin (**Figure 1.48d** and **e**).

Power stroke

Myosin heads pull on the actin in an action called the *power stroke*. The trigger of this power stroke is due to the release of the single phosphate molecule from the myosin. Actin is attached to the sarcomere at each end so as the power stroke pulls the myosin over the actin, the sarcomere shortens (**Figure 1.48f**). Following the power stroke all the energy is used up and the ADP molecule uncouples from the myosin head. However, the cross-bridge remains firmly interlocked and the only way for the actin and myosin to uncouple is for another molecule of ATP to bind to the myosin head.

> If there is a lack of ATP, the myosin head can become stuck in the cross-bridge. Clinically this is apparent as rigor mortis and the muscle will neither contract nor relax.

Termination

The cross-bridge cycling process happens repeatedly until either all the Ca^{2+} or ATP is used up. To terminate a contraction Ca^{2+} needs to be removed from the sarcomere. This can occur by stopping the release of Ca^{2+} from the sarcoplasmic reticulum and by actively pumping the Ca^{2+} back into the sarcoplasmic reticulum. The reverse

sequence occurs as calcium is actively pumped away, resulting in the troponin C becoming inactive and tropomyosin goes back to its normal resting position, blocking the binding of myosin and actin.

1.14.11 Muscle control

Muscles are able to generate powerful contractions by causing more of the fibres to contract at one time. However, if all the motor units were to fire at the same time, the power generated could tear the tendons away from their bony attachments. The contraction is therefore regulated so only some of the motor units contract while others rest; they then rotate around so the contraction can be maintained for longer. Golgi tendon organs are proprioceptive sensors that monitor muscle tension; they are present at the junction of muscles and tendons. Golgi tendon organs regulate the tension in muscles by a sensory feedback loop via afferent nerves to the spinal cord. If too much tension is felt in the muscles, then efferent nerves signal for the contraction to cease, thus protecting the muscle from tearing (see inverse myotatic reflex, *Section 1.16.3*).

1.15 Tendons and ligaments

Tendons and ligaments attach to bone and either help initiate or restrict movement (**Table 1.18**).

■ **Tendons** attach muscle to bone and are long and thin, so the muscle bulk is out of the way

when the muscle contracts and the joint is moving. They normally act in synchronous pairs of opposite movements and thus also help with joint stability.

Table 1.18 *Properties of tendons and ligaments*

	Ligaments	Tendons
Attachments	Bone to bone	Bone to muscle
Function	Joint stabilisation	Transfer movement to bones
Water	More water	Less water
Collagen	Less collagen Type I 70%	More collagen Type I 85% Type III 0–5%
Elastin	More elastin 5–10%	Less elastin 2%
Proteoglycan	More proteoglycan 5–10%	Less proteoglycan 1–5%
Fibroblasts	Rounder fibroblasts	Elongated fibroblasts

- **Ligaments** attach bone to bone. Their primary role is to prevent excessive movements of the joints. They also function as a check rein as they have an ability to feed back proprioceptive information.

1.15.1 Microstructure

Matrix

Structurally, ligaments and tendons are made from the same constituents, as they both have an extracellular matrix of mostly collagen and contain fibroblast cells. The matrix also has smaller amounts of elastin and proteoglycan. Similar to articular cartilage, water follows the negative charge of the proteoglycans and collagen, making the matrix absorb water.

Collagen and elastin

Ligaments contain more elastin than tendons, whereas tendons contain more collagen. Elastin allows the ligaments to stretch and recoil, which is useful to resist joint movements, but the maximum strength of elastin is lower than collagen. The arrangement of the collagen and elastin fibres in a criss-cross fashion gives

ligaments an extra advantage (**Figure 1.49**) as it allows movement to be restrained in multiple directions. This is in contrast to tendons, where the collagen is layered in parallel bundles. Tendons are long and straight and their main function is to resist tensile stretching forces and the parallel arrangement of the more inelastic collagen fibres is key to this function. In summary, when tendons are stretched along their axis they are stronger than ligaments, but ligaments can resist strain in multiple directions. In structures such as menisci they are arranged like a lattice and also resist compression forces.

1.15.2 Bursae

Bursae are synovial membrane-lined fluid-filled sacs that protect tendons from wear and tear when they move over joints. They act like a cushion, allowing the tendon to glide over them with little friction. Most large joints have bursae surrounding them: commonly the knee, shoulder, elbow and hip. They are prone to inflammation due to overuse or degeneration of adjacent tendons (see *Section 7.10*).

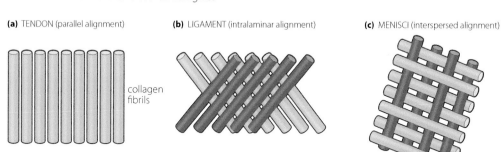

(a) TENDON (parallel alignment)   **(b)** LIGAMENT (intralaminar alignment)   **(c)** MENISCI (interspersed alignment)

collagen fibrils

Figure 1.49 The collagen fibres in (a) tendon; (b) ligaments; (c) menisci.

1.16 Locomotion

Locomotion is the movement of the body from one place to another. The human body is able to do this in many ways, from crawling as a child to walking, running, swimming and jumping. Each of these movements requires a sequence of muscle contractions to move the bones and joints against gravity. The brain and spinal cord regulate these movements consciously and unconsciously.

1.16.1 Planes and arcs of movement

Movements are complicated and can occur in multiple directions, so standardised nomenclature is used to describe these movements (**Figure 1.50**). Three anatomical planes exist and are based on the arms being externally rotated,

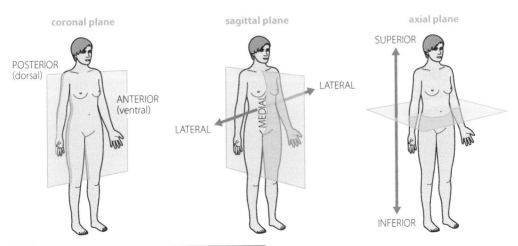

Figure 1.50 The anatomical position and axis planes.

with palms, feet and head facing forwards (the anatomical position) (**Table 1.19**):

- coronal (frontal)
- sagittal (median)
- axial (transverse).

These planes are used in cross-sectional imaging such as CT and MRI to describe which plane you are looking at. The images are orientated from the viewpoint of you standing at a patient's feet.

Movements and limb position are standardised and are referenced towards the midline or to the closest joint. Movements always work in couples, so for every movement there will be an opposite.

The middle digit only ABducts as it can't ADduct towards itself.

Specialist movements

In the spine and neck lateral flexion is bending to one side away from the midline in the frontal plane, e.g. ear onto shoulder.

In the foot joint, the terms eversion and inversion are used to describe a simple movement of tilting the sole of the foot towards (inversion) or away (eversion) from the midline in the sagittal plane (**Figure 1.51**).

Other specialist movements occur in the forearm, known as pronation and supination.

Plane	Description	Example
Coronal	ABduction – away from the midline ADduction – towards the midline	In the hands and feet ABduction and ADduction occur in relation to the middle digit
Sagittal	Flexion – joint curls towards the centre of body Extension – joint is straight and away from the centre of the body	In the wrist, extension is often call dorsiflexion and true flexion named palmar (palm of the hand) flexion Similarly, in the foot extension is termed dorsiflexion and plantar (sole of the foot) flexion is true ankle flexion
Axial	Internal rotation – towards the midline External rotation – away from the midline	In a fractured hip the limb externally rotates due to the muscle attachments of the external hip rotator muscles that attach to the greater trochanter

Table 1.19 *Description and examples of the anatomical planes of movement*

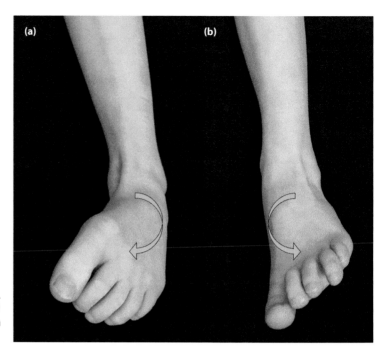

Figure 1.51 (a) Inversion or supination; (b) eversion or pronation.

Pronation is an inward (medial) rolling, while supination is an outward rolling along the long axis of the bone (see **Figure 1.23**).

> Think of **sup**ination as holding a bowl of **soup** and **pro**nation as playing **pro** basketball.

In the foot, pronation and supination are more complicated and are a triplanar combination of movements. Supination is a combination of plantarflexion, inversion and adduction. Pronation is the combination of dorsiflexion, eversion and abduction.

Limb alignment

Alignment of the limb is also important biomechanically, because abnormal stresses on the bones can lead to joint wear and tear. The knee is a classic example as people are often described as being bow-legged or having knocked knees. This alignment of the limb can be described as varus or valgus, respectively.

> Va**L**gus describes when the most distal part of the limb deviates **laterally** and away from the midline.

1.16.2 Normal motion

Normal motion is a combination of multiple processes, from the conscious thought to the muscle contracting, sensory feedback and fine adjustments. This all happens in an instant and some as a reflex without conscious thought.

Muscle length and contraction

Muscles contract when activated, but that doesn't always mean they shorten. For example, if you hold a dumbbell out in front of you with your arm straight but without moving it, your biceps muscle – which flexes your elbow – is resisting the downward force of gravity by creating tension in the muscle, but the muscle does not change its length. This is an isometric contraction, as the length of the muscle does not change despite tension being exerted through the muscle. If you were to then bend your elbow up towards you, the muscle will still be under tension but the muscles will be shortening. This is called a concentric contraction and the opposite movement is an eccentric contraction (**Figure 1.52**). So, when the dumbbell is lowered from full flexion to extension it is controlled by the biceps

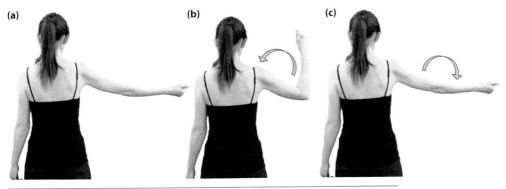

Figure 1.52 Types of muscle contraction: (a) isometric; (b) concentric; (c) eccentric.

muscle and tension in the muscle is generated whilst the muscle is lengthening.

1.16.3 Balance

Proprioception
Balance is controlled by proprioceptors in muscles, tendons and joint capsules that feed back position sense. The muscles' spindles and Golgi tendon bodies can sense when they are being stretched and therefore are able to send afferent signals to the spinal cord and, if appropriate, up the dorsal columns to the brain. Most balance and proprioceptive mechanisms are unconscious and form a reflex arc which only incorporates the spinal cord and does not communicate with the brain. An example of this in clinical practice is the testing of muscle reflexes such as the knee jerk.

Knee jerk reflex
The knee jerk is a motor reflex response to a stretch in the patellar tendon. The reflex arc is monosynaptic, which is the most simplistic reflex, only existing with one sensory and one motor neuron (**Figure 1.53a**). The resultant action is to

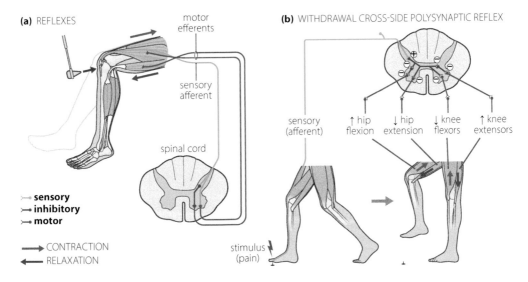

Figure 1.53 Cross-section of the spinal cord showing the afferent and efferent pathways of a reflex: (a) myotatic reflex; (b) withdrawal and cross-synaptic reflexes.

try to overcome the stretch by contracting the quadriceps muscles that act to extend the knee.

When the tendon hammer strikes the patellar tendon, **muscle spindles** sense this **stretch** in the muscle fibres of the quadriceps muscle. This information is transmitted through the afferent fibres to the dorsal horn of the spinal cord at the L4 level. An efferent motor neuron directly synapses with this sensory neuron in the ventral horn and sends a signal to the quadriceps muscle to contract.

As well as this excitatory motor neuron there is also an inhibitory signal sent from the ventral horn to the hamstring muscles that flex the knee, making them relax. The resultant movement is an uninhibited extension swing of the knee.

Withdrawal and crossed extensor reflex

Similar reflexes occur in response to pain but this time the peripheral receptor is a nociceptor. On the ipsilateral limb the same process occurs, but this time the knee flexes to withdraw from the painful stimulus and the extensor muscles are inhibited.

The crossed extensor reflex is polysynaptic, as it contains an interneuron which connects the sensory and motor neurons. If you were to stand on something sharp such as a nail, you would feel pain as sensed by the nociceptor. As with the withdrawal reflex, this is relayed up through the afferent fibres to the dorsal horn. In the dorsal horn this time they synapse with an interneuron which passes to the contralateral ventral horn to synapse with the efferent motor neurons to the contralateral limb. The extensor muscles contract and flexors relax to shift the weight to the opposite foot and protect the foot that has stood on the nail (**Figure 1.53b**).

Inverse myotatic reflex

This reflex protects the muscles and tendons from overload. During muscle contraction tension is felt in the muscles and tendons. **Golgi tendon** bodies are the peripheral sensors that activate if there is too much **tension** in the muscle and, to overcome this, they inhibit the overstretched muscle as a protective mechanism. This is the opposite of the stretch reflex, the peripheral sensors of which are the muscle spindles.

1.16.4 Normal gait patterns

The gait cycle describes a smooth transition from one foot to another while propelling the body forwards. It occurs in two main phases: when the foot is in contact with the floor (stance phase) and when the foot is in the air (swing phase). When describing the gait cycle, it is conventional to refer to one limb at a time.

Stance phase

Initial contact with the ground in the normal gait is with a heel strike on the lateral border. The weight is transferred forwards to mid-stance with a roll of pronation from the lateral border of the foot to the foot being flat on the floor. As the weight continues to move forward, the foot plantarflexes so that the big toe is the last contact with the floor – known as toe off (**Figure 1.54**).

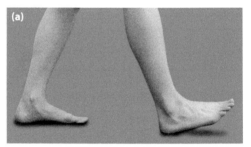

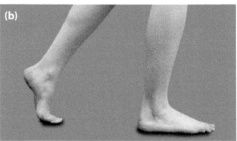

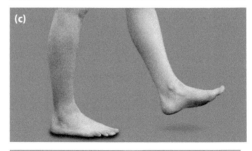

Figure 1.54 The gait cycle: (a) heel strike; (b) toe off; (c) swing.

Swing phase

In swing phase the hip starts in full extension and flexes forwards to continue with another heel strike. For the foot to be able to clear the ground during swing phase, the hip needs to rise on the ipsilateral side.

Force couple

Muscle groups work in pairs to control movements as a force couple. A force couple is when two equal and opposite forces exert a rotation force. Most muscles work synergistically and rarely in isolation. The control for the muscles around the hip and their resultant movements during normal gait is complex.

Hip movements

The muscles in the anterior hip are the hip flexors called iliacus, psoas and rectus femoris. They attach to the transverse processes of the lumbar spine and onto the lesser trochanter. The extensor muscle of the hip is the gluteus maximus but it is also helped by the hamstring muscles, known as the biceps femoris, semitendinosus and semimembranosus, which attach to the pelvis and cross both the hip and knee joint. Both these muscle groups act together during walking as a force couple. When your leg swings forwards under the action of the hip flexors, your hip extensors work to slow down the movement towards the end of swing phase.

Pelvic tilt

During the swing phase the contralateral hip abductor muscles – gluteus medius and minimus – that attach to the iliac wing of the pelvis and to the greater trochanter of the femur are activated. As the contralateral limb is connected to the ground, the abductive force raises the ipsilateral hip, allowing the foot to clear the ground. Hip adductors on the ipsilateral side keep the swinging foot in the midline (see Trendelenburg test, *Section 2.3.4*).

1.16.5 Abnormal gait

Altered gait patterns can occur due to muscle weakness, pain, spasticity or nerve injury (**Table 2.6**).

1.17 Answers to starter questions

1. Red marrow, which is full of newly formed blood cells, is mostly found in flat bones such as the sternum, pelvis and skull. Bone marrow biopsies are taken with a large needle which needs to pierce bone. The sternum and the iliac bone of the pelvis can be felt just underneath the skin and access to these bones is relatively easy.

2. The secondary ossification centres (see **Figure 1.6**) of the distal humerus are, in order of appearance and fusion: **C**apitellum; **R**adial head; **I**nternal (medial) epicondyle; **T**rochlea; **O**lecranon; **L**ateral epicondyle; hence the mnemonic **CRITOL**. They form at around 2, 4, 6, 8, 10 and 12 years of age, respectively, although they form a little earlier in girls.

3. Fingers and toes are formed by the advancing of the apical ectodermal ridge to form a flat plate. Apoptosis (programmed cell death) of the cells in the web spaces forms the digits. Failure of these separations can lead to syndactyly, in which fingers and toes are webbed or stuck together.

4. The growth plate is cartilage made up of collagen matrix and full of chondrocyte cells. As the chondrocytes grow and move up towards the metaphysis they become calcified. Only calcified bone can be seen on radiographs, as it absorbs the photons from the X-ray beam, whereas non-calcified bone does not.

5. Most, but not all autoimmune conditions are more common among women. It is thought this is due to gender differences in the immune system, driven by hormones. For example, in pregnancy some autoimmune conditions improve significantly, probably due to the relative state of immunosuppression led by regulatory T cells; an example is rheumatoid arthritis.

6. In the development of atherosclerosis, there is an inflammatory process within vessel walls which causes injury, preceding the deposition of cholesterol and resulting in the formation of a plaque. In rheumatoid arthritis, systemic inflammation can accelerate such processes.

7. In west Africa, the incidence of SLE is rare. However, a person of west African descent is at increased risk of SLE compared to a Caucasian person living in Europe or the USA. Theories of why this should occur include loss of a protective satisfactory vitamin D level (vitamin D has immunomodulatory function) and less exposure to malaria or parasitic infections, which may skew the immune response.

8. If you have a normal healthy diet, then increasing dietary calcium does little to increase the amount of calcium in your bones. Calcium is under tight regulation in the blood by calcitonin and parathyroid hormone (PTH) released by the thyroid and parathyroid glands, respectively. PTH upregulates the activity of osteoclasts to release calcium from bone in the presence of low calcium. Conversely, in high plasma calcium, although osteoclast activity is down-regulated in the presence of high calcium due to calcitonin, more calcium is not deposited in the bones if sufficient is already present and it is instead excreted in the urine.

9. Reaming inside the medullary canal for fracture fixation destroys the endosteal blood supply; the heat from the drill increases this process. Care must be taken not to also damage to the periosteal blood supply, to prevent a fracture non-union (when the bone fails to heal).

10. Stressing a bone by bearing weight through it increases its bone mineral density. Stress from mechanically loading bone activates stretch ion channels on osteocytes, triggering the expression of genes that mediate bone growth and resorption.

11. Lumbar punctures are usually performed between L3 and L4 vertebrae but can be placed at the L4/5 space or the L2/3 space. This level is chosen as it is after the spinal cord has ended, usually at level L1 or L2 and divided into the terminal spinal roots.

12. A hemi transection of the spinal cord would clinically present as Brown-Séquard syndrome. Brown-Séquard syndrome presents with weakness and numbness on the ipsilateral (same) side of the body and loss of pain and temperature on the contralateral (opposite) side. This is due to the spinothalamic tracts that transmit pain and temperature decussating at the level of the spinal cord. The lateral corticospinal tracts (motor) and dorsal columns (vibration and proprioception) decussate at the level of the medulla.

13. Botulinum toxin (Botox) prevents the SNARE proteins from binding the ACh vesicles to the presynaptic membrane. Inhibiting the ACh entering the synaptic cleft prevents muscle contraction, producing paralysis. Botox is used to treat children with cerebral palsy suffering with spasticity and also used in the cosmetic industry to relax the facial muscles.

14. Muscle strains occur when the muscle is pulled under tension, causing breaking of the actin and myosin bonding. In severe strains, when the muscle is quickly stretched beyond its resting length, part of the muscle may rupture.

15. Rhabdomyolysis is a condition in which muscle is broken down, resulting in high levels of myoglobin in the blood. Myoglobin is present in skeletal muscle cells and is an oxygen-binding protein, depending on the amount of oxygen bound to the deep red colour of muscle. Myoglobin is a large globular protein similar to haemoglobin and when levels are high can cause damage to the kidneys, resulting in renal failure.

16. Joint stability can be constrained by both dynamic and static stabilisers. Static stabilisers include the bony shape of the joint and the static ligaments surrounding the joint restraining movement. Dynamic stabilisers are the muscles and they only stabilise the joint when they are activated.

17. Gait can be assessed by clinical examination, watching a patient walk and noting down the range of movement, muscle patterning and foot position. More accurate and reproducible methods are now available in the clinical laboratory which include using force plates to assess what part of the foot is contacting the ground and with how much force. Video analysis using optoelectrics (a method of localising joints in a space) can measure range of movement.

18. Below-knee amputation increases energy expenditure while ambulating, and the body tries to compensate for this higher energy expenditure. On the prosthetic limb side, hip extensors are working hard in stance phase and in swing phase on the unaffected limb. Ultimately the mechanical work that is absent shifts up the kinetic chain to the trunk. Increasing the momentum in the trunk compensates for the loss of power from the prosthesis.

Chapter 2
Clinical essentials

Starter questions

Common symptoms and how to take a history

1. In which musculoskeletal conditions is a family history important?
2. What type of pain is a red flag symptom?

Common signs and how to examine the patient

3. Which unusual sites may give clues to diagnoses that are commonly missed when examining the musculoskeletal system?
4. Is it necessary to fully undress a patient for a musculoskeletal examination?

Investigations

5. Why doesn't everybody with rheumatoid arthritis test positive for rheumatoid factor?
6. Why are plain radiographs still used when CT and MRI are available?

Management options

7. Why does one patient with RA get benefit from a treatment but another doesn't?
8. What risks does immunosuppression carry?
9. Should patients exercise a painful joint?
10. When is acupuncture indicated?

Answers to questions are to be found in *Section 2.12*.

Patients presenting with musculoskeletal symptoms come from a diverse demographic. Male, female, young and old are all affected by joint disease, and subsequent disability can have profound effects on function and quality of life. Joints themselves can be disrupted due to an isolated trauma or a systemic or chronic illness. Extra-articular features are common, and tissues ranging from bones and tendons to blood vessels and skin can be affected. This can make taking a history and performing an adequate examination challenging; it is nevertheless important in order to narrow down the possible diagnoses. Likewise, investigations are varied and becoming increasingly complex in order to support timely diagnosis of conditions which now have more sophisticated but successful treatments.

2.1 How to take a history

Many musculoskeletal conditions can be diagnosed following a thorough clinical assessment. Epidemiological factors such as age, sex and ethnicity can predispose to certain conditions. Has something happened to the patient such as injury or trauma? Have they been recently unwell, e.g. infection? Have they had recent surgery? Are there any predisposing medical or surgical problems?

History taking in cases of trauma or sepsis needs to be focused. You do not have time to take a detailed history but pertinent questions are essential to the emergency management of an acutely unwell patient (see *Section 2.5*).

2.1.1 Age, sex and ethnic origin

The age, sex and ethnic origin of the patient give significant pointers in some disorders. For example, conditions such as osteoarthritis, osteoporosis, polymyalgia rheumatica and multiple myeloma are all more common in older patients, usually over the age of 50 years. Inflammatory arthritis, autoimmune disease and primary bone tumours are more common in a younger population.

Conditions such as rheumatoid arthritis (RA), systemic lupus erythematosus (SLE), osteoporosis and anterior cruciate knee ligament injuries are more common in females, whereas axial spondylitis (ankylosing spondylitis) and gout are more common in males.

SLE is more common in Afro-Caribbean populations, whereas RA is more common in Caucasian or native American populations.

2.1.2 Patient's problem list (presenting complaint)

This is the list of problems or symptoms that the patient either declares or that come to light following questioning. It should be presented as a list of simple words or phrases, e.g. knee pain, stiffness in the hands, unable to walk. It is important to note if the patient is left- or right-handed.

2.1.3 History of presenting complaint

Ask more detailed information about the patient's problem list or presenting complaint; this can be divided into the biomedical and patient perspective.

Biomedical perspective

This is detailed medical information about the patient's problem or problems. It should include the setting and context of the assessment (e.g. GP surgery, hospital outpatient clinic, emergency department); a clear sequence of events and timeline; a thorough analysis of symptoms (using e.g. the 'SOCRATES' acronym for pain – see *Section 2.2.1*); and an appropriate review of other relevant body systems. For example, if you suspect an inflammatory joint condition such as rheumatoid arthritis, are there any extra-articular multisystem manifestations in other organs?

Patient perspective

It is important to establish the patient's thoughts and opinions. The 'ICE' acronym of Ideas, Concerns and Expectations is useful here:

- **I**deas: has the patient any idea what the cause of the problems may be?
- **C**oncerns: does the patient have any particular worries or concerns as to what might be happening and if so, what is the basis for these views?
- **E**xpectations: what is the patient expecting to happen next?

Also establish to what extent symptoms are affecting the patient's life. For example, can they work, is their mobility affected, can they perform their activities of daily living, are they sleeping (**Table 2.1**)? Patients attending musculoskeletal services may normally be very active, either through hobbies or work. The effects of musculoskeletal disease are antagonistic: the less a joint is used, the weaker it becomes. The less confident individuals are at mobilising, the greater the risk of falls.

Table 2.1 *The impact of musculoskeletal disease*	
Consequences of pain	**Consequences of loss of joint function and disability**
Depression	Depression
Sleep disturbance	Reduced confidence
Reliance on medication, with associated side-effects	Falls
	Social isolation
	Relationship problems
Reduction in mobility	Employment problems (sick leave and unemployment) and financial difficulty
Relationship problems	
Employment problems (sick leave and unemployment) and financial difficulty	
	Difficulty in caring for young children or other dependants

Keep in mind that there is often a close relationship between physical, psychological and social factors that have an impact on musculoskeletal symptoms. For example, acute psychological stress can manifest as a worsening of physical musculoskeletal symptoms. Alternatively persistent musculoskeletal pain which disturbs sleep can increase fatigue, worsen depression and further exacerbate musculoskeletal symptoms.

2.1.4 Background information

Past medical history

A clear list of any past medical or surgical musculoskeletal problems should be gathered, including dates and whether the issue remains active (e.g. ongoing symptoms or treatment) or is now inactive. Any history of previous similar problems and treatments, prior injury or fractures, joint surgery or replacement, or infections may be particularly relevant. Many disorders of other systems are associated with musculoskeletal manifestations (**Table 2.2**). Asking about these conditions in your history taking can be enlightening. For example, patients may not think a past uveitis can be an important clue to the cause of their joint symptoms.

Table 2.2 *Conditions associated with musculoskeletal disease*	
Condition	**Association**
Uveitis	Seronegative arthropathies, e.g. axial spondyloarthritis, psoriatic arthritis
Inflammatory bowel disease: ■ Crohn's ■ ulcerative colitis	Sacroiliitis, axial spondyloarthritis, arthralgia, inflammatory mono- and oligoarthritis
Coeliac disease	Osteoporosis
Chronic kidney disease	Gout
Skin rash, e.g. psoriasis	Psoriatic arthritis
History of other autoimmune disease, e.g. Hashimoto's thyroiditis	General predisposition to other autoimmune disease

Medication history

Taking an accurate drug history, including asking specifically about over-the-counter medication, is vital. It can tell you how much pain the patient is suffering and prevent you from prescribing a drug that may interact with a pre-existing medication.

Record current medications, including name, dose, indication and duration of treatment. As well as prescription drugs, don't forget to ask about over-the-counter preparations, particularly analgesics such as paracetamol or ibuprofen, dietary supplements, alternative or complementary therapies, and physical therapies such as physiotherapy or manipulation. Record whether the patient has responded to the treatment: this may help to confirm the diagnosis, e.g. an inflammatory problem is more likely to respond to non-steroidal anti-inflammatory drugs (NSAIDs) or corticosteroids. Ask if there have been any side-effects. An allergy history, including allergen and response, is also very important because there can be cross-reactivity with some drugs; for example, those with an allergy to aspirin will be allergic to sulfasalazine (*Section 2.8.4*). Remember to consider whether the medication could be contributing to the patient's problems, e.g. diuretics in gout (see *Section 3.8*). Ask about substance abuse, which may increase the risk of unusual infections such as hepatitis, HIV and tuberculosis; these can affect the musculoskeletal system and pose increased risks for immunosuppressive therapies.

Family history

There is a genetic basis to a number of musculoskeletal conditions, e.g. osteoporosis and hip fracture. Disorders related to HLA-B27 (see *Section 1.7.1*) include:

- axial spondyloarthritis
- psoriatic arthritis
- inflammatory bowel disease
- reactive arthritis
- anterior uveitis.

Be specific about this and draw out a family tree of at least first-degree relatives, i.e. parents, siblings and offspring (**Figure 2.1**). Record if they are still living, cause and age of death if not, and any musculoskeletal or specific medical problems. This provides a record for the notes and helps you to track inheritance patterns.

Social history

Occupation and the nature of work can increase the risk of musculoskeletal illness per se or be relevant to a patient's ability to perform necessary duties. Manual work increases the risk of injury, and the incidence of conditions such as osteoarthritis is greater with repetitive movements, heavy lifting and load bearing in specific joints over time. Lifestyle factors such as obesity, smoking and alcohol may be relevant. Hobbies and interests such as sports can be relevant to both cause and effect, e.g. tendinopathy (see *Section 7.13*). Establishing a patient's home situation – whether they live alone, have a local support network, the type of accommodation they live in, etc. – influences plans for ongoing care, rehabilitation and recovery.

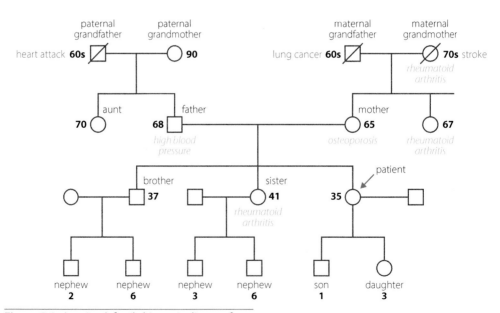

Figure 2.1 A patient's family history in diagram form.

2.2 Symptoms of musculoskeletal disease

Pain is a common presenting symptom and a thorough analysis of its site, onset, character, radiation, associations, time course, exacerbating and relieving factors can be revealing. The number and pattern of joint involvement can identify the type of arthritis. Joint stiffness and swelling are useful pointers towards inflammatory joint disease and the site of symptoms provides important clues. A refined diagnostic shortlist can then be confirmed with further investigations.

2.2.1 Pain

Pain is the most common musculoskeletal symptom. Gather as much detailed information as possible about the nature of a patient's pain. The 'SOCRATES' acronym provides a helpful framework to gather this information:

- **S**ite
- **O**nset
- **C**haracter
- **R**adiation
- **A**ssociations
- **T**ime course
- **E**xacerbating/relieving factors
- **S**everity

Site

Where is the pain? Or where is the maximal site of the pain? Which anatomical structure is involved – is it a joint, bone, tendon or other soft tissue structure? Pain from joints is termed 'arthralgia' and pain from muscles and other soft tissues 'myalgia'. Is the pain at more than one site? Does the pain differ between sites? Can the patient point to the site with one finger? Be as precise as you can when describing the site, e.g. left proximal femur, or right third proximal interphalangeal joint. If the pain is diffuse and involving many soft tissue structures then the patient may have a muscular problem, pain syndrome or fibromyalgia. The pattern of joint involvement may be a useful clue to the diagnosis, e.g. thumb carpometacarpal and distal interphalangeal finger joints in osteoarthritis. Don't forget to ask about other sites of pain, as the patient may only be describing the most painful area.

Onset

When did the pain start, and was it sudden or gradual? Did anything happen at the time, e.g. physical trauma? Include whether it is getting worse or better.

Character

What is the pain like, e.g. ache, stabbing, sharp?

Radiation

Does the pain radiate or move anywhere? Which direction, e.g. proximal or distal? Remember that joint pain can radiate distally and proximally, so always consider the pain could come from the joint above or below and make sure you assess adjacent joints and structures.

Associations

Are there any other symptoms or signs associated with the pain? For example, swelling, erythema (redness) and stiffness may suggest an inflammatory problem. Look for other features, e.g. numbness or loss of sensation may suggest a nerve problem.

Time course

Does the pain follow any pattern? Acute vs. chronic; speed of onset; worse with rest or use? Record the timings.

Exacerbating/relieving factors

Does anything change the pain? Is it worse with rest or use? For example, pain in inflammatory arthritis may be better with use and exercise and may respond well to NSAIDs such as ibuprofen. Conversely, pain in osteoarthritis often gets worse with use and activity. Lateral epicondylitis ('tennis elbow'; see *Section 7.14*) will be worse on extending the wrist.

Severity

How bad is the pain? Although somewhat subjective, getting the patient to quantify their pain using a pain scale of 0 ('no pain') to 10 ('worst pain you can imagine') can be useful and also provides a point of comparison for subsequent assessments.

2.2.2 Swelling

Similar to pain, there are a number of characteristic features of swelling which should be established.

Site

You should try to determine which anatomical structure is swollen – is it a joint, bone, tendon or other soft tissue structure?

Onset

Ask when the swelling started, and whether it was sudden or gradual. Did anything happen at the time – was there a precipitating or associated event or change? Ascertain whether it is getting worse or better.

Character

Ask what the swelling is like. Is it soft (implying an inflammatory element) or hard (suggesting a bony origin)?

Associations

Check if there are any associated inflammatory symptoms such as warmth or redness.

Time course

Determine whether the swelling follows any pattern. Did it appear suddenly or over a longer period? What was the speed of onset? Did anything happen at the time? Does it disappear or is it constant? Does it ease if a particular activity is avoided?

Pattern

Record which joints are affected or have been affected. The joints affected can change in inflammatory arthritis, so you need to know which joints have ever been involved, not just the present problematic ones. The pattern may be very characteristic, e.g.:

■ monoarthritis – a single swollen joint, e.g. septic arthritis
■ oligoarthritis – two to four swollen joints, e.g. psoriatic arthritis
■ polyarthritis – many swollen joints, e.g. RA.

In the latter two, note whether the pattern is:

■ symmetrical, or
■ asymmetrical.

Finally, check the distribution of joint involvement, for example:

■ small or large joints
■ distal or proximal joints
■ axial arthritis (spine and sacroiliac joints).

The pattern and distribution will often provide a good idea of the diagnosis (**Figure 2.2**). Patients present with different patterns of arthritis; for example, not every joint will be affected in

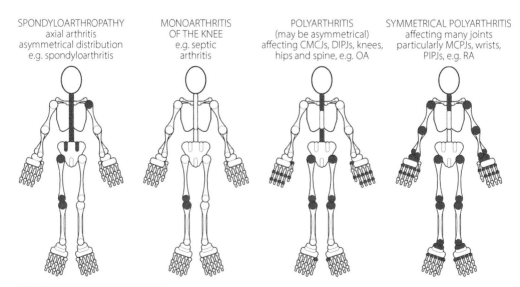

SPONDYLOARTHROPATHY
axial arthritis
asymmetrical distribution
e.g. spondyloarthritis

MONOARTHRITIS
OF THE KNEE
e.g. septic
arthritis

POLYARTHRITIS
(may be asymmetrical)
affecting CMCJs, DIPJs, knees,
hips and spine, e.g. OA

SYMMETRICAL POLYARTHRITIS
affecting many joints
particularly MCPJs, wrists,
PIPJs, e.g. RA

Figure 2.2 Patterns of arthritis.

rheumatoid arthritis but the pattern (mainly MCP and PIP joints) with a symmetrical distribution gives a clue. Tender and swollen joints need to be confirmed on examination.

> Arthritis in load-bearing joints of the hips, knees, spine, thumb bases, DIPJs and great toe MTP joints is a characteristic pattern of OA.

2.2.3 Stiffness

Prolonged stiffness (>30 minutes) in joints or muscles, particularly after rest and in the early morning, suggests an inflammatory problem. Typical patterns are:

- stiffness in the proximal muscles of the arms and pelvis in a patient over 60 years (polymyalgia rheumatica)
- stiffness in symmetrical hand and wrist joints (rheumatoid arthritis)
- stiffness mainly localised to the spine in a young adult (axial spondyloarthritis)
- stiffness lasting <30 minutes after rest, evening stiffness or stiffness after exercise or activity (more suggestive of a degenerative problem, e.g. osteoarthritis).

Osteoarthritis stiffness will typically get better with rest, whereas rest usually results in increasing stiffness in inflammatory disease. Note that it is common for a localised area to become stiff after injury or unaccustomed exercise.

2.2.4 Differentiating between inflammatory and degenerative conditions

Table 2.3 outlines different aspects of the history that help to differentiate between inflammatory and degenerative conditions. These characteristic symptoms can give you clues very early on in the history taking to the cause of the patient's presenting complaint.

2.2.5 Loss of function

An acute injury may result in loss of function. Inability to move a joint suggests a significant problem. The effect of the patient's symptoms is

Table 2.3 *Symptoms of inflammatory and degenerative (osteo-) arthritis*

Inflammatory	Degenerative
Can occur anytime in life but peak years of onset 30–60 (children can be affected)	Older patients (>50–60)
Boggy swollen joints	No/minimal/cool swelling
Multiple joints affected, symmetrical pattern	One or more joints affected, varying patterns, load-bearing joints
Pain worse in morning/after rest	Pain worse in evening/ following activity
Significant response to NSAIDs or corticosteroids	Less response to NSAID or corticosteroid therapy
Rapid onset	Slow onset
Early morning stiffness >30 minutes	Early morning stiffness <30 minutes
Systemic symptoms including fatigue, weight loss, fever	Systemic symptoms uncommon
Extra-articular symptoms, e.g. skin rashes, lung disease, neuropathy	Extra-articular symptoms not present

often what is most important to them, and they will probably report this without prompting. However, it is also essential to establish any functional difficulties during history taking. Consider any change in mobility, e.g. walking distance, stairs. A limp in a child is likely to be significant and should be investigated. Are activities of daily living (ADL) affected, e.g. washing, dressing, going to the toilet, cooking, shopping and cleaning? Are there any occupational effects, e.g. are they able to go to work and perform their daily duties normally?

2.2.6 Muscle weakness

Muscle weakness may be a sign of primary muscle pathology (e.g. polymyositis) or could relate to injury or disuse with secondary wasting. To differentiate between causes it is best to identify the location of the symptoms:

- Are proximal or distal muscles affected? Inflammatory muscle disease usually affects large muscle groups, so proximal muscles tend to be affected. Distal symptoms may suggest a neurological problem.
- Are multiple muscles or a single muscle affected? Involvement of a single muscle suggests a localised problem.
- Is there associated pain? Subjective muscle weakness may be caused by pain or stiffness and can be associated with inflammatory conditions such as polymyalgia rheumatica. Injury to a muscle or joint can lead to subsequent deconditioning of surrounding muscles.

2.2.7 Symptoms of fracture

Focal bony tenderness, reduced range of movement and deformity can all indicate fracture. Obtaining a clear history and mechanism of any injury is important in confirming the type, location and severity of any fracture.

> **Don't discount the possibility of a fracture** in a patient with sudden onset pain but no history of trauma. Osteoporosis can lead to fractures without a traumatic mechanism of injury.

2.2.8 Mechanical symptoms

A range of symptoms may indicate a mechanical problem within or adjacent to a joint. The main problem often relates to damage to the joint cartilage.

Crepitus (grating)

Patients are likely to describe crepitus as 'grating'. They may hear a scraping or grinding noise as their joints move or they may feel a clicking sensation. The most common cause is rough cartilage and bone rubbing together in a joint, usually caused by degenerative arthritis or joint injury. In the knee this may be associated with pain at the front of the knee, made worse on going up and down stairs and getting up from and down onto the floor (patello-femoral osteoarthritis).

Locking

Locking of the joint occurs most commonly in the knee: the leg gets stuck in flexion and the patient is unable to straighten the leg. Often the patient reports having to wiggle the knee around, or they must adopt a certain position before the joint can loosen and move again. It is usually caused by a physical block to extension of the knee, usually due to a meniscal tear. Sometimes pain can be so severe in a joint that it can cause 'pseudo-locking'; i.e. there is no physical block to the hinge mechanism, but the joint is too painful to extend.

Giving way

Giving way is a term for when a joint buckles unexpectedly. A joint giving way suggests instability or more severe muscle weakness. In the knee this could represent a ligament injury, meniscal tear or osteoarthritis. A knee can also give way if pain causes a reflex where the quadriceps tendon is inhibited.

2.2.9 Extra-articular features

Many diseases that affect the musculoskeletal system also affect other organ systems. Examples of multisystem diseases include RA and SLE. Perform a review of systems assessment to detect any additional symptoms by systematically moving through each organ system asking additional questions about skin rashes, mouth ulcers, breathlessness, paraesthesia, etc. (**Table 2.4**). Equally, it is also important to look for systemic disease that may be the cause of or associated with musculoskeletal problems.

> **Don't forget the possibility of genitourinary disease producing musculoskeletal symptoms.** In a patient presenting with acute arthritis, ask about conjunctivitis and vaginal or urethral discharge. A sexual history is important because reactive arthritis can be associated with *Chlamydia* and gonococcal infection.

Table 2.4 *Systems review in musculoskeletal history taking; the symptoms you may enquire about depend on the presenting complaint*

Symptom	Possible significance
Recent malaise or prodromal event	Some infections can trigger musculoskeletal symptoms, e.g. reactive arthritis
Weight loss	Significant inflammation, e.g. severe arthritis or vasculitis Cancer
Shortness of breath	Vasculitis, sarcoidosis, interstitial lung disease (relating to rheumatoid arthritis or connective tissue disease)
Indigestion	Connective tissue disorders
Mouth ulcers	SLE, Behçet's disease, inflammatory bowel disease
Hair loss	SLE or autoimmune alopecia
History of miscarriage	SLE or primary antiphospholipid syndrome
Fever	Infection, malignancy, vasculitis, adult onset Still's disease
Tingling/ numbness	Nerve entrapment, e.g. prolapsed disc, tumour, inflammation of surrounding soft tissue, peripheral neuropathy
Fatigue	A common symptom present in inflammatory arthritis, connective tissue disease, vasculitis, fibromyalgia
Dry eyes and mouth	Sjögren's syndrome
Diarrhoea	Inflammatory bowel disease
Skin rash	Vasculitis, psoriatic arthritis

2.2.10 Red flags

Red flag symptoms potentially signify severe life- or organ-threatening disease such as vasculitis, infection or cancer. You must always enquire about systemic illness, weight loss, fever and pain at night which disturbs sleep. Unremitting progressive symptoms should prompt urgent further assessment. Sometimes the patient can be non-specifically unwell without any focal symptoms, so persistent constitutional symptoms such as fatigue and exhaustion should also be taken seriously.

Localised bone pain

Localised bone pain should alert you to the possibility of malignancy. However, patients can sometimes present with musculoskeletal pain and stiffness as part of a paraneoplastic syndrome, caused by a primary malignant process elsewhere in their body. A thorough history, including a review of systems, may identify other problems. Primary bone cancer is rare, whereas secondary metastasis to bone is more common (see *Section 10.3*).

Constant and/or night pain

Unremitting 24-hour pain is a worrying symptom. Pain disturbing patients significantly at night is also a red flag. Whilst some inflammatory arthritides are extremely severe, the level of pain usually varies to some extent during the day.

Unintentional weight loss

Unintentional weight loss indicates an unexpected increase in the body's metabolic rate. This often signifies rapidly dividing cells. This may be due to excessive inflammation (and the subsequent increase in energy demands of the immune system) or rapidly dividing cancer cells.

Neurological deficit

Neurological deficit can indicate:
- nerve entrapment due to a serious pathology requiring surgery, e.g. severe spinal stenosis or disc disease in the spine
- a tumour encroaching on either central or peripheral nerves, e.g. Pancoast tumour of the lung affecting the nerve roots of the brachial plexus

- inflammation so severe that nerves are compressed, e.g. carpal tunnel syndrome in inflammatory arthritis
- damage to the blood supply of nerves, e.g. vasculitis.

These pathologies can cause significant morbidity and mortality if undiagnosed or left untreated.

Cauda equina syndrome is an emergency presentation caused by damage to the nerves at the distal end of the spinal cord. It may present with loss of bowel or bladder function, loss of sensation in the perineum ('saddle area'); there may be lower back pain and progressive paraplegia. See *Section 9.5* for a more detailed review.

Fever

Fever in terms of musculoskeletal conditions usually indicates infection, vasculitis or malignancy.

Septic arthritis is a medical emergency because infection in a joint can cause rapid destruction of cartilage, bone and soft tissue structures. It usually presents with relatively sudden onset of pain, swelling, redness, warmth and inability to move a joint (e.g. the patient is unable to stand on the affected leg). A single joint (monoarthritis) is the more common pattern and the knee joint is most commonly affected. Septic arthritis is discussed in detail in *Section 8.1* and *Case 11.3*.

2.3 How to examine the musculoskeletal system

Basic observations and a full physical examination are paramount when examining the musculoskeletal system. Straightforward measurements are useful for initial assessment but also as a record for assessing response to treatment. Certain signs are pathognomonic of specific conditions, whilst basic observations build a picture of the patient and help to recognise the unwell patient (**Table 2.5**).

From the history, it is likely that you will have identified one or more joints as the focus for your examination. Ideally, all joints should be examined and it is certainly good practice to examine the joints above and below the affected

Table 2.5 *The relevance of basic observations in the musculoskeletal clinic*	
Observation	**Relevance**
Body habitus	Height, weight and body mass index (BMI) are recorded; this tells you if the skeletal frame and muscles are overloaded or if someone is at risk of osteoporosis due to low BMI
	Patients with high BMI have greater risks of surgical complications, both in terms of the surgery itself and the anaesthetic
Urine dipstick	Urinalysis is performed to look for kidney pathology causing proteinuria or haematuria, which can be present in a patient with vasculitis or connective tissue disease
	Patients on immunosuppressive therapy are at increased risk of infections and a urinary tract infection causes white blood cells and nitrites on dipstick testing
Blood pressure	High blood pressure is important when considering the overall health of a patient or when commencing medication that can exacerbate hypertension (e.g. leflunomide, etoricoxib)
	Low blood pressure in an acutely unwell patient may represent infection or sepsis
Temperature	In someone presenting with either new joint pain or an exacerbation of existing joint pain, a high temperature should alert you to a potential diagnosis of septic arthritis
	Cyclical pyrexia can be seen in adult onset Still's disease

joint to ensure referred pain is not responsible for the presenting complaint. At all times during an examination, the patient must feel comfortable and secure. Therefore, it is good practice to ask the patient whether any joint or muscles currently hurt and ask them to tell you if you cause them discomfort. Reminding them throughout the examination will help to build rapport. Keep reassuring them with phrases such as:

- "Which area(s) is most painful today? I will come to that last."
- "I will try to look at your face when I'm examining your joints but this isn't always possible. So please do tell me if I'm causing you discomfort".
- "OK, I'm moving round to look at your back now; please let me know if anything I do causes you pain."

A distracting injury is one that distracts the examiner from assessing more important injuries. This is particularly prevalent in cases of trauma. For example, after a fall, a patient is brought to the Emergency Department with a bloodied limb caused by an open fracture. The team work on this without top-to-toe assessment and miss a neck injury that requires immediate stabilisation.

2.3.1 General inspection

The examination starts as soon as you see the patient. Note their build, whether they are in pain, what type of gait they have.

It is helpful to have the patient undress down to their underwear for a thorough musculoskeletal assessment. The patient's consent must be sought. It is appropriate to seek a chaperone, e.g. a nurse of the same sex as the patient, to put the patient at ease. Patients should be covered with a sheet when concentrating on individual joints, to minimise their exposure and to respect their dignity.

A general inspection is the first part of any system examination and the following points are quick to observe:

- Does the patient look systemically well? Take note of the basic observations (**Table 2.5**).
- Does the patient look in pain?
- Did you see them walk into the examination room? Is there any abnormality in gait?
- Can they undress/dress independently?
- Is there any obvious abnormality or asymmetry of joints, muscle bulk, spine curvature, etc.? (**Figure 2.3**)
- Are there any obvious red and swollen joints?
- Is there a rash?

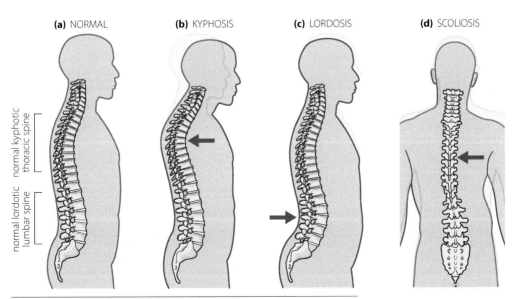

Figure 2.3 Spinal curves: (a) normal; (b) kyphosis; (c) lordosis; (d) scoliosis.

- Are there any scars? Commonly, scars are often not visible until you are in close proximity to the patient.
- Do any limbs look to be at an unusual angle – e.g. shortened and externally rotated leg in neck of femur fracture? (**Figure 6.1**).
- Look top-to-toe for any abnormality including the eyes, skin and scalp.

2.3.2 The GALS assessment

The GALS (gait, arms, legs, spine) tool is a screening assessment that provides a structured approach to assessing the musculoskeletal system via brief questions and a general examination. Once an abnormality has been detected, there can be a more thorough assessment of that specific area.

The patient is asked three questions:

- Do you have any pain or stiffness in your muscles, joints or back?

- Can you dress yourself without any difficulty or help?
- Can you walk up and down stairs without difficulty?

> **The GALS screening tool** will need to be amended according to the patient's ability to perform the tests.

This is followed by a general examination in four areas:

Gait

Ask the patient to walk both towards you and away from you so that you can assess the front and back of the patient. Look for abnormalities in their gait (**Table 2.6**), for muscle and joint asymmetry from top to toe, and for presence of foot arches (**Figure 2.4**). Flat feet can be part of a normal spectrum or related to hypermobility.

Table 2.6 *Types of gait, their features and causes*

Gait	Feature	Cause
Antalgic	Shortened stance phase on the affected leg reducing the standing time and pain endured	Painful lesions of the hip, knee, ankle or foot
High stepping	To overcome foot drop the knee needs to be brought higher; the foot often slaps on the ground due to the inability to heel strike first	Foot drop after common peroneal nerve injury
Scissor	Legs cross while walking	Cerebral palsy
Short leg	Patients with a short leg will often lean towards the side of the longer leg when they are walking	Limb shortening (congenital or acquired)
Stiff hip	No flexion at hip	Hip pathology, including infection and tuberculosis
Quadriceps	Limping gait with hand on knee	Poliomyelitis
Trendelenburg	Weak hip abductors cause the pelvis to dip on the contralateral side; the body is thrown to the ipsilateral side causing the whole body to tilt so the foot can clear the ground in swing phase	Weakness of the abductor muscles caused by chronic osteoarthritis
Calcaneal	No push-off	Calf weakness
Stiff knee	Pelvis raised during swing phase	Stiff knee
Ataxic	Wide-based gait, unsteady	Cerebellar disease

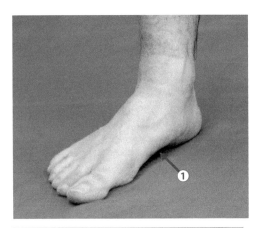

Figure 2.4 A normal foot arch is observed when there is a visible gap between the foot and the surface of the floor ①.

Arms

This can be performed with the patient sitting on the edge of a bed or standing. Inspect for deformity then test function from shoulder to fingers, as follows:

- Shoulder – "Put both your hands behind your head"
- Shoulder external rotation – "Put your hands behind your back as high as you can"

- Elbow – "Place both arms straight in front of you"
- Forearms – "Tuck your elbows tight into your side and turn your arms so the palms are facing upwards, and now the other way" (**Figure 2.5**)
- Grip strength – "Make a tight fist"
- Wrist flexion and finger extension – "Make a prayer sign" (**Figure 2.6**); a negative prayer sign is where the patient brings their

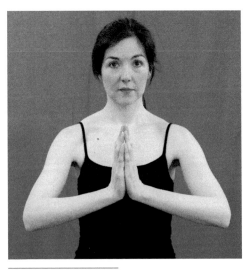

Figure 2.6 Prayer sign.

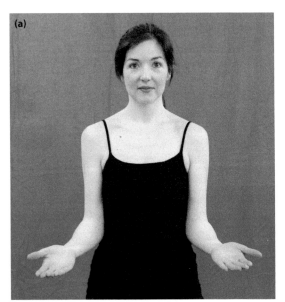

Figure 2.5 Movements of the forearm: (a) supination; (b) pronation.

hands together with no gaps on the palmar surface. There will be gaps if there are flexion deformities, and the sign is then positive.

■ Fine motor – "With each finger on your left hand in turn, touch your thumb on your left hand"; repeat on the right hand

■ Hand tenderness – squeeze the metacarpal area by gripping the lateral and medial aspects of the hand (**Figure 2.7**); if a patient experiences tenderness when the hand is squeezed in this area it raises suspicions of synovitis here.

Legs

Ask the patient to stand. Inspect again for any deformity. Then ask the patient to lie on an examination couch.

■ Feel each knee for warmth or swelling. If there is swelling, check for a patellar tap (**Figure 2.8**).

■ Flex each knee as far as possible, feeling for crepitus (**Figure 2.9**).

■ Rotate each hip joint, checking for restriction or tenderness (**Figures 2.9** and **2.10**).

■ Squeeze across the metatarsal area of both feet (**Figure 2.11**).

■ Check the soles of the feet for injury or callus formation.

Spine

With the patient standing, inspect from the front, back and side. Look specifically for normal spinal curvature; cervical lordosis, thoracic kyphosis and lumbar lordosis (**Figure 2.3**).

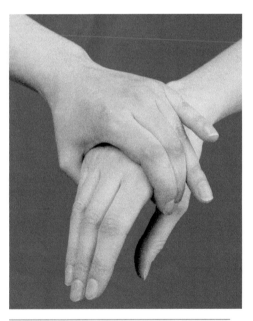

Figure 2.7 Metacarpophalangeal squeeze test.

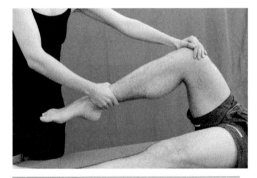

Figure 2.9 Hip movement: internal rotation. On bending the knee, feel for crepitus.

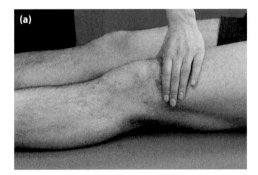

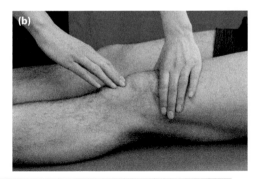

Figure 2.8 Patellar tap: (a) first fluid is milked distally from the suprapatellar pouch; (b) using the other hand, the patella is pressed down. If a large amount of fluid is present, there will be a tap as the patella strikes the femur.

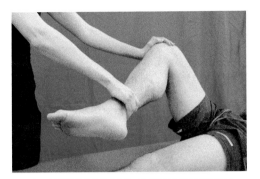

Figure 2.10 Hip movement: external rotation.

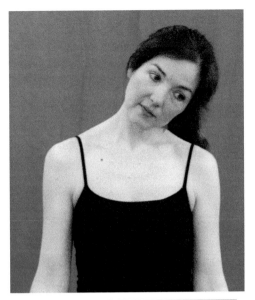

Figure 2.12 Lateral flexion of the cervical spine.

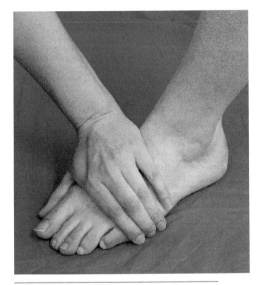

Figure 2.11 Metatarsophalangeal squeeze test: tenderness on palpation suggests synovitis.

- Test spinal flexion – "Can you please touch your toes?"
- Test lateral flexion of the C-spine – "Can you put your ear to your shoulder? And now your other ear to your other shoulder?" (**Figure 2.12**). Normal range of motion is up to 45°.
- Test rotation – "Now look over to your right, and now to your left" (**Figure 2.13**). Normal range of motion is up to 80°.

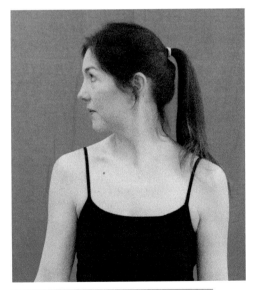

Figure 2.13 Rotation of the cervical spine.

2.3.3 Examination of specific joints

The standard approach for joint assessment is the same for all joints. However, each joint is unique in terms of its range of movement, functionality and special tests that can be performed. Always compare joints from both sides.

Look

Many abnormalities in the musculoskeletal system are obvious on sight alone, for example:
- limb deformity or gross swelling as a result of fracture or dislocation

- pathognomonic patterns of joint swelling arising in inflammatory arthritis (**Figures 2.2, 2.14, 2.15, 2.16** and *Chapter 3*)
- rashes that are instantly recognisable 'from the end of the bed' in conditions such as psoriasis and vasculitis (**Figure 2.17** and *Sections 3.3 and 4.13*)
- tophi associated with gout (**Figure 2.18**).

Some musculoskeletal abnormalities have eponymous names but if you are able to describe the deformity you see, e.g. fixed flexion of the elbow, lateral deviation of the great toe, then this is more useful and informative.

Feel

Feel around the individual joints. Examine finger joints with both hands (**Figure 2.19**) to assess swelling. When feeling a joint, consider the following questions:

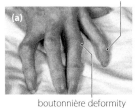
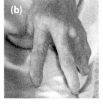

swan-neck deformity

boutonnière deformity

Figure 2.14 Small joint deformities associated with RA: (a) boutonnière and swan-neck deformities; (b) Z deformity of the thumb. These deformities are becoming less common with modern treatments.

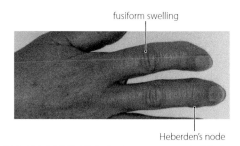

fusiform swelling

Heberden's node

Figure 2.15 Joint deformities associated with OA: Heberden's nodes of the index and middle finger and fusiform swelling of the fingers.

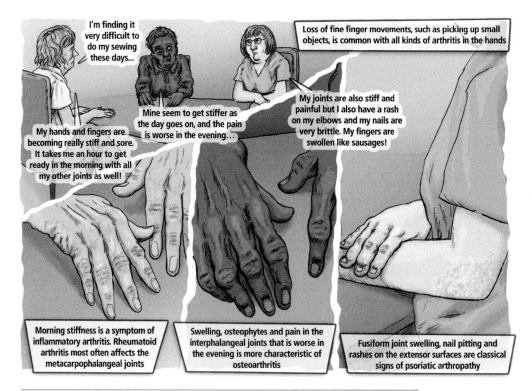

Figure 2.16 Typical symptoms and hand deformities in OA, RA and psoriatic arthritis.

- Is the joint warm?
- Is there a swelling? Is it hard (bone) or soft (soft tissue)?
- Is this an effusion (an increased amount of fluid within a synovial joint)? Is the swelling liquid/fluctuant? Is the patellar tap positive?
- Is it synovitis? Synovitis feels like a boggy swelling around a joint which is tender to touch.
- Am I causing the patient pain? Some patients will have chronic swelling or bony swelling of the joints but it is non-tender. Patients with acute synovitis or effusion will have significant tenderness on examination.

Move

Movement of joints consists of active movement (the patient moves their joints) or passive movement (the clinician moves the patient's joints). Active movement is helpful as it tells you something about day-to-day function that the patient feels comfortable managing. It is easiest to face the patient and ask them to copy you for the majority of the movements, rather than instructing them which can become confusing. Simply ask them to move a joint in the planes of movement expected to be achieved. When conducting passive movements, you can feel for crepitus over the joint and look for pain. Crepitus is often felt over the patella when the knee is flexed and extended; this is highly suggestive of osteoarthritis affecting the patellofemoral joint.

Examples of passive and active movements are shown in **Figures 2.20** and **2.21**. There can be a wider increased range of movement in those

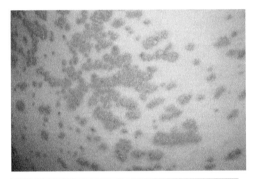

Figure 2.17 Skin psoriasis can take many forms: multiple small plaques or isolated large plaques.

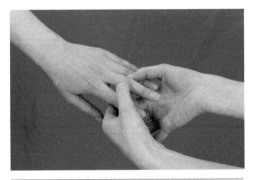

Figure 2.19 Bimanual palpation of the small joints of the hand, using the tips of both thumbs.

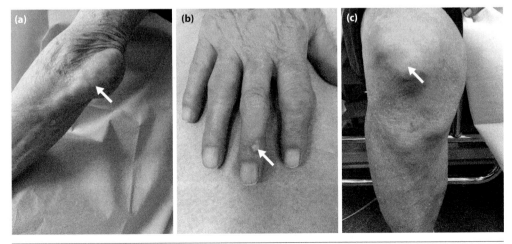

Figure 2.18 Gouty tophi are collections of monosodium urate crystals (always check the helix of the ear): (a) elbow; (b) fingers; (c) knee.

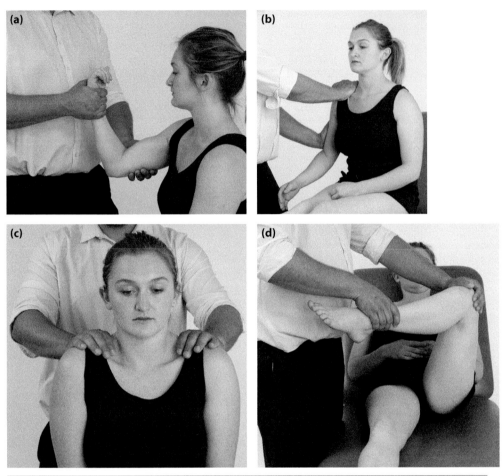

Figure 2.20 Joint movements: (a) elbow flexion and extension; (b) shoulder abduction and adduction; (c) shoulder elevation and depression; (d) hip internal and external rotation.

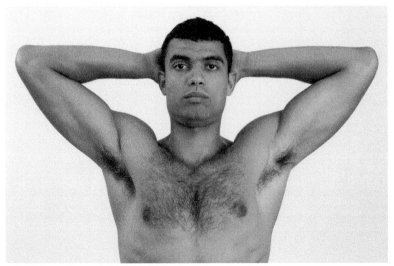

Figure 2.21 Testing movement of the shoulder and elbow.

patients with ligament disruption, connective tissue disease or hypermobility (see *Chapter 4*).

2.3.4 Special tests

Because of the number of joints involved in the musculoskeletal examination, all with their different functions, there are numerous special tests that can be performed, depending on the clinical scenario. The ones most useful in a general musculoskeletal examination are noted here.

> **The McMurray test**, which appears in many orthopaedic and rheumatology publications, assesses the knee for a meniscal tear. It is not described here because it is no longer thought to have a high diagnostic yield and can exacerbate damage to the joint.

Shoulder

Scarf test
The examiner moves the patient's arm across their body horizontally (**Figure 7.6**). In a positive test, pain is felt at the acromioclavicular joint.

Wrist

Finkelstein's test
By holding the thumb tucked into the palm and introducing sudden ulnar deviation of the wrist, symptoms of de Quervain's tenosynovitis (pain

over the radial aspect of the wrist) can be elicited (see **Figure 7.13**).

Phalen's and Tinel's tests
These two tests are used to assess for median nerve compression. A common problem at the wrist is carpal tunnel syndrome (see *Section 9.8*). The tests are positive if the symptoms of pain and paraesthesia are reproduced by holding the hands in a reverse prayer sign (Phalen's test, **Figure 2.22**) or by tapping over the volar aspect of the wrist (Tinel's test, **Figure 2.23**). Tingling occurs

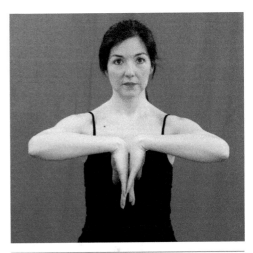

Figure 2.22 Phalen's test. Holding the hands in this position for 1 minute elicits pain and/or paraesthesia if there is median nerve compression.

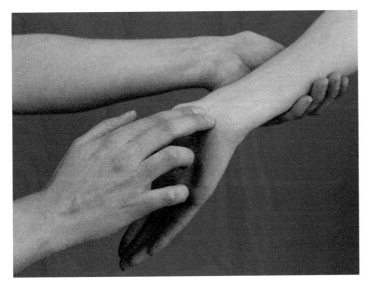

Figure 2.23 Tinel's test elicits pain and/or paraesthesia if there is median nerve compression.

in the palm in the distribution of the median nerve (usually the palmar aspect of thumb, index, middle finger and radial half of the ring finger).

Spine

The modified Schober's test

This assesses the extent of lumbar flexion. It is a particularly useful test when monitoring the progression of conditions such as axial spondyloarthritis. With the patient standing, the skin is marked at the point of the spine between the iliac crests. A mark is placed 5cm below and 10cm above this point (**Figure 2.24a**). When

the patient bends down to touch their toes, the distance between the upper and lower mark should increase by more than 5cm for it to be considered normal (**Figure 2.24b**).

Straight leg raise test

This is used to assess for sciatic nerve root irritation, most commonly due to a disc prolapse. With the patient lying flat, the leg is raised to 90°; usually the clinician needs to help lift the leg to reach this position. In a positive test, pain is felt in the posterior thigh. Bending the knee relieves the pain (**Figure 2.25**).

10 cm above iliac crest

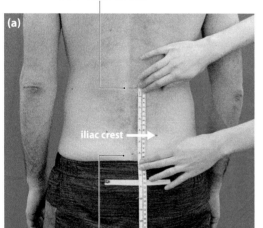

iliac crest →

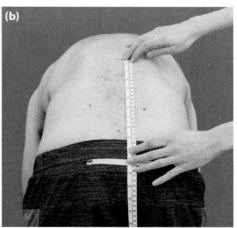

5 cm below iliac crest

Figure 2.24 The modified Schober's test: (a) marks being placed; (b) position during test.

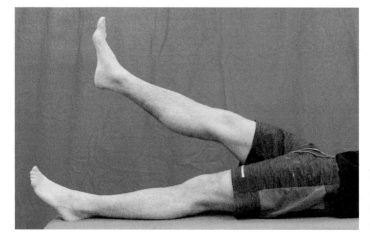

Figure 2.25 Straight leg raise: the patient's leg here is almost at 30° on active movement.

Hip

Thomas' test

This is used to test for fixed flexion deformity. The patient lies on their back on the examination couch. Ask them to bring both of their knees to their chest, i.e. flex their knees. Then ask them to lower one of their legs onto the examination table (**Figure 2.26a**); the hand under the patient's back ensures that it isn't lifting off the table. If they are unable to place the leg down straight, this is known as a positive Thomas' test and suggests a fixed flexion deformity (**Figure 2.26b**).

Trendelenburg test

This is used to test for hip and gluteal muscle weakness. With the patient standing, ask them to raise their leg whilst you observe from behind. The test is negative if the line of the hips remains relatively neutral when one leg is raised. If, however, the pelvis drops to the side of the raised leg, then there is a weakness on the contralateral side; this is a positive test. Repeat on the opposite side (**Figure 2.27**).

Knee

All of the tests on the knee are performed with the patient lying supine. Effusions can be tested for either by the patellar tap or looking for a bulge sign.

The patellar tap

This is positive if the patella is ballotable (bounces back up to the examiner's hand once

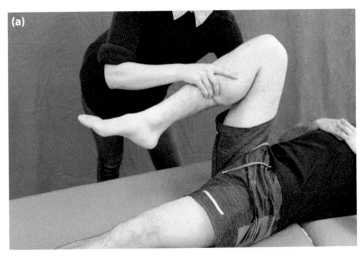

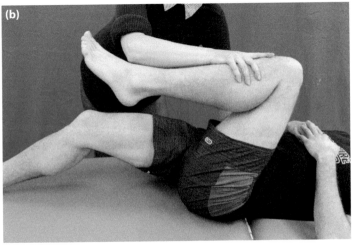

Figure 2.26 Thomas' test: (a) negative; (b) positive.

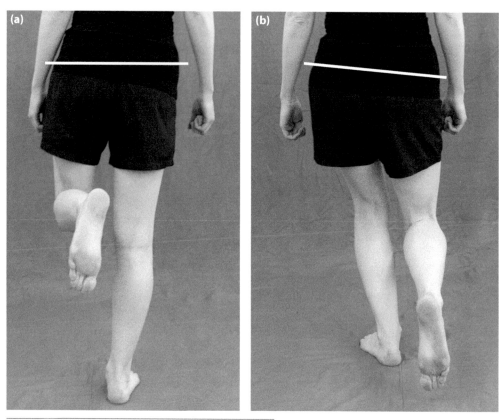

Figure 2.27 Trendelenburg test: (a) negative; (b) positive.

pushed down). One hand milks fluid down into the suprapatellar pouch while the other hand attempts to bounce the patella gently over the fluid (**Figure 2.8**).

The bulge sign

This is most effective if the effusion is small. Fluid is milked (pushed) from the medial compartment of the knee. Then pressure is applied quickly in

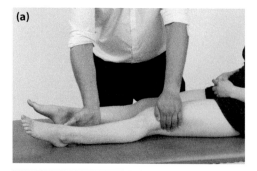
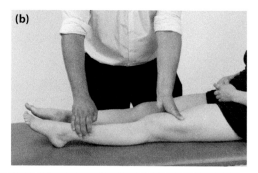

Figure 2.28 Assessing collateral ligament stability: (a) a valgus stress is placed on the knee in 15° of flexion to assess the medial collateral ligament; (b) a varus stress is placed on the knee in 15° of flexion to assess the lateral collateral ligament.

a smooth sweeping motion superiorly and then laterally. A bulge may appear on the medial side as fluid reaccumulates here.

Collateral ligament stability

This is tested by flexing the knee to 15–20° and stressing one side and then the other by applying gentle force (**Figure 2.28**).

Anterior drawer test

The cruciate ligaments are assessed by the anterior and posterior drawer tests (**Figure 2.29**). The knee to be tested is flexed to 90°. You can sit lightly on the patient's foot to give stability. Place hands behind the knee on the tibia, with thumbs either side of the patella; draw the tibia towards you slowly. If the tibia moves significantly there is ACL damage. If there is a posterior sag in the tibia when the knee is flexed to 90°, this can indicate PCL damage.

2.3.5 Function

Function is a test of whether a patient can perform day-to-day activities with their affected joint. Common examples are fastening and unfastening a button, picking up a coin (pincer grip), holding a pen and assessing grip strength. The function of larger joints tends to be assessed during the examination where the patient is asked to move joints, e.g. putting hands behind their head will assess their ability to wash their hair or remove a sweater. Examining gait gives you an idea of how mobile they are (**Table 2.6**).

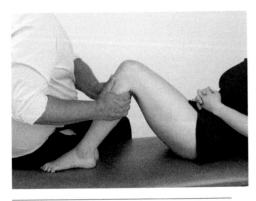

Figure 2.29 The anterior drawer test to assess ACL stability.

2.3.6 Additional examinations

When completing your musculoskeletal examination, always consider performing a neurological and vascular examination because of the potential for abnormalities in neighbouring structures. This is important in the orthopaedic setting, because trauma can cause damage to specific nerves and vessels. Documenting the patient's neurovascular status is essential prior to any intervention.

Nerve innervation of dermatomes and reflexes is shown in **Figure 2.30** and **Table 2.7**. Test power of individual muscle groups and record them according to a universal scale (**Table 2.8**). In the trauma setting, test individual nerve supply to the injured area to be more specific about damaged structures (**Table 2.9**). Feel for pulses around the site of an injury and on the contralateral side.

Table 2.7 *Deep tendon reflexes*	
Reflex	**Spinal level**
Biceps	C5–C6
Triceps	C7–C8
Supinator (brachioradialis)	C5–C6
Patellar/knee jerk	L3–L4
Achilles/ankle jerk	S1–S2

Table 2.8 *Grading muscle power: the UK Medical Research Council scale*	
Grade	**Description**
0	No movement
1	Flicker of muscle contraction
2	Movement only with gravity eliminated
3	Can overcome gravity but no resistance
4	Some resistance but can be overcome by examiner
5	Normal strength

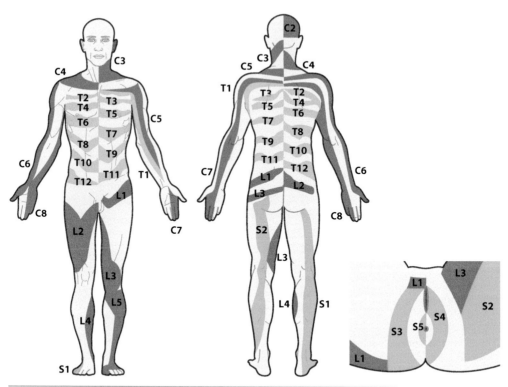

Figure 2.30 Dermatome map: each dermatome represents a spinal sensory nerve.

Table 2.9 *Peripheral nerves*			
Peripheral nerve	**Components of nerve**	**Peripheral nerve**	**Components of nerve**
Radial	C5–C8	Sciatic	L4–S2
Median	C6–T1	Tibial	L4–S2
Ulnar	C7–T1	Common peroneal	L4–S1
Axillary	C5–C6	Femoral	L1–L4
Musculocutaneous	C5–C7	Obturator	L2–L4

In the presence of pain, the assessment of power is unreliable. However, it should still be recorded in order to monitor deterioration or improvement.

2.4 Signs of musculoskeletal disease

The signs of musculoskeletal disease vary from obvious abnormalities that can be spotted as the patient walks into the examination room, or from the end of the bed, to special tests performed on clinical examination. Here we summarise some of the important signs and how to interpret them.

2.4.1 Tenderness

Tenderness is pain that is elicited on palpation; usually only light touch is required. It tends to be a sign of inflammation in response to injury or a disease process. This can be around a joint if there is a fracture or synovitis, or on palpation of inflamed muscle, tendon or ligaments. It can be a useful way to pinpoint the specific structure involved. For example, a patient complains of ankle pain. When you examine them, the joint appears normal but there is tenderness when the Achilles tendon is palpated, suggesting inflammation here.

2.4.2 Swelling

Joint swelling is an objective finding that is often easy to identify when examining joints. This is because for most joints there is a joint on the other side for comparison and the asymmetry may be obvious. However, subtle swelling, particularly in an overweight patient, may be more difficult to detect.

It is important to establish how localised the swelling is; for example, is the whole limb swollen – as can occur in lymphoedema – or are there definite discrete areas of joint swelling, suggesting an effusion? Swelling associated with increased warmth and erythema (redness) suggests an inflammatory process, whereas cool, non-erythematous, hard swelling is likely to be bony, e.g. osteophyte formation in OA.

For patients with inflammatory arthritis, the number of tender and swollen joints are recorded at each appointment. This information can be used:
- in scoring systems to assess disease activity, e.g. inflammatory arthritis
- to satisfy criteria for prescribing certain medications, e.g. biologic disease-modifying antirheumatic drugs (DMARDs) in RA
- to assess response to treatment in an objective way.

Site
Swelling over a joint often indicates an effusion, the main causes being arthritis or infection. However, other possibilities include bony swelling,

tumour, crystal arthropathies and fracture. Swelling over soft tissue structures may indicate ligament or tendon damage.

Severity
The size of the swelling does not always correlate with the nature of the underlying pathology. Accurate history, examination and investigations are more useful to determine this.

2.4.3 Reduced range of movement

A patient who is in pain will have reduced movement of the affected joint. Other factors can also contribute to a reduced range of movement such as fixed flexion deformities (patient unable to fully extend joint, e.g. due to severe osteoarthritis), acute injury including dislocation, or abnormalities of surrounding joint structures, e.g. in 'frozen shoulder' (adhesive capsulitis) where there is thickening and inflammation of the glenohumeral capsule. A damaged nerve supply or reduced muscle strength will also contribute to a reduced range of movement, and pain may or may not be present in these scenarios.

2.4.4 Joint deformity

Joint deformity can be caused by destruction of the joints themselves or damage to their surrounding supporting structures (tendons, ligaments, etc.) via various insults including injury or systemic inflammatory processes.

Keep in mind that deformities can also be congenital, e.g. lower limb abnormalities such as club foot in children, or caused by muscular or neurological disorders such as Charcot–Marie–Tooth disease. An accurate history will usually identify the cause.

Common examples of joint deformity are listed in **Table 2.10**. This table does not list individual deformities that are caused by trauma because these are unique to each individual case and should be described as seen.

The hand is an important place to look for patterns of joint swelling and deformities. These characteristic changes can help to diagnose a particular condition. Hand deformities in RA are demonstrated in **Figure 2.14** and those in OA

Table 2.10 *Common orthopaedic and rheumatological deformities*

Region	Sign	Definition
Spine and neck	Torticollis	Twisting of the neck to one side
	Scoliosis	Lateral spinal curvature in the coronal plane
Upper limb	Winging of the scapula	Abnormal protrusion of the scapula
Hand and wrist	Bouchard's node	Osteoarthritic bony enlargement of the PIP joint
	Heberden's node	Osteoarthritic bony enlargement of the DIP joint
	Mallet finger	Isolated flexion at the DIP joint
	Claw hand	Extension at the MCP joints with flexion at the DIP and PIP joints
	Swan-neck deformity	Hyperextension at the PIP joint and flexion at the DIP joint
	Boutonnière deformity	Flexion of the PIP joints with hyperextension of the DIP joints
	Ulnar deviation of the fingers	Medial deviation of the fingers in the direction of the ulna, usually at the level of the MCP joints
	Caput ulna	Prominence of the ulna at the wrist as a result of subluxation and palmar translation of the radius at the distal radio-ulnar joint
Hip	Fixed flexion deformity	Inability of the affected hip to reach full extension
Knee	Genu valgum	A knocked knee deformity; valgus deviation of the tibia
	Genu varum	A bow-legged deformity; varus deviation of the tibia
Foot and ankle	Hindfoot varus	Angling of the heel towards the midline, as viewed from behind
	Hindfoot valgus	Excessive angling of the heel away from the midline, as viewed from behind
	Pes planus	Loss or flattening of the medial arch
	Pes cavus	Exaggeration of the medial arch
	Hallux valgus (bunion)	Lateral deviation of the great toe at the MTP joint
	Hallux rigidus	Stiffness of the great toe MTP joint
	Claw toe	Hyperextension at the MTP joint with flexion at the PIP and DIP joints
	Hammer toe	Flexion at the PIP joint
	Mallet toe	Flexion at the DIP joint

DIP, distal interphalangeal; MCP, metacarpophalangeal; MTP, metatarsophalangeal; PIP, proximal interphalangeal

are demonstrated in **Figure 2.15**. **Figure 2.16** illustrates the differences in the pattern of hand joint involvement in OA, RA and psoriatic arthritis.

2.4.5 Signs of fracture

Signs of a fracture include:
- pain at rest or on slight movement of the affected area
- tenderness (may be the only sign, e.g. stress fracture)
- swelling or bruising over the bone
- bone protruding from the skin, in the case of open fracture
- deformity of the affected limb
- patient unable to use the affected limb, e.g. unable to bear weight.

2.4.6 Muscle weakness

Muscle weakness is difficult to interpret because it is greatly affected by pain. A thorough neurological assessment is helpful to grade the muscle strength (**Table 2.8**).

2.4.7 Muscle wasting

Muscle wasting should be assessed with muscle strength. If a muscle is wasted, it suggests that it is not being used or not receiving adequate nerve stimulation. Again, pain will stop a patient using a particular limb and the degree of muscle wasting can give clues to the chronicity of the condition.

2.4.8 Extra-articular signs

Looking at the patient as a whole gives vital clues to the underlying disease process; extra-articular signs can give vital clues to the cause of joint swelling or deformity. The examination therefore must include a top-to-toe assessment, taking into account eyes, skin, hair and nails as well as including a full system-based physical examination. **Table 2.11** lists some common examples seen in the musculoskeletal clinic. Others are discussed throughout the book as individual conditions are described.

Tissue	Signs
	Table 2.11 *Important extra-articular signs of musculoskeletal disease*
Skin	Rashes, e.g. vasculitic rash (**Figure 4.15**), psoriasis (**Figure 2.17**), dermatomyositis (**Figure 4.11**)
	Gouty tophi (look over the joints but also the olecranon and ear lobe) (**Figure 2.18**)
	Calcinosis in systemic sclerosis (**Figure 4.6**)
	Skin tightening in scleroderma (**Figure 4.7**)
	Erythema nodosum in sarcoidosis
	Malar rash in SLE (**Figure 4.4**)
	Mouth ulcers in inflammatory bowel disease or Behçet's disease (**Figure 4.9**)
Nails	Psoriatic nail changes including nail pitting, onycholysis and subungual hyperkeratosis (**Figures 3.12** and **3.13**)
	Splinter haemorrhages in antiphospholipid syndrome (APLS; see **Figure 4.13**)
	Nailfold capillary abnormalities in connective tissue disease (**Figure 4.9**)
Eyes	Uveitis or scleritis in inflammatory arthritis
	Cataract formation due to steroid use
	Dry eyes in patients with Sjögren's symptoms
	Blue pigmentation of sclera in osteogenesis imperfecta
Hair	Alopecia in connective tissue disease
	Scalp psoriasis

2.5 Assessing the acutely unwell patient

An unwell patient needs rapid and streamlined assessment. Delays to treatment risk poor outcomes. Assessment and treatment run concurrently. Protocols are used to ensure swift optimal decision making and management. Sepsis and trauma are the most common emergency presentations concerning the musculoskeletal system (see also *Chapters 8* and *11*).

> **Algorithms** are used in clinical situations that are time critical. They promote efficient team working and reduce diagnostic and treatment errors.

2.5.1 Sepsis

Sepsis in the rheumatology or orthopaedic patient can occur following septic arthritis, surgery, trauma or due to any infection exacerbated by immunosuppression, e.g. pneumonia in a patient taking immunosuppressive medication. Initial information from the patient or their relative/carer should include:

■ Are there any symptoms to suggest a source of infection, e.g. cough, acute joint swelling?
■ Is the patient taking any medication? Are they on steroids? Are they immunosuppressed?
■ Has there been any change to the patient's mental state?
■ Has their urine output been normal?
■ Have they had any recent surgery or other medical intervention?

Clinical suspicion, with or without abnormal basic observations, triggers a pathway to help identify the source of the infection whilst treating the patient. Once the patient is stabilised, a more thorough review can be conducted. The initial, emergency investigation and treatment of suspected sepsis is known as the "sepsis six" bundle and comprises:

1. Giving oxygen
2. Taking blood cultures
3. Giving intravenous antibiotics
4. Giving intravenous fluids
5. Checking serial lactate
6. Measuring urine output.

> **Medications can prevent a patient mounting a typical reaction to trauma or sepsis,** e.g. beta blockers prevent tachycardia, anti-inflammatories prevent pyrexia.

2.5.2 Trauma

Orthopaedic doctors are part of a team assessing trauma patients in the Emergency Department. Primary surveys are conducted with the aim of resuscitating the patient and developing an overview of the injuries. Secondary surveys allow a more detailed review to establish the full extent of the injuries.

Primary survey

Detect and react to any immediate threats to life.
■ C-spine: immobilise in hard collar.
■ Airway: does the patient have a patent airway? Use adjuncts if necessary.
■ Breathing: is the patient able to breathe for themself? Is it normal? Are their oxygenation levels satisfactory? Give oxygen.
■ Circulation: are blood pressure and pulse normal? Correct with blood products and fluids as necessary.
■ Disability: check blood sugar. Is the patient alert?
■ Exposure: undress the patient. Are there any obvious wounds?

Secondary survey

Perform a top-to-toe examination of the patient to identify any likely fractures or wounds. Stabilise as necessary. Organise appropriate initial investigations, e.g. CT scans, chest X-ray. Prioritise the most urgent intervention.

2.6 Investigations

Specialised investigations narrow down diagnoses and give clues to the severity of a condition and the immediacy of management necessary. Caution should be taken in ordering appropriate tests and interpreting the results – you should only order tests that are relevant to the patient's presentation and that will help answer a specific clinical question.

Investigations can throw up incidental findings, so every investigation needs to have a solid rationale. Unnecessary investigations can lead to undue risk and stress to the patient.

2.6.1 Biochemical tests

Blood tests help with the diagnosis of musculoskeletal disease and are used in monitoring response to treatment. They are often not specific, so they need to be interpreted within the context of the patient's clinical presentation. Always check local reference ranges as these can vary.

2.6.2 Full blood count

A full blood count (FBC) includes:
- the numbers of red cells, white cells and platelets
- the breakdown of white blood cells into specific populations, e.g. neutrophils, lymphocytes and eosinophils
- the concentration of haemoglobin.

In musculoskeletal disease the FBC is useful in the following ways:
- A raised white blood cell count and high platelet count suggest inflammation or infection.
- A normochromic, normocytic anaemia indicates anaemia of chronic disease caused by chronic inflammation.
- Neutrophil count: this is carefully monitored when patients take disease-modifying therapies because it can drop rapidly due to effects on the bone marrow, leaving the patient prone to infection. A raised neutrophil

count can indicate inflammation or infection, or corticosteroid treatment.

2.6.3 Inflammatory markers

There are three common serum parameters that become elevated when there is inflammation of any cause, including inflammatory arthritis, trauma, malignancy and infection. Several different inflammatory markers can be measured in the initial assessment of a patient and are also used to monitor their response to therapy. CRP is the most commonly used and the useful measure of acute inflammation.

C-reactive protein
C-reactive protein (CRP) is a protein produced by the liver in response to a stimulus which activates the immune response (**Figure 2.31**). It rises and falls rapidly in response to the presence and then absence of a stimulus (**Figure 2.32**). For example, in the initial presentation of inflammatory arthritis it may be high but then come down to normal with treatment.

Erythrocyte sedimentation rate
The erythrocyte sedimentation rate (ESR) is a measurement of how quickly red cells fall through a column of blood. This is affected by the quantity of large proteins (e.g. immunoglobulins) within the blood which cause red blood cells to stick together, hence becoming heavier and falling more quickly. ESR naturally increases with age, in females and in anaemia (greater protein to red blood cell ratio). Its response in the presence of inflammation is more graduated (**Figure 2.32**) so may be less useful in the assessment of response to treatment in the acute setting.

Plasma viscosity
Plasma viscosity (PV) can be more predictive of a change in disease activity than ESR. It is a measurement of how sticky the blood is (by measuring what force is required to move blood along a surface). Like ESR, it can be affected by other proteins in blood plasma.

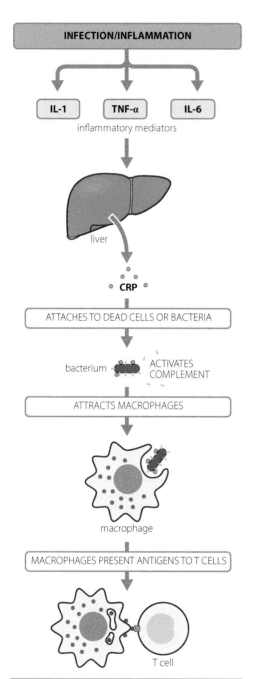

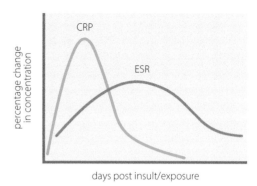

days post insult/exposure

Figure 2.32 CRP and ESR response: CRP rises and falls more quickly than ESR.

Some patients with inflammatory conditions do not have a standard measurable response to inflammation, i.e. their CRP does not go up and down as predictably with disease or treatment. Therefore, a clinical assessment of symptoms and signs must take precedence over blood tests in informing management decisions.

2.6.4 Bone profile

A typical bone profile test consists of plasma levels of
- calcium
- phosphate
- alkaline phosphatase (ALP).

Calcium, phosphate and ALP fluctuate according to bone turnover, and the pattern of abnormalities in these changes points towards specific metabolic bone diseases (see **Table 2.12**, *Section 1.9* and **Table 5.2**). ALP is not specific to bone and is produced by the kidney, placenta, liver and small intestine. ALP isoenzyme testing can be used to differentiate the organ of origin.

Parathyroid hormone

When calcium levels are found to be abnormal, the levels of parathyroid hormone (PTH) can point towards a cause (see *Section 1.9*).

Primary hyperparathyroidism is usually caused by a tumour in the parathyroid glands. Excess PTH is secreted, causing serum calcium to rise.

Figure 2.31 CRP is made in the liver and initiated by mediators such as IL-1, IL-6 and TNF-α.

Table 2.12 *Variations in bone profile due to abnormalities in skeletal turnover*

	Osteoporosis	Osteomalacia	Paget's disease	Acute fracture*
Calcium	normal	low/normal	normal	increased
Phosphate	normal	low/normal	normal	increased
ALP	normal	increased	increased	increased

*Bone profile markers vary significantly according to the elapsed time following fracture

Secondary hyperparathyroidism is a physiological response to low serum calcium, most commonly due to chronic kidney disease. However, sometimes it is due to low vitamin D (which can also occur in chronic kidney disease). Replacing vitamin D can help regulate calcium levels and lower PTH.

Tertiary hyperparathyroidism occurs when the parathyroid glands continue to secrete PTH even when calcium levels are corrected.

Vitamin D

In musculoskeletal medicine, serum vitamin D levels are measured when osteomalacia or rickets are suspected (see *Section 5.3*).

Vitamin D deficiency is important not only in bone mineralisation but also in multiple sclerosis, some cancers, diabetes and asthma. Supplementation is now recommended for at-risk groups, including pregnant or breastfeeding women, those aged under 5 and over 65 years, and people who may not make enough vitamin D in the skin, e.g. because of covering up or dark skin.

2.6.5 Protein electrophoresis

Serum protein electrophoresis is a laboratory technique which separates serum protein into subsets according to their size, shape and electrical charge. A discrepancy in the proportion of subsets of these proteins can point to certain conditions. Albumin is the largest plasma protein component and is reduced in a wide variety of disorders, including burns, infection and inflammation.

Of the globulins, the gamma globulins are most commonly abnormal, increasing in rheumatoid arthritis, connective tissue diseases, multiple myeloma, Hodgkin's disease and amyloidosis.

2.6.6 Virology

Viral infection can result in arthralgia or myalgia (**Table 2.13**). Common examples include parvovirus B19, hepatitis B and C.

Table 2.13 *Common and important viral illnesses causing myalgia, arthralgia and arthritis; consider whether the patient has had an infectious prodrome*

Virus	Presentation
Parvovirus B19	Febrile illness followed by arthritis and arthralgia
	IgG to the virus present in patient's serum
Hepatitis (B and C)	Malaise, jaundice
	Arthralgia in hepatitis C; arthritis more common in hepatitis B
	Patients will have antibodies to surface antigens of the hepatitis virus
Epstein–Barr virus	Myalgia more common than arthritis
	Follows typical symptoms of infectious mononucleosis – fever and pharyngitis
Human immunodeficiency virus (HIV)	Uncommon to present with arthritis, but consider in at-risk patient with history of recent flu-like episode

2.6.7 Uric acid

Serum uric acid or urate is measured in the biochemistry department using a blood sample. Urate is the end product of purine metabolism. Increased metabolism (e.g. increased dietary intake of purines from red meat or beer, or systemic diseases such as cancer leading to increasing cell turnover) or reduced excretion (e.g. in chronic kidney disease) can cause plasma urate to be elevated (hyperuricaemia). This predisposes to the development of gout which is a localised inflammatory reaction to uric acid crystals entering a joint. Measuring serum uric acid is useful in the diagnosis of gout and monitoring response to treatment with urate-lowering therapies (see Section 3.8).

> Paradoxically in the acute presentation of gout, a normal serum urate should not exclude the diagnosis as the excess uric acid is mobilised to the affected tissues, giving a falsely low serum level.

2.6.8 Creatine phosphokinase

Creatine phosphokinase (CPK) or creatine kinase (CK) is found in skeletal muscle and cardiac muscle, and in the brain, bladder, stomach and colon. Blood levels become elevated after strenuous exercise, muscle injury, myocardial infarction or acute kidney injury. It is raised in muscular dystrophy and is also used to monitor polymyositis (see Section 4.9), as it is a useful disease activity marker of inflammatory muscle disease.

2.6.9 Ferritin

Ferritin is an acute phase reactant and can be elevated in any inflammatory process. Very high levels can be due to adult onset Still's disease or haemochromatosis.

2.6.10 Renal function

Renal function tests – urea and electrolytes (U&Es) – are measured in blood serum and usually comprise:

- urea
- creatinine
- sodium
- potassium.

The laboratory can also calculate the estimated glomerular filtration rate (eGFR), which is a measure of kidney function.

Renal function may be affected by systemic complications of rheumatological conditions, e.g. SLE, scleroderma and vasculitis. It is measured routinely as part of routine disease monitoring and more frequently during disease flares. Renal function should be considered when assessing suitability for drug treatments or surgery and as part of regular side-effect monitoring of DMARDs.

The urine dipstick test is an essential clinic or bedside test: the presence of haematuria or proteinuria may indicate acute kidney injury or chronic damage in connective tissue disease, or the presence of white cells or nitrites may indicate infection.

2.6.10 Liver function

A laboratory request for liver function tests will provide the following serum measurements:

- alanine aminotransferase (ALT)
- aspartate aminotransferase (AST)
- alkaline phosphatase (ALP)
- bilirubin
- albumin
- +/− gamma glutamyl transferase (GGT).

In addition, clotting studies, e.g. prothrombin time and international normalised ratio (INR) are an important marker of liver function, because clotting factors are produced by the liver.

An isolated rise in ALP may be due to fracture, metabolic bone disease or inflammation. Increased ALT is a marker of hepatocyte damage and can be caused by toxic effects of drug treatments; it is included in routine monitoring protocols for most DMARDs.

2.6.11 Autoantibodies

Autoantibodies can be detected in the blood but they are not definitive or diagnostic tests for specific conditions. Specificities and sensitivities vary. Rather, they are a useful tool to build a picture of the probability of a diagnosis. The Immunology section in *Sections 1.4–1.8* is a useful refresher for the terminology used below.

> Pitfalls in autoantibody testing are that false positives are common and most autoantibodies are not specific to a particular condition. Always ensure that a positive autoantibody test is interpreted and explained to the patient in the context of their clinical presentation.

Rheumatoid factor

Rheumatoid factor (RF) is an antibody (usually IgM but can be any isotype) bound to the Fc portion of an IgG antibody. Bound together, they form an immune complex which contributes to tissue damage. RF is associated with rheumatoid arthritis 'seropositive' but not everyone with a clinical diagnosis has a positive RF: such patients are termed 'seronegative'. Those who are positive for RF are more likely to develop aggressive disease with joint damage and extra-articular systemic manifestations.

RF can also occur in people without RA with other conditions, e.g. infection, malignancy or other inflammatory conditions.

Anti-citrullinated protein antibody

Anti-citrullinated protein antibody (anti-CPA; ACPA) or anti-CCP (cyclic citrullinated peptide) is a more recently discovered autoantibody which is much more specific to RA than RF. It may also be positive several years before symptoms develop and be a more reliable prognostic factor for the severity of disease. Between 60 and 80% of patients with RA will be ACPA positive.

Antinuclear antibody

Antinuclear antibody (ANA) targets intracellular components (cytoplasmic and nuclear) within the body's own cells. Cells are fixed onto a slide and, if antibodies are present within a blood sample, they will attach to these cells. A second antibody, labelled with a dye and directed towards human antibodies, is washed over this slide. If positive, there will be visible staining and this pattern is recorded. The sample is then diluted until the

lowest concentration at which staining can still be seen. This is the ANA titre.

ANA positivity can occur in the population without an associated disease. ANA is not specific to any particular condition but can be seen in SLE, scleroderma, drug-induced lupus, RA, thyroid disease, viral infections, and with certain medications.

Extractable nuclear antigens

Should the ANA result be positive, the blood sample is then processed for extractable nuclear antigens (ENAs). Individual components of the cell nucleus are presented to the patient's serum to check for specific antibodies. Along with the clinical presentation, the pattern of ENA positivity allows for closer correlation with a particular disease pattern (**Table 2.14**). These are diagnostic tests and tend not to be used for monitoring disease activity.

Table 2.14 *ENA-associated conditions*

ENA	Condition
Anti-RNP	Mixed connective tissue disease, SLE
Anti-Sm	SLE
Anti-SSA (Ro)	Sjögren's disease, SLE
Anti-SSB (La)	Sjögren's disease, SLE
Scl-70	Scleroderma
Anti-Jo1	Polymyositis

Anti-double-stranded DNA

When ANA is positive, antibodies towards double-stranded DNA (dsDNA) are tested, particularly if SLE is suspected. This can also be useful as a monitor of disease activity.

Complement

Complement levels, particularly C3 and C4, can be useful in monitoring disease activity in SLE. It is thought that complement activation leading to tissue injury occurs in SLE and the lower the serum complement levels, the more active the disease.

Antiphospholipid antibodies

A positive antiphospholipid antibody test is a major criterion for antiphospholipid syndrome (see *Section 4.11*) and can also be seen in other autoimmune conditions. Antiphospholipid antibodies include

- lupus anticoagulant
- anticardiolipin

- anti-beta2-glycoprotein 1.

Lupus anticoagulant and anticardiolipin are the most commonly tested. Just one alone needs to be positive but they need to be found in the patient's blood on two separate occasions at least 3 months apart. They can also be present transiently in other situations, including drug exposure and infection.

2.7 Imaging

Musculoskeletal imaging identifies structural abnormalities caused by congenital conditions, inflammation, trauma or malignancy. This information can inform diagnoses and provide objective data on the efficacy of treatment.

Interpretation of imaging is not always straightforward and it is often helpful for imaging and clinical specialists to meet in a musculoskeletal radiology conference, as clinical correlation with imaging findings is important to make accurate diagnostic and management decisions.

2.7.1 X-ray (plain radiograph)

X-rays are easily accessible, quick and inexpensive. A beam of X-rays is targeted onto a particular body area. Body tissues of different properties absorb X-rays at different rates. Those X-rays that are not absorbed pass through the body and register onto X-ray sensitive film. Bone absorbs X-rays well, hence they look white compared to darker surrounding tissue that does not absorb so well.

X-rays in the orthopaedic and rheumatology departments are used to detect bone-based pathology including:

- fractures (see **Table 2.15** for a guide to how to describe them)
- erosions and deformity of inflammatory arthritis (which have different patterns according to the disease) (**Figure 2.33** demonstrates RA deformities on X-ray)
- joint space narrowing, bone cysts, subchondral sclerosis and osteophyte formation in osteoarthritis (**Figure 2.34b**).

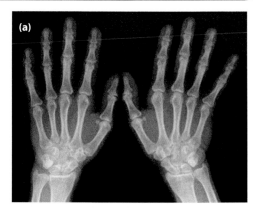

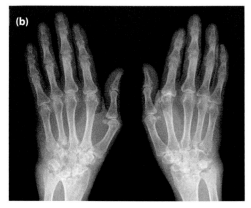

Figure 2.33 Progressive radiographic changes in RA. X-rays demonstrate progressive erosive joint damage in a patient with severe active RA over 5 years: (a) = baseline; (b) = 5 years later. Note the development of erosions and change in shape of the second metacarpal joints and the moth-eaten appearance of the carpal bones and disruption of the normal anatomy with progressive erosions, joint space loss and bone remodelling.

Table 2.15 *Radiographic description of fractures*

Which part of the bone?	Diaphysis	Shaft of the bone
	Metaphysis	Between the shaft and the end of the bone
	Epiphysis	At the end of the bone near or around the joint
How many fractures?	Simple	Only one fracture line
	Multi-fragmentary	Multiple fragments and fracture lines
What shape is the fracture?	Transverse	Fracture line straight across the bone, usually a high energy direct blow
	Oblique	Fracture line diagonal across the bone caused by a slanted force to the bone
	Spiral	A spiral shape formed from a twisting injury
	Butterfly	A wedge of bone in the shape of a triangle
	Buckle	An incomplete fracture in which the cortex is compressed in children
Does it involve the joint?	Intra-articular	Involves the joint surface
	Extra-articular	Does not involve the joint surface
Describe any displacement (lateral/medial or volar/dorsal)	Angulation	Angle of the distal part of the fracture in relation to the proximal part of the fracture in degrees
	Translation	The percentage overlap of the distal part of the fracture in relation to the proximal part of the fracture compared to the width of the bone
	Rotated	The angle of the distal part of the fracture in relation to the proximal part of the fracture, in degrees
Other features or mechanism	Fracture dislocation	An incongruent joint associated with a fracture
	Avulsion	Small fragment of bone associated with a tendon or ligament insertion that has pulled from the bone under tension
	Crush	Compression fracture usually multi-fragmentary and seen in digits and in the spine

Rarely, other pathologies such as primary or secondary malignancy may be detected.

It is common to take baseline hand and foot X-rays on diagnosis of an inflammatory arthritis, so that response to treatment or progression of disease can be monitored over time (**Figure 2.33**). X-rays pre- and post-orthopaedic intervention are quick and invaluable tools, for example, in order to confirm correct re-alignment of fractures. Soft tissue swelling can often be observed but detailed visualisation of soft tissue structures is not possible.

2.7.2 Ultrasound

Ultrasound imaging is an accessible and safe tool. The equipment emits high frequency sound waves which bounce back from tissue onto the transducer within the ultrasound probe to enable the computer to build a picture on

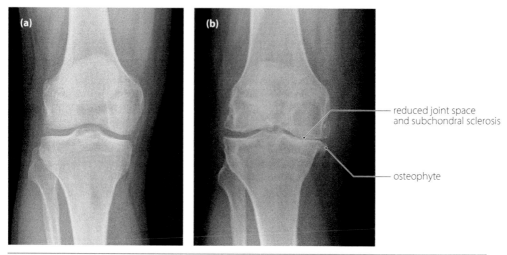

Figure 2.34 Radiographic changes in OA: anterior–posterior (AP) radiographs of (a) normal right knee; (b) right knee showing OA changes in the medial tibiofemoral compartment, including subchondral sclerosis, joint space narrowing and osteophytes.

screen. Ultrasound provides good visualisation of the soft tissues and cortical bone surface. In musculoskeletal disorders the principal roles of ultrasound are:

- detecting joint effusion, synovitis, enthesitis, erosions and new bone formation in inflammatory arthritis; to look for tendon, ligament or muscle tears, foreign bodies, soft tissue masses, and to aid infant hip assessment in the orthopaedic department
- as an interventional tool to guide aspiration (and/or therapeutic injection) of a joint or fluid-filled space.

2.7.3 Magnetic resonance imaging

Magnetic resonance imaging (MRI) uses magnetic fields and radio waves to build a picture of the part of the body being examined. Different settings can be used to highlight specific tissues and pathologies.

It is useful for in-depth assessment of the musculoskeletal system (**Figure 2.35**). The presence of joint inflammation as well as soft tissue and bone marrow abnormalities can be detected. MRI imaging of the spine is very sensitive for assessing disc disease, spinal cord and nerve root compression and inflammation.

Contraindications for MRI include significant claustrophobia, certain pacemakers, insulin pumps, implanted hearing aids, metallic bodies in the eye, joint replacements and metallic valves. However, modern medical devices are often designed to be MRI-safe.

2.7.4 Computed tomography

In computed tomography (CT) scanning, multiple X-rays are emitted from various angles and the images are processed by computer. This allows creation of virtual 'slices' of the area being examined. CT is excellent at providing good anatomical detail and in particular, detecting cortical bone injury. When a fracture is suspected clinically but plain X-ray is unhelpful, CT is often used to provide a more detailed assessment (**Figure 2.36**).

2.7.5 Dual energy X-ray absorptiometry

Dual energy X-ray absorptiometry (DEXA) scans are primarily used for assessment of bone density. X-rays at two distinct energy peaks are passed through representative bones, e.g. hips, wrists

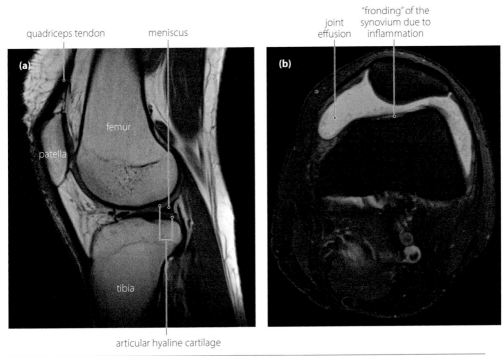

Figure 2.35 Musculoskeletal MRI: (a) a T1 sagittal view MRI of a normal knee showing normal articular cartilage, quadriceps and patellar tendon as well as the cruciate ligaments and meniscus; (b) T2 weighted coronal view MRI of the right knee showing synovitis (fluid is bright on T2 weighted MRI).

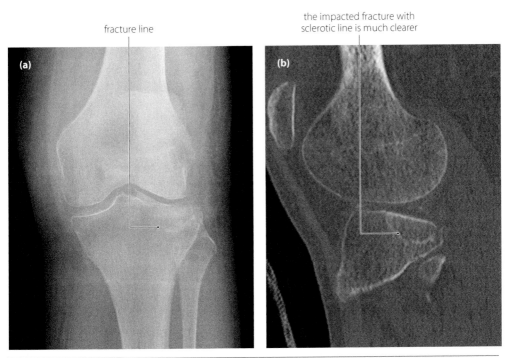

Figure 2.36 Imaging used in trauma: (a) an AP radiograph of the left knee showing an undisplaced tibial plateau fracture; (b) a sagittal CT view showing the fracture more clearly.

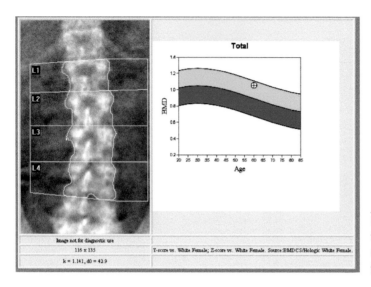

Figure 2.37 DEXA scan of the lumbar spine showing normal bone mineral density for a 60-year-old patient.

and vertebrae. A detector calculates how much of the X-rays have been absorbed by the bones (one X-ray peak will be better absorbed by bone, one by soft tissue). A score which compares the individual to a reference population is then used.

Bone mineral density (BMD) is referred to using a T or Z score:

■ T scores represent the number of standard deviations the patient's results are above or below the average BMD of a young person of the same sex
  □ a T score of <−2.5 is diagnostic of osteoporosis
  □ a T score of −2.5 to −1 is diagnostic of osteopenia
■ Z scores represent the number of standard deviations above or below the average BMD in an age-matched population.

Figure 2.37 shows you what the images in DEXA reports look like. However, it is the data and scores that are important rather than the images themselves. Information from serial scans can be used to assess progression and response to treatment.

2.7.6 Isotope bone scan

An isotope bone scan is sometimes called a nuclear medicine bone scan. It uses the radioactive substance technitium-99 combined with methylene diphosphonate (a bisphosphonate) to highlight areas of bone turnover, e.g. arthropathy, bone metastasis and trauma. The isotope or radiotracer is injected into the patient's bloodstream through a vein in the hand or arm. Nuclear gamma cameras are then used to trace where these have gone to in the body. The tracer is attracted to areas of damage or inflammation (**Figure 2.38**). Bone scans can be useful in the assessment of bone pain, some primary bone malignancies or metastatic disease. They are also used for the assessment of arthritis and infection. They are sensitive for detecting pathology but not specific, so any abnormality is likely to require further imaging using a different modality.

2.7.7 Positron emission tomography

Positron emission tomography (PET) scans are most often used by oncology teams for the diagnosis and assessment of malignancy. They are carried out in the nuclear medicine department. A relative of glucose, fludeoxyglucose (FDG), labelled with a radioactive tracer, usually fluorine-18 (18F), is injected intravenously. This molecule is attracted to areas of high metabolism.

PET scanners tend to be combined with CT scans (PET-CT). This allows a three-dimensional image to be created to assess structural anatomy as well as metabolic activity. PET-CT is

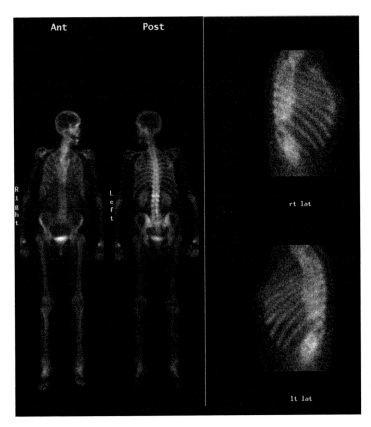

Figure 2.38 Isotope bone scan.

available at regional centres so often requires patients to travel and there are also larger costs involved. Therefore, whilst PET-CT can give a musculoskeletal assessment and can be used to identify subclinical inflammatory disease, it is not yet widely used other than in research and in difficult cases of vasculitis (**Figure 2.39**).

2.7.8 Joint aspiration

Joint aspiration is the removal of a quantity of synovial fluid from a joint, using a needle and syringe. It is performed for diagnostic and therapeutic reasons:

- All cases of suspected septic arthritis should have the swollen joint urgently aspirated and the sample sent for microscopy and culture.
- Joint fluid can be useful to diagnose crystal arthritis (e.g. gout and calcium pyrophosphate arthropathy) and haemarthrosis (haemorrhage into the joint).

- In a patient with a significantly swollen joint, aspiration can provide instantaneous symptom relief with a reduction in pressure.
- In a patient with recurrent joint swelling and a confirmed diagnosis, aspiration is often performed routinely, with subsequent injection of therapeutic corticosteroid.
- In instances when a joint is small, inaccessible or hard to access (e.g. hip), ultrasound-guided aspiration is used.

Joint aspiration is usually well tolerated with a low likelihood of complications, but there is a low risk of bleeding (particularly if a patient is on anticoagulant medication) and infection.

Results and diagnosis

The macroscopic appearance of joint fluid can provide clues as to the diagnosis (**Figure 2.40**). Normal synovial fluid is clear and straw-coloured. In severe crystal arthropathy it looks almost like milk. In inflammatory disorders, the fluid looks more

(a)

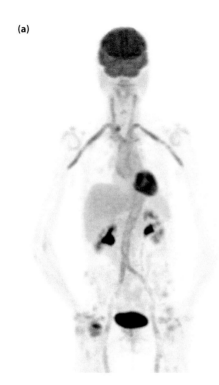

(b)

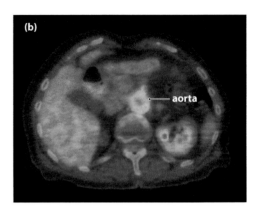

Figure 2.39 (a) a PET-CT using the radiolabelled tracer 18F-FDG; (b) the vessel wall of the ascending aorta shows increased uptake of the tracer, demonstrating vasculitis.

(a)

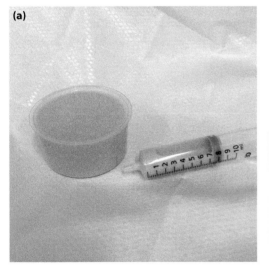

(b)

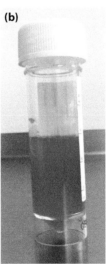

(c)

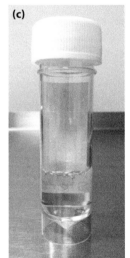

Figure 2.40 Appearances of synovial fluid: (a) gout or septic arthritis – the aspirate can appear like pus, or thick or chalky in sepsis or severe crystal arthropathy; (b) joint fluid – more often the fluid is straw-coloured or darker in inflammatory conditions; (c) normal synovial fluid – light straw colour.

yellow or turbid. Septic fluid is generally cloudy and purulent but, if clinical suspicion is high, a normal-looking aspirate should not discount septic arthritis until the microscopy and culture results are known. Often fluid can be assessed immediately by the naked eye but the laboratory is crucial in confirming specific conditions.

Laboratory examination of the fluid provides strong indicators of inflammation, presence of crystals and, crucially, infection (**Table 2.16**).

In a patient in whom septic arthritis is suspected but cultures are negative, other infections such as tuberculosis should be suspected and joint fluid tested for acid-fast bacilli.

2.7.9 Nerve conduction studies

Nerve conduction studies (NCS) are useful in situations in which a patient complains of paraesthesia or weakness and a problem with the peripheral nervous system is suspected, e.g. carpal tunnel syndrome.

An electrical impulse is applied to skin over a peripheral nerve. A nerve action potential is then recorded further down the nerve and a muscle action potential can be recorded at the target muscle site. The quality and speed of the nerve transmission can be assessed.

2.7.10 Electromyography

Electromyography (EMG) is often done in conjunction with NCS. In this test, a needle is inserted directly into a muscle. The patient is asked to contract the muscle and electrical activity is recorded. By comparing the NCS and EMG results, the neurophysiologist can infer whether there is a problem at the nerve, muscle or neuromuscular junction.

Table 2.16 *Synovial fluid characteristics*			
Diagnosis	**Appearance**	**Cell count**	**Other findings**
Normal	Colourless or clear straw-coloured	<2000WBC/mm^3	Gram stain negative Culture negative No crystals
Inflammatory arthritis (with no superadded infection)	Straw-coloured or cloudy, reduced viscosity	<100 000WBC/mm^3	Gram stain negative Culture negative No crystals
Gout	Cloudy/milky	<200 000WBC/mm^3	Gram stain negative Culture negative Monosodium urate crystals
Pseudogout	Cloudy/milky	<200 000WBC/mm^3	Gram stain negative Culture negative Calcium pyrophosphate crystals
Septic arthritis (sample required prior to antibiotics for accurate result)	Turbid	>50 000WBC/mm^3 >90% neutrophils	Gram stain positive Culture positive
Haemorrhagic (can occur in trauma or bleeding disorders)	Red or brown	<10 000WBC/mm^3 RBCs present	Gram stain negative Culture negative No crystals

WBC, white blood cell; RBC, red blood cell

2.7.11 Tissue biopsy

Tissue biopsies are useful in cases of diagnostic uncertainty and involve obtaining a sample of tissue, often guided by imaging or during surgery for histopathological assessment. Examples include:

- excision of a soft tissue mass to analyse for infection, cancer or other pathology
- excision of bone when infection or bone cancer is suspected
- a sample of muscle for diagnosis of myositis or genetic disorders affecting muscle, e.g. muscular dystrophy
- temporal arteritis, where a portion of the temporal artery is excised to look for infiltration of inflammatory cells – including giant cells – into the artery wall
- skin biopsy in a patient presenting with a rash which may suggest vasculitis or connective tissue disease
- sampling or excision of an enlarged lymph node, e.g. malignancy or sarcoidosis.

2.8 Medications

The aim of treatment is to relieve pain, preserve function, slow and if possible stop progression of disease, prevent disability and maintain quality of life. This is achieved by an appropriate combination of medications, surgical procedures, physical therapies, patient education and self-management facilitated by a multidisciplinary team approach.

2.8.1 Analgesia

Analgesia or painkilling medications are often taken long term by patients who have chronic pain, or in short bursts during flares of disease or peri-operatively. They do not alter the course of disease but provide relief of symptoms.

Paracetamol

Mode of action
Paracetamol (also known as acetaminophen) is a painkiller and an anti-pyretic (reduces fever). Its mode of action is not fully understood but there is general consensus that it acts to reduce prostaglandin synthesis, reducing pain perception, and may have an inhibitory effect on cyclooxygenase (COX) enzymes (see *Section 2.8.2*). It has little anti-inflammatory effect.

Indications
Paracetamol can be bought over the counter and is often the first-line analgesic. It can be given safely in combination with most other drugs. Care must be taken when people are prescribed combination drugs such as co-codamol, which has paracetamol incorporated. Many cold and flu remedies also contain paracetamol.

Adverse effects
Paracetamol is one of the safest analgesics when used at the recommended dosage but the threshold for toxicity is low. As it is readily available it is often used in drug overdoses, both accidental and intentional. When metabolised, paracetamol produces small amounts of a toxic metabolite (*N*-acetyl-*p*-benzoquinone imine, or NAPQI). The liver can normally process this by glutathione conjugation, which detoxifies this metabolite. If the dose of paracetamol exceeds the stores of glutathione the liver is at risk of damage. Those with lower levels of glutathione stores are most at risk, e.g. in alcohol excess or malnourishment.

In general, paracetamol rarely causes side-effects; however, in the short term allergy can develop and overdose results in liver toxicity. *N*-acetylcysteine (NAC) can be given as an effective antidote in overdose to prevent permanent liver damage.

Take care when prescribing paracetamol for children: the dose is based on age and weight. Also take care when prescribing for adults who weigh less than 50kg: the dose may need to be reduced.

Opiates and related medications

Drugs in this group

Opiates are natural substances derived from the opium poppy plant, with properties similar to morphine. Opioid is a more general term, which also includes synthetic versions that are created chemically, e.g. fentanyl. The most commonly used opioids are listed in **Table 2.17**.

Mode of action

Opioids act on receptors within the nervous system. There are four subtypes of receptor; MOP (mu), DOP (delta), KOP (kappa) and NOP (nociceptin). The MOP receptor is the predominant target for opioid drugs. Activation of central opioid receptors causes reduction in cell excitability and the transmission of nociceptive impulses. However, activation of peripheral opioid receptors leads to many of the characteristic side-effects of opioid drugs, e.g. reduced gastrointestinal (GI) motility, leading to constipation.

Indications

Opioids are not used as first-line analgesia other than in acute severe pain, e.g. trauma or peri-operatively. When commenced for chronic pain, they should be titrated according to effect. The side-effects that patients experience with these drugs often limit their use.

Adverse effects

The most common adverse effects with opiates are:

- nausea and vomiting
- sedation
- euphoria or confusion
- constipation
- rash and pruritus
- respiratory depression.

In cases of severe adverse effects, e.g. respiratory depression, naloxone (an opioid antagonist) can be used to reverse opioid toxicity.

2.8.2 Non-steroidal anti-inflammatory drugs

NSAIDs are amongst the most commonly prescribed drugs, and certain preparations can also be bought over the counter, e.g. ibuprofen. They are of particular use in musculoskeletal conditions in which inflammation is the dominant cause of pain, for example in inflammatory arthritis, and during the peri-operative period.

Drugs in this group

There are many NSAIDs and they are classified according to their mode of action (**Table 2.18**). Aspirin is an NSAID, but at the standard dose of 75mg per day it is insufficient to inhibit COX enzymes (see below). Instead, at this dose it works to reduce thromboxane A_2, preventing platelet aggregation.

Mode of action

NSAIDs are COX inhibitors. They inhibit the cyclooxygenase enzyme which is present in two

Table 2.17 *Commonly used opioids and their characteristics*

Drug	Relative strength	Delivery
Morphine (naturally occurring)	Strong	Intravenous Patch Tablet Intrathecal (spinal)
Fentanyl (synthetic)	Strong	Patch IV (e.g. patient-controlled devices)
Buprenorphine (semi-synthetic)	Intermediate	Patch
Codeine	Weak	Tablet

Table 2.18 *NSAIDs according to the type of COX inhibition*

Type of COX inhibition	Examples
Non-selective	Salicylates, e.g. aspirin
	Diclofenac
	Ibuprofen
	Naproxen
COX-2 selective	Meloxicam
	Celecoxib
	Etoricoxib

main isoforms; COX-1 and COX-2. COX-1 facilitates the production of prostaglandins. These act to maintain renal blood flow and regulate gastric acid secretion and platelet aggregation, and have a 'housekeeping' role. COX-2 is produced in response to tissue injury and triggers an inflammatory and pain response. Many NSAIDs block both COX-1 and COX-2. The potential advantage of COX-2 specific inhibitors is that they block the COX-2 inflammatory response, whilst maintaining the physiological COX-1 effects and so reducing the risk of side-effects.

Indications

Anti-inflammatory medications are useful for many situations where analgesia is required. They can be used in combination with paracetamol or opioid drugs. They can be administered via oral, rectal, topical intramuscular or intravenous routes.

Adverse effects

Adverse effects limit the use of NSAIDs (**Table 2.19**). COX-2 inhibitors generally have a safer profile with reduced gastric side-effects, but other side-effects are similar to traditional non-selective NSAIDs. To counter gastric effects, proton pump inhibitors (PPIs) are prescribed. NSAIDs should be used in short-term courses and should be avoided in patients with kidney disease, as they can reduce renal blood flow.

2.8.3 Corticosteroids

Steroids are produced in the human body by the adrenal cortex in two forms; glucocorticoids (hydrocortisone) and mineralocorticoids (aldosterone). Glucocorticoids, commonly referred to as corticosteroids, are anti-inflammatory and immunosuppressive.

Drugs in this group

Synthetic versions of glucocorticoids have been produced to mimic these effects and examples include:

Table 2.19 *Adverse effects of NSAIDs*

System affected	Pathogenesis
Gastric irritation	Prostaglandins act to reduce acid secretion and promote production of a protective lining; when this is disrupted, erosions and ulcers can develop
Renal impairment	NSAIDs can reduce renal perfusion and can cause acute kidney injury in a susceptible individual and exacerbate chronic kidney disease
Hepatic impairment	Uncommon, but liver function tests may be transiently abnormal during their use
Asthma exacerbation	NSAIDs can worsen asthma control due to excess leukotriene production, leading to bronchospasm
Cardiovascular effects	Increased blood pressure, increased risk of bleeding (thromboxane inhibition), increased risk of clots (prostacyclin inhibition)
Drug interactions	e.g. patients on warfarin or lithium will have the effects of these drugs potentiated, as NSAIDs displace them from protein binding sites

- short-acting, e.g. hydrocortisone
- intermediate-acting, e.g. prednisolone, methylprednisolone
- long-acting, e.g. dexamethasone.

Mode of action

Corticosteroids act in multiple ways to reduce inflammation. Primarily this is achieved by suppressing gene expression of inflammatory markers. This leads to effects such as limiting cytokine production, reducing cell oedema, reducing the number and impairing the abilities of innate and adaptive immune system cells, including macrophages and T cells. These multiple effects enable synthetic steroids to be the most powerful and rapid-acting anti-inflammatory agents. However, their heterogeneous effects also provide a long list of side-effects.

Indications

Steroids are useful in a broad spectrum of conditions across medical specialties including asthma, ulcerative colitis, eczema, idiopathic thrombocytopenic purpura and croup. In musculoskeletal conditions their primary use is in the inflammatory mediated conditions including rheumatoid arthritis, lupus and vasculitis. Such rheumatological conditions are the main reasons for long-term steroid use, as opposed to short-lived illnesses like croup where short courses are administered. Steroids are injected into joint spaces to alleviate local inflammation and pain.

Adverse effects

Steroids are infamous for their long list of side-effects. These are important to know and easy to remember if you learn a couple per body system (**Table 2.20**). As well as their anti-inflammatory and immunomodulatory effects, corticosteroids also have metabolic actions including:

- increased protein catabolism – leads to muscle wasting
- stimulation of gluconeogenesis – causes hyperglycaemia and can lead to diabetes
- heightened bone catabolism – causes osteoporosis
- mineralocorticoid activity – responsible for fluid retention and hypertension.

Table 2.20 *Adverse effects of steroids*

System	Examples
Cardiovascular	Hypertension, heart failure
Musculoskeletal	Muscle wasting, osteoporosis
Endocrine	Cushing's syndrome, adrenal suppression, irregular periods
Central nervous	Mood disturbance, sleep disturbance
Gastrointestinal	Gastric irritation, ulcers
Immune	Immunosuppression, leucocytosis
Ophthalmic	Cataracts, glaucoma
Metabolic	Diabetes, truncal obesity
Skin	Thin skin, easy bruising, striae

Addisonian crisis can be caused if patients abruptly stop steroids when they have been on high doses or taking them for longer than 3 weeks. Patients must be informed about risks of stopping steroids abruptly.

Steroids and DMARDs all cause immunosuppression to various degrees. Patients must be warned about the risks of infection and advised what to do with their medication should they develop an infection.

2.8.4 Non-biologic disease-modifying antirheumatic drugs

A disease-modifying drug is one which changes the processes that underlie the symptoms and signs of a disease and slows down disease progression. For the inflammatory autoimmune musculoskeletal diseases there two types of disease-modifying antirheumatic drug (DMARD): biologic (bDMARD) and non-biologic (nbDMARD). The nbDMARDs are first-line disease-modifying therapy; bDMARDs are used if there is inadequate response or side-effects to nbDMARDs.

nbDMARDs can be used singly or in combination for optimum effect. All have slightly different modes of action and significant side-effects. They are initiated under the supervision of a consultant rheumatologist. Regular blood tests are required for most of them (unless stated otherwise below). *Section 1.4* describes normal immune system processes which will help you to understand the mechanism of action of these drugs. Indications listed are musculoskeletal but many of the drugs are used in other settings, e.g. gastroenterology for inflammatory bowel disease or dermatology for cutaneous psoriasis.

> The aim of treatment with disease-modifying therapy is to send the inflammatory arthritis into remission, so that the patient is symptom-free with no tender or swollen joints.

Methotrexate

Methotrexate (MTX) slows the growth of rapidly dividing cells and was originally used to treat cancer. Subsequently it was discovered that it was beneficial to patients with inflammatory arthritis and psoriasis, and also that it halted growth of ectopic pregnancies (an unlicensed indication). As an agent for inflammatory arthritis, it is usually given in tablet form, once a week. However, subcutaneous injections that patients can administer themselves are available and helpful to reduce GI side-effects and improve efficacy, as MTX is poorly absorbed from the gut.

Mode of action

MTX inhibits dihydrofolate reductase, meaning that folic acid is not reduced to tetrahydrofolate. Tetrahydrofolate is required for synthesis of purine and pyrimidine, the precursors of DNA and RNA. Hence the ability for cell turnover is markedly reduced by MTX. The theory is that cells of the immune system are thus unable to proliferate in the same way when provoked by an inflammatory response (see *Section 1.4*).

Indications

MTX is a first-line DMARD in many types of inflammatory arthritis. It can be used in combination with other DMARDs and with bDMARDs. There is some evidence to suggest that taking MTX alongside bDMARDs can prevent the immune system creating antibodies towards the biologic drugs, thereby allowing the patient to keep taking them for longer, and for them to be more effective. MTX is also licensed for use in skin psoriasis, without associated arthritis.

Adverse effects

Common side-effects of MTX include nausea (especially on the day after taking the medication) and mouth ulcers. These can be reduced by taking folic acid supplements. These act to prevent folic acid being depleted so much that healthy cell division, e.g. gut lining replacement, is impaired. Usually it is sufficient to take folic acid once per week, but those with side-effects may need more frequent dosing up to 6 times a week, but not on the same day as MTX. MTX can have significant adverse effects on sperm and the developing embryo. Therefore, contraception is mandatory and both men and women who are considering starting a family need to stop MTX for 3–6 months prior to conception. Other less common but serious side-effects include hepatotoxicity, myelosuppression and pneumonitis.

Sulfasalazine

Sulfasalazine is another popular first-line treatment for rheumatoid and psoriatic arthritis.

Mode of action

This remains unclear but is thought to be due to the inhibition of transcription of inflammatory molecules.

Indications

Indications include rheumatoid arthritis, psoriatic arthritis, and arthritis and enthesitis associated with inflammatory bowel disease.

Adverse effects

Sulfasalazine most commonly causes GI disturbances or a rash. Dizziness and headache can also develop. More seriously, bone marrow depression and hepatotoxicity can occur. In men, sperm count can drop but overall the drug can be continued in pregnancy and when breastfeeding. It is contraindicated in patients with aspirin or sulphonamide sensitivity.

Hydroxychloroquine

Originally used as an anti-malarial drug, it is most commonly now used to treat SLE or as a part of combination therapy strategy in RA. It can also be used to treat inflammation in OA. It alleviates a multitude of symptoms including joint pain and fatigue. Initially, chloroquine was used but hydroxychloroquine is its safer derivative. It is a milder DMARD and best regarded as an immunomodulatory, as it does not have a significant immune system-suppressing action.

Mode of action

Hydroxychloroquine alters the pH within cells, disrupting protein secretion, reducing cytokine production and altering the antigen-presenting ability of monocytes (see *Section 1.4*).

Indications

RA, SLE, inflammatory OA.

Adverse effects

Hydroxychloroquine is well tolerated. GI disturbance and skin rash or pruritus are the predominant adverse effects. No regular blood tests are required. There is a low risk of corneal deposits and macular pigmentation, therefore patients should be reviewed annually by an optician. Ocular toxicity risk is low, and much lower risk than chloroquine.

Leflunomide

Leflunomide is less commonly prescribed and is most often used if other DMARDs have failed. It is less effective than MTX and has a long half-life so, if side-effects are encountered, it takes a while for the drug to be completely metabolised.

Mode of action

Leflunomide inhibits dihydroorotate dehydrogenase which affects pyrimidine synthesis and reduces lymphocyte proliferation, dampening the immune response.

Indications

RA and psoriatic arthritis.

Adverse effects

GI effects, particularly diarrhoea; however, these can resolve with time. Other side-effects include skin rash, hair loss, hypertension, hepatotoxicity and myelosuppression, the risk of which increases when taken in combination with MTX. It is contraindicated in pregnancy and there needs to be a long period free from the drug before it is safe to conceive. In cases of significant adverse effects, leflunomide washout can be performed using cholestyramine.

Azathioprine

As with MTX, azathioprine was originally a drug used in the treatment of cancer due to its cytotoxic effects. However, it is now used as an immunosuppressant.

Mode of action

Azathioprine is metabolised to 6-mercaptopurine. This resembles a purine nucleotide and competes with host purine molecules during normal cell replication. In this way it acts to reduce cell proliferation, including cells of the immune system.

Indications

RA, SLE, polymyositis.

Adverse effects

People with a constitutional depletion of thiopurine methyltransferase (TPMT) are at increased risk of toxicity with azathioprine, because they are less able to metabolise the drug. Serum levels are checked in patients before commencing treatment, and a lower dose or alternative treatment is considered for patients with low TPMT levels. Co-administration of allopurinol reduces metabolism of azathioprine and increases its immunosuppressive and bone marrow suppressive effects. Hypersensitivity reactions can occur and GI effects are relatively common. Bone marrow suppression can be significant, as can hepatotoxicity. Men and women who are trying to conceive can take the drug and it can be continued in pregnancy.

Mycophenolate

Mycophenolate is mainly used to prevent transplant rejection. Its use in rheumatology is less frequent but it can be effective in treating autoimmune connective tissue diseases. However, it is ineffective in treating inflammatory arthritis.

Mode of action

Mycophenolate inhibits inosine monophosphate dehydrogenase which affects a different route of nucleotide synthesis to azathioprine. Proliferation of B and T cells is reduced.

Indications

SLE, dermatomyositis, polymyositis.

Adverse effects

GI side-effects, hypertension and metabolic and electrolyte disturbances can occur. Monitoring for neutropenia should occur. It is avoided in pregnancy.

Cyclophosphamide

Predominantly used as chemotherapy for cancer, in musculoskeletal disorders cyclophosphamide tends to be reserved for situations where potent immunosuppression is required in the context of severe multisystem inflammatory disease.

Mode of action

Cyclophosphamide metabolites form DNA cross-linkages which lead to cell apoptosis. Immune cell numbers are depleted.

Indications

SLE, RA with systemic complications, vasculitis.

Adverse effects

Side-effects traditionally associated with chemotherapy occur, including hair loss, nausea and vomiting, and bone marrow suppression. Haemorrhagic cystitis and cancers (e.g. leukaemia, bladder cancer) can also occur. It must be avoided in pregnancy and can cause both male and female infertility.

Ciclosporin

Like cyclophosphamide, this is a potent immunosuppressive drug which has significant adverse effects. It is used uncommonly to treat musculoskeletal inflammatory disease.

Mode of action

Ciclosporin is a calcineurin inhibitor which suppresses T-cell activation. Calcineurin normally facilitates the production of pro-inflammatory cytokines including IL-2 and TNF-α. These cytokines activate T cells and promote their proliferation.

Indications

In RA, ciclosporin is only used when other options are ineffective. It can also be used to treat psoriasis and psoriatic arthritis; again, when other options have failed.

Adverse effects

Nausea and vomiting, hirsutism, tremor, gingival hypertrophy, photosensitivity, neuropathy, kidney injury, hypertension, secondary malignancy. Avoid in pregnancy.

2.8.5 Biologic disease-modifying antirheumatic drugs

Biologic DMARDs (bDMARDs) or 'biologics' are used in inflammatory arthritis, autoimmune connective tissue disease and vasculitis that is particular severe; or where conventional nbDMARD therapy has failed. Despite them being very effective drugs that have significantly improved disease outcomes, they are expensive and their use is subject to satisfying various criteria. For nbDMARD therapy to be deemed a failure usually requires inefficacy or intolerance of at least one or two nbDMARDs. Some biologics are IV infusions for which patients have to attend hospital; others are subcutaneous injections that patients can give themselves, and there are some new oral agents. The mode of administration often affects which drug patients choose.

The side-effects listed are not exhaustive. Before any patient is started on a medication like this, they need to be appropriately counselled. Screening is performed for pathogens at risk of reactivation, e.g. hepatitis and tuberculosis (TB).

Anti-TNF drugs

These include:

- adalimumab (subcutaneous injection)
- etanercept (subcutaneous injection)
- infliximab (intravenous infusion)
- certolizumab (subcutaneous injection)
- golimumab (subcutaneous injection).

Mode of action

Anti-TNF drugs inhibit the actions of the pro-inflammatory cytokine TNF-α. Usually they are prescribed in combination with MTX, which has a synergistic effect.

Indications
- Rheumatoid arthritis (adalimumab, etanercept, infliximab, certolizumab, golimumab)
- Psoriatic arthritis (adalimumab, infliximab, certolizumab, golimumab)
- Axial spondyloarthritis (infliximab, certolizumab, golimumab, adalimumab).

Adverse effects
Risks include minor and more severe infections, e.g. septicaemia, TB and hepatitis B reactivation. Others include injection site reactions, infusion reactions (usually treatable), blood disorders (e.g. anaemia, pancytopenia) and worsening of heart failure. Despite the theoretical risk in view of their mode of action, long-term studies have shown that these drugs do not increase the risk of cancer.

Rituximab
Rituximab blocks the effect of B cells and is administered by intravenous infusion in a hospital ward or day-case unit.

Mode of action
It is an anti-CD20 monoclonal antibody which binds to the surface of B cells. These B cells are then destroyed by cellular and complement responses. It is therefore most useful in patients with high levels of autoantibodies.

Indications
RA, SLE, ANCA-associated vasculitis (see *Sections 3.3, 4.4* and *4.17*).

Adverse effects
Infection risk including septicaemia and reactivation of TB and hepatitis B, although the risk may not be as great as with other biologic agents. Hypersensitivity reactions to the infusion are common. Nausea, abdominal pain and cytopenias can occur.

Tocilizumab
Tocilizumab is an intravenous infusion or subcutaneous injection given every 4 weeks that blocks IL-6, a potent pro-inflammatory cytokine. It can be particularly effective at reducing direct IL-6-mediated effects; for example, it can reduce CRP and improve anaemia and fatigue.

Mode of action
It is an antibody which competitively binds the IL-6 receptor. By reducing the binding of IL-6 to its receptor, the recruitment of B and T cells is reduced.

Indications
RA, large vessel vasculitis, adult onset Still's disease.

Adverse effects
Tocilizumab should be avoided in patients with a history of diverticular disease due to risk of intestinal perforation. Other risks include infection, leucopenia, neutropenia and mouth ulcers.

Abatacept
Abatacept is given as an infusion fortnightly for three doses, and then every four weeks.

Mode of action
It binds to antigen-presenting cells, inhibiting T-cell response.

Indications
RA.

Adverse effects
Most common side-effects include infusion reactions, headache or dizziness. Infection and blood disorders can occur.

JAK inhibitors
Janus kinase (JAK) inhibitors are new oral medications demonstrating good efficacy for RA and psoriatic arthritis and in trials for other conditions. Examples are baricitinib, tofacitinib and upadacitinib.

Mode of action
JAK inhibitors block cell signalling pathways essential for cytokine activity, and so moderate their pro-inflammatory effects.

Indications
RA and psoriatic arthritis.

Adverse effects
Infection, e.g. herpes zoster, GI upset and cytopenia. There has been a small increased risk

of thromboembolic events in clinical trials using high dose preparations.

IL-17 and IL-23 inhibitors

IL-17 and IL-23 are cytokines which act together, particularly in the development of inflammation. Secukinumab is an example of an IL-17 inhibitor; ustekinumab is an example of an IL-23 inhibitor.

Indications

Psoriasis and psoriatic arthritis. Secukinumab is also used in axial spondyloarthritis.

Adverse effects

There is an increased risk of infection and malignancy. Arthralgia, back pain and diarrhoea are common side-effects.

> As patents for biological therapies expire, different pharmaceutical companies manufacture drugs that are structurally similar but not identical, called **biosimilars**. These are already in clinical use, particularly biosimilar anti-TNFs. This creates greater competition in the market and a reduction in drug costs, resulting in cost savings and potentially greater patient access.

2.8.6 Drugs used in osteoporosis

There are several different drugs for the management of osteoporosis. These should be used in addition to lifestyle measures including diet and exercise (see *Section 2.11.1*). The aim of any treatment is to reduce further bone loss and prevent fractures. Hormone replacement therapy is also an option for women who are peri-menopausal.

> **Always ask patients if they are taking their bisphosphonate.** It is common for patients to not take oral bisphosphonate due to the weekly dosing causing them to forget, the care required when ingesting the medication and its side-effect profile.

Bisphosphonates

The most commonly used bisphosphonates are:
- alendronic acid (oral, weekly dose)
- zoledronic acid (IV infusion yearly)

- pamidronate (IV infusion, variable frequency).

Mode of action

Bisphosphonates attach to the bone surface and prevent bone resorption by osteoclasts.

Indication

Bisphosphonates are used in the treatment of osteoporosis or its prevention in at-risk populations, e.g. long-term steroid use. Zoledronic acid is used when patients are intolerant of oral bisphosphonate. Pamidronate is licensed for hypercalcaemia, bone pain and Paget's disease.

Adverse effects

Dyspepsia is common with alendronic acid and the main reason for intolerance. Patients should take their bisphosphonates first thing in the morning on an empty stomach with a large volume of water and sit upright for 30 minutes after taking their dose to reduce oesophageal irritation. Rarely, bisphosphonates can cause atypical fractures or osteonecrosis, e.g. of the jaw. Patients are advised to have a full dental check-up and complete any dental work prior to commencing a bisphosphonate to reduce this risk.

Denosumab

Denosumab is a subcutaneous injection given six-monthly.

Mode of action

It is a monoclonal antibody which blocks RANKL and prevents normal osteoclast maturation and function.

Indication

Denosumab is indicated when bisphosphonate therapy is not tolerated and patients meet specific criteria, including severity and risk factors for fracture. It is generally started on the advice of a hospital specialist but can be administered in the community.

Adverse effects

Hypocalcaemia must be corrected prior to receiving denosumab, as hypocalcaemia can be fatal. GI upset may occur. Atypical fractures and osteonecrosis are rare but important to discuss with the patient before commencing treatment.

Teriparatide

Mode of action

Teriparatide is a synthetic parathyroid hormone which stimulates new bone formation by activating osteoblasts.

Indication

It is indicated in severe osteoporosis with very low bone mineral density and recurrent fractures. It requires specialist recommendation.

Adverse effects

Arthralgia, GI upset, hypercalcaemia.

2.8.7 Drugs used in gout

The aim of gout therapy is to reduce symptoms in an acute attack, control pain and lower uric acid levels to reduce the frequency and severity of episodes. Common initial acute therapy comprises NSAIDs, corticosteroids or colchicine. The choice generally depends on the patient's comorbidities. Common urate-lowering therapies are allopurinol and febuxostat. The doses should be titrated up until the serum urate level is below 300μmol/L. Canakinumab and rasburicase can be used for severe recurrent gout.

Colchicine

Mode of action

Colchicine modulates multiple inflammatory pathways, including the migration of inflammatory cells and the production of cytokines.

Indications

Acute flare of gout.

Adverse effects

Diarrhoea is the most recognised side-effect. This is usually dose-dependent, so is less common now that standard dosing is used. Previously the dose was titrated up until the patient experienced diarrhoea. Nausea and vomiting can also occur.

Allopurinol

Mode of action

It inhibits xanthine oxidase, which normally metabolises hypoxanthine and xanthine (nucleic acids) to uric acid in the purine metabolic pathway.

Indications

Repeated gout attacks, usually two or more in a 12-month period.

Adverse effects

Rashes or GI upset are the most common side-effects.

> **Starting allopurinol treatment can induce a flare of gout due to mobilisation of uric acid.** However, the drug should not be stopped in this situation; just treat the acute attack in the usual way. Similarly, if a patient with a flare of gout is already on allopurinol, this drug should not be stopped but the acute attack should be treated.

Febuxostat

Mode of action

Febuxostat is a more potent and non-purine inhibitor of xanthine oxidase.

Indications

Recurrent gout where allopurinol is unsuitable.

Adverse effects

Patients may experience GI upset, rash and deranged LFTs. Cardiac conditions, e.g. heart failure, may be exacerbated.

2.8.8 Antibiotics

In musculoskeletal disease, antibiotics are crucial:
- in the peri-operative patient
- in the patient with septic arthritis (see *Section 8.1*).

Commonly used antibiotics include:
- benzylpenicillin
- flucloxacillin
- clindamycin
- cefalexin.

However, local microbe resistance should always be taken into account. Hospitals have their own policies regarding which antibiotics to use and these should be followed, and cases should be discussed with the local microbiologist.

2.8.9 Chemotherapy

Several chemotherapeutic drugs originally used for cancer management now have applications in non-malignant musculoskeletal disease, e.g. MTX and cyclophosphamide. For malignant disease of the musculoskeletal system (see *Section 10.1.6*), chemotherapeutic drugs are used for a different effect.

Cancer of bone marrow cells, i.e. the haematopoietic cells, is managed by haematologists. In cases of myeloma, there are different treatment options including the CTD regime which comprises:

- cyclophosphamide (causes cell death)
- thalidomide (causes cell death, halts cell growth, prevents angiogenesis)
- dexamethasone (high-dose steroid).

For solid bone tumours, e.g. Ewing's sarcoma, chemotherapy can be used to shrink tumours prior to surgery and radiotherapy, and afterwards to destroy any remaining cancer cells. Chemotherapy is supervised by an oncologist and can involve several of the following agents, which prevent cell growth:

- vincristine
- ifosfamide
- doxorubicin
- etoposide
- cyclophosphamide
- actinomycin.

2.8.10 Radiotherapy

Radiotherapy treatment, supervised by a clinical oncologist, has two major uses in the management of musculoskeletal malignancy:

- It is used to shrink primary bone tumours prior to surgery; intensity-modulated radiation therapy (IMRT) allows a high dose to be given in a targeted way to a tumour to minimise damage to surrounding healthy tissue.
- Palliative radiotherapy in both primary and secondary bone malignancies allows tumours to shrink enough to relieve pressure on structures such as nerves, reducing pain.

2.9 Surgery

2.9.1 Fracture management

The basic principles of fracture management are discussed below. *Section 6.1.8* discusses trauma in more detail. The aims of fracture management are:

- to realign bone
- to hold (immobilise) the bone in place while it heals
- to prevent infection
- to reduce pain and deformity and restore function (rehabilitation).

In simple fractures, immobilisation can be achieved with casting. Casting involves using a thin wool bandage that is applied close to the skin which is overlapped with a roll of either fibreglass or plaster of Paris (POP). The rolls of POP and fibreglass are initially malleable until they are dipped in water and activated. The casting material will turn hard in an exothermic reaction in which heat is emitted. Casts often need to immobilise the joint above and below the fracture and so cause stiffness of these joints. Closed reduction of the fracture (realigning the bone ends by pulling, manipulation or gradual traction) is sometimes required prior to cast application. Surgery is required when bone cannot be held in adequate alignment with casting techniques (**Figure 2.41**; **Table 2.21**).

2.9.2 Arthroplasty

Trauma or arthritis causing damage to the joint can be addressed by several surgical techniques that aim to improve pain and/or function (**Table 2.22**).

Arthroplasty is the replacement of joints with a prosthetic implant that is fixed to the bone using cement or cementless techniques. Arthroplasty may be offered for joints damaged by osteoarthritis, inflammatory arthritis, fracture and congenital abnormalities, transforming lives by giving patients pain-free movement. The knee and hip are the most commonly replaced joints. However, the bearing surfaces do wear out and the implants can loosen with time. Improvements in prosthetic implants, bearing surfaces and

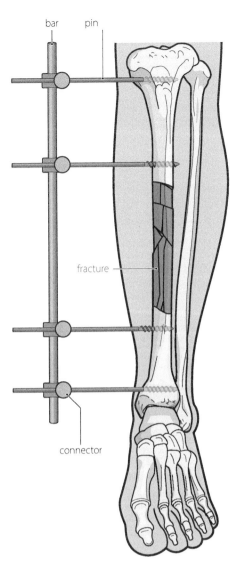

bar   pin

fracture

connector

cementing techniques have increased the time before implants wear out and they can now last up to 20 years. Joint replacements are now being offered to younger patients with joint disease due to these improvements, as well as the development of techniques to successfully revise worn implants.

A total arthroplasty is the most common joint replacement, in which both joint surfaces are replaced (**Figure 2.42**). Replacing both joint surfaces increases the time before it wears out. Hemiarthroplasty is where only one half of the joint surface is replaced. Hemiarthroplasty is most commonly used when the joint is not expected to wear out, e.g. in non-weight-bearing joints (shoulder or digits) or in elderly patients with lower life expectancy, e.g. following hip fracture (see *Section 6.5*).

2.9.3 Arthrodesis

Arthrodesis is the surgical fusion of a joint. It is used in the small joints of the digits, tarsal and carpal bones where arthroplasty techniques are not yet sophisticated enough to offer a good chance of success (**Figure 2.43**). When these

Figure 2.41 External fixation for a multifragmentary tibial fracture: pins are inserted into the bone and are connected to rods to form a stable construct.

Table 2.21 *Surgical techniques used in the management of fractures*

Type	Explanation	Description
Open reduction and internal fixation	Plate and screws	The fracture is exposed through an incision in the skin and realigned. A plate is placed flat to the bone and secured with screws.
Closed reduction and pinning	K wires	Fracture is manipulated and realigned. Wires inserted through the skin and bone go across the fracture to fix in place.
Intramedullary fixation	Intramedullary nail	A rod which is either solid or flexible is inserted inside the bone canal and across the fracture. Solid nails are fixed at either end with bolts.
External fixation	Circular or linear frames	Pins are inserted into the bone through the skin distant to the fracture site. The fracture is then aligned and rods are connected to the pins to form a rigid construct (**Figure 2.41**).
Arthroplasty	Replacement of the joint	If the fracture involves the joint surface and cannot be reconstructed, an option is to replace or partially replace the joint, e.g. fractured neck of femur.

Table 2.22 *Surgical procedures used in the treatment of arthritis*

Type	Explanation	Description	Action
Arthroplasty	Replacement of the joint	Both surfaces of the joint are replaced with a prosthetic implant	Joint surfaces are realigned and not rubbing, reducing pain and improving movement
Fusion	Fusion of the joint	The damaged joint surfaces are excised and compressed, and held until the bones have healed together	The exposed bone heals and does not permit movement
Osteotomy	Realignment of the joint	Pressure placed on one side of the joint is realigned by cutting a wedge in the bone	Transfers stress away from the worn side of the joint, reducing pain

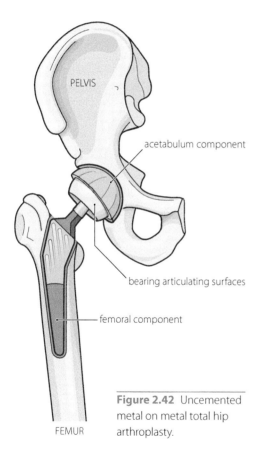

Figure 2.42 Uncemented metal on metal total hip arthroplasty.

PELVIS

acetabulum component

bearing articulating surfaces

femoral component

FEMUR

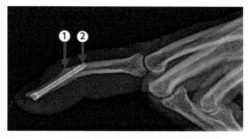

Figure 2.43 Joint fusion for OA: an example of a distal interphalangeal joint fused using an intramedullary screw. ① distal interphalangeal joint fused; ② intramedullary screw.

function, therefore patients are usually willing to sacrifice some function for pain relief.

In some instances, fusion puts strain on other areas of the body and may worsen OA in other joints. Patients need to be counselled prior to surgery that this may occur.

2.9.4 Osteotomy

Osteoarthritis, deformity or trauma can damage the joint surface unevenly, wearing one side of the joint more than another; an example of this is the knee. It is common for sportsmen, especially sprinters, to have a varus deformity of the tibia (bowed legs) causing wear on the medial part of the knee. It is unknown whether the varus deformity gives the person advantage in sprinting or whether the deformity is a result of the person training and sprinting while they are growing and

joints are fused there is no movement. However, as there are other multiple small joints that compensate, function is often not compromised. The main indication for this procedure is ongoing pain. Patients with severe pain have compromised

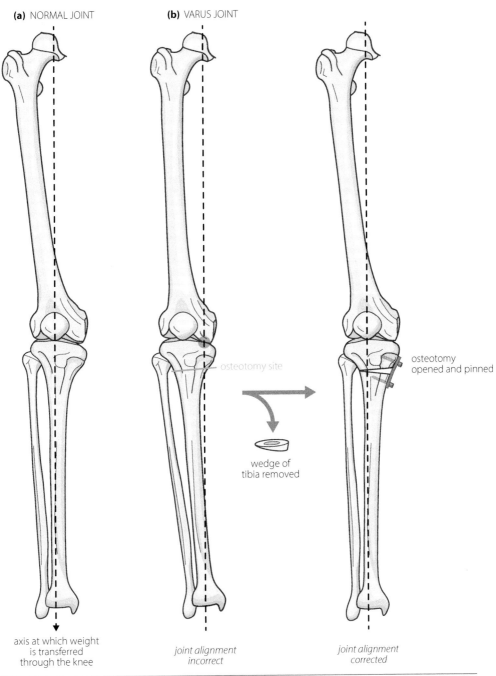

(a) NORMAL JOINT

(b) VARUS JOINT

osteotomy site

osteotomy opened and pinned

wedge of tibia removed

axis at which weight is transferred through the knee

joint alignment incorrect

joint alignment corrected

Figure 2.44 Medial open wedge tibial osteotomy of the knee: (a) the majority of the force is entering through the medial side of the knee in this varus knee; (b) opening up the medial side with an osteotomy transfers the force to the lateral side of the knee – the osteotomy is secured in place with a plate.

thus developing the deformity, although it is likely to be the latter. Osteotomy translates from Latin as a bone cut. In this example a cut is made on the medial aspect of the tibia and opened up as a wedge. This redistributes the forces produced when weight-bearing to the lateral part of the knee, reducing pain (**Figure 2.44**).

Osteotomies are used when there is a deformity that can be corrected and to extend the time before a joint replacement is needed.

2.10 Physical therapies

Both the orthopaedic and rheumatology departments rely heavily on the services of allied health professionals. These teams see people within hospital who may be recovering from an operation, or inflammatory flare, or in the outpatient department to help treat other acute or chronic presentations. They can offer good preventative measures to help with self-management of conditions and prevention of further joint damage. The lines between the services are blurred, in the sense that sometimes a service can be provided by either a physiotherapist or an occupational therapist, e.g. provision of hand splints, or advice on function. A patient may be referred to one or all of these services depending on their needs and what is available in a specific locality.

2.10.1 Physiotherapy

Physiotherapists provide a wide range of services in the musculoskeletal department. Following their assessment of a patient they can offer:
- tailored exercise programmes
- group exercise sessions
- hydrotherapy
- educational sessions
- local joint steroid injections
- manual therapy
- acupuncture (**Figure 2.45**)
- taping (**Figure 2.46**)
- electrotherapy (**Figure 2.47**).

2.10.2 Occupational therapy

The role of occupational therapists in musculoskeletal disorders is to:
- assess a patient's physical and functional abilities and limitations
- assess a patient's environment to determine what adaptations are needed to allow the patient to live and work within it
- provide education and self-management plans for patients.

Their services include providing tailored splints, home and work visits to assess equipment or adaptations and providing education relating to disease management including joint protection, pacing and sleep hygiene. **Figure 2.48** illustrates

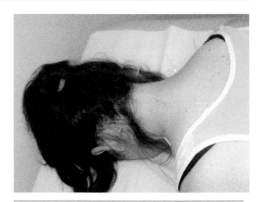

Figure 2.45 Acupuncture: needles are placed in specific locations for different indications.

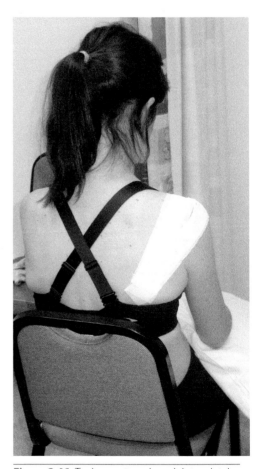

Figure 2.46 Taping or strapping a joint maintains it in a position to rest an injury or to educate the patient with regard to correct posture or movement.

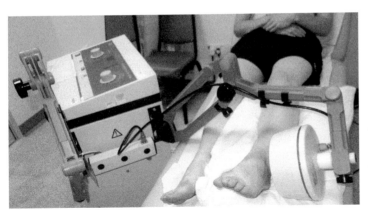

Figure 2.47 Electrotherapy or pulsed shortwave therapy is thought to encourage healing processes.

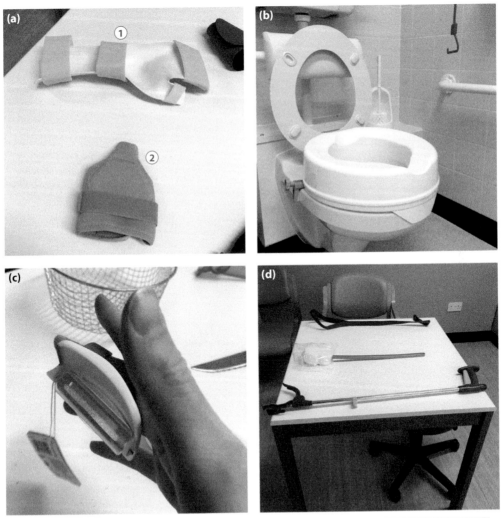

Figure 2.48 Occupational therapy aids: (a) wrist splint ① and thumb splint ②; (b) toilet raise, useful for patients recovering from hip replacement; (c) kitchen aids – potato peeler and sieve, in which food can be cooked to avoid the need to drain heavy pans; (d) grabbers, sock and stocking aids.

some of the equipment which can be provided to patients; such aids can be life-changing in recovering from surgery or living with a disabling chronic condition.

2.10.3 Podiatry

Podiatrists specifically assess and treat conditions affecting the lower leg, ankle and foot. Through direct assessment of the foot, lower limb and via gait analysis they assess biomechanical and skin surface problems, e.g. ulcers in diabetes. They can request imaging and offer appropriate management. Common treatments offered include insoles and orthotics that can be made bespoke to the patient's individual requirements, as well as exercise-based treatments.

Insoles/orthotics

A supportive boot to reduce weight-bearing or a brace can be provided for Achilles tendon pathology, healing fractures, plantar fasciitis or posterior tibialis tendinitis (**Figure 2.49**). Insoles, which are used to accommodate and also correct deformities, vary in levels of support (**Figure 2.50a**); their aim is to spread the body weight more evenly across the foot. They can be provided 'off the shelf' or custom-made after taking impressions of a patient's feet, where the patient stands in an oasis box; a plaster of Paris

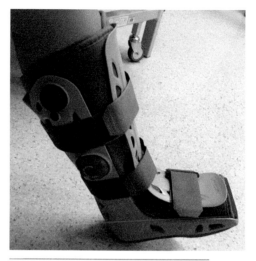

Figure 2.49 A 'moon boot' is used to help stabilise the ankle joint in simple fractures and sprains, and is easy to remove.

cast is taken of their foot shape and bespoke insoles created which are individual to the patient (**Figure 2.50b**). Podiatrists will often also provide advice on appropriate footwear. Provision of special shoes for patients with advanced deformities is rare, given advances in medical treatment of arthritis, but these can be provided if necessary.

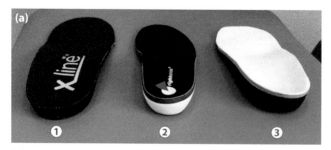
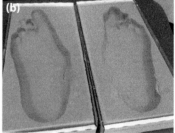

Figure 2.50 (a) Insoles vary in levels of support, ranging from ① minimal to ③, which is aiming to bridge the gap between the feet and the floor – sometimes required in fixed deformities where there is little movement in the feet; (b) casting of feet to make tailored insoles.

2.11 Self-management

Self-management is a fundamental part of treatment in all musculoskeletal conditions. Empowering patients with the tools to have

some control over their disease can have positive emotional and physical effects. However, tasks such as achieving and maintaining a healthy weight, changing dietary habits and incorporating regular exercise into day-to-day life can be challenging for patients.

> A reminder during clinic appointments regarding weight management or smoking cessation has been shown to positively change patients' behaviour.

2.11.1 Lifestyle

A patient's lifestyle can have a profound impact on their disease progression, response to injury or recovery from surgery.

Diet

Patients should be advised to maintain a healthy diet and weight, particularly as obesity can cause and exacerbate musculoskeletal conditions, as well as to prevent or control diabetes and other metabolic disorders. There have been many diets suggested to be beneficial, particularly for RA, but there is no strong evidence to support a particular regime. Rather, patients should be advised to follow a diet which is balanced. Patients with osteoporosis should receive advice on calcium and foods rich in vitamin D, whilst patients with gout need information on how to avoid excessive purine intake.

Many food supplements have been suggested to have beneficial effects on the musculoskeletal system, including omega 3 fish oils, glucosamine, cider vinegar and honey. However, there is a lack of consistent scientific data to prove these effects, but patients may report benefit. They should be advised that they can take supplements if they wish, provided they keep their general practitioner and specialist up to date with what they are taking, particularly as some supplements can have adverse effects and interactions with drug treatments, e.g. glucosamine can interfere with anticoagulants and increase their potency.

Weight

A higher body weight can have several effects on the musculoskeletal system (**Table 2.23**). Of note, a very low body weight predisposes to osteoporosis.

Exercise

Exercise is used to prevent and manage conditions. Exercise has a multitude of beneficial effects on bones and muscles, as well as positive psychological effects which can reduce pain perception:

- Weight-bearing exercise improves bone mineral density.
- Actively participating in physiotherapy post-arthroplasty increases range of movement and reduces pain.
- Aerobic and weight-bearing exercise builds endurance and improves balance, reducing the risk of falls and injury.

Table 2.23 *Complications of obesity for the musculoskeletal system*

Mechanical	Added pressure to joints can cause pain due to the mechanics of an abnormal load, and also increased cartilage wear and pressure on adjacent soft tissue structures
Muscular	A patient's ability to exercise is impaired, reducing muscle strength which can further exacerbate joint pain
Operative	Complications peri-operatively include increased risk of wound infection, increased risk of thrombosis, reduced ability to rehabilitate, reduced longevity of a joint replacement and anaesthetic complications
Inflammatory	More fat cells may lead to an increased concentration of cytokines which perpetuate inflammation (CRP may be elevated on blood tests)
Pharmaceutical	Patients who are overweight or obese may not respond as well to DMARD or biologic therapy

- Strengthening muscles around a joint and increasing flexibility can vastly reduce the pain experienced in arthritis.
- Strengthening muscles around joints in hypermobility reduces symptoms.

Pilates and yoga are often recommended to patients for core muscle strengthening.

A very painful joint may need to be rested and patients require education on the right balance of rest and exercise for their condition. Physiotherapists and occupational therapists can educate patients on how to recognise when to push themselves and when to rest.

Smoking

In addition to its general health hazards, smoking causes specific orthopaedic and rheumatological problems in the following ways:

- There is a higher risk of cardiovascular disease in inflammatory conditions, which is increased much further if a patient smokes.
- The risk and severity of rheumatoid arthritis is increased in smokers.
- The risk of lung disease associated with either rheumatological conditions or the medications used to manage these conditions, is increased if the patient smokes.

- Smoking increases the risk of osteoporosis.
- Smoking is a major risk factor in surgery. The anaesthetic risks (e.g. pneumonia, thromboembolism) are increased, as is the risk of poor wound healing.
- Smoking cessation support can be offered to patients at outpatient clinics, during hospital admissions or through primary care.

Alcohol

Drinking alcohol in moderation appears to have a protective effect against inflammation and cardiovascular disease. However, drinking heavily can lead to harm including osteoporosis, high risk of falls, gout attacks, poor wound healing and an increased risk of hepatotoxicity when a patient is taking certain disease-modifying drugs. Asking about alcohol use in the consultation can enable the clinician to provide the patient with support.

2.11.2 Complementary and alternative therapies

Sometimes patients wish to try alternative therapies ranging from scented oils to manual therapy such as spinal manipulation. **Table 2.24**

Table 2.24 *Alternative and complementary therapies in musculoskeletal disease*		
Type	**Mode of action**	**Risks**
Acupuncture	Not clear – postulated to reprogramme pain signal perception	Local reaction to needle placement, infection
Homeopathy	Unknown – postulated that exposing a patient to a small quantity of a drug that could trigger a disease in high doses can cure the same disease	Minimal due to low concentrations of active ingredient
Aromatherapy	Oils used to create relaxation through inhalation, massage – no evidence of curative effect	Local sensitivity reactions
Chiropractic manipulation or osteopathy	Physical movements are used with the intention of correcting subtle deformities and relieving stiffness	Stroke and spinal cord injury are rare but catastrophic
Herbal medicine	e.g. devil's claw, rosehip; mixtures are tailored to the patient's needs	Interactions with other medication as well as side-effects of their own; patients should be advised to only use registered products

lists some of the common therapies tried by patients with arthritis. Some studies show small short-term benefits and, if they are not harmful and make the patient feel better, there may be positive health benefits. However, an over-reliance on these methods in a patient with a significant arthritis requiring immunosuppression or surgery can lead to poor outcomes, e.g. progressive joint damage and disability.

2.12 Answers to starter questions

1. A family history should be taken in any patient presenting with joint pain unrelated to trauma. Most rheumatological conditions have some genetic susceptibility.

2. Pain that is constant and affects patients at night needs further investigation.

3. The ears, scalp and natal cleft are common areas to miss during examination. These should be looked at when examining a patient suspected to have an inflammatory arthritis, as a psoriatic rash or tophi may be found here.

4. Patients should ideally be undressed down to their underwear to examine them adequately. Deformities, rashes and muscle wasting may otherwise be missed. Patients should be adequately covered following general examination.

5. One-fifth of patients with clinical rheumatoid arthritis will be negative for rheumatoid factor. They tend to have milder disease. The exact role of rheumatoid factor in the pathogenesis of RA is not clear. It may be that patients with negative rheumatoid factor may represent a group with a distinct type of inflammatory arthritis.

6. Plain radiographs are cheap and accessible. They expose the patient to lower doses of radiation than CT. Often it provides an answer more quickly. Once a plain radiograph has been performed, the patient may go on to have CT or MRI.

7. It isn't clear why patients with the same disease respond to disease-modifying and biologic drugs in different ways. It may be due to the way individuals metabolise the drug or the disease variant that the individual is experiencing.

8. Immunosuppression carries numerous risks. The most severe are infection; patients can be badly affected by infections which normally go unnoticed or diseases can be activated, e.g. TB. Infections in the immunocompromised can be life-threatening. There is a higher risk of cancer due to reduced immunosurveillance.

9. Patients should continue to exercise unless the pain is severe and following expert advice from physiotherapists and occupational therapists. If the joint goes unused, the surrounding muscle will atrophy, causing further pain as the support for that joint has been diminished.

10. Acupuncture is used in physiotherapy as a tool to relieve pain such as lower back pain. It is considered an adjunct for other aspects of physical therapy rather than a stand-alone treatment.

Chapter 3
Arthritis

Starter questions

1. How do we ensure that inflammatory arthritis is identified early?
2. Why is prompt treatment of inflammatory arthritis important?
3. Do we know why rheumatoid arthritis is more common in women?
4. How do we make an accurate diagnosis of crystal arthritis?
5. How long can a hip or knee prosthesis last?

Answers to questions are to be found in *Section 3.10*.

Arthritis is a broad term that encompasses a variety of specific medical conditions affecting joints and surrounding tissues. There are over a hundred different types of arthritis, and they can be broadly divided into inflammatory and degenerative categories, reflecting the underlying pathological processes.

Inflammatory arthritis can be categorised as:

■ **seropositive arthritis**, i.e. there are circulating antibodies associated with rheumatoid arthritis
■ **seronegative arthritis**, i.e. antibodies are absent.

An alternative grouping is **spondyloarthropathy** or **spondyloarthritis**, indicating spinal involvement, as opposed to peripheral arthritis which specifies that only joints in the limbs are affected; this can be further subdivided into large joints (e.g. hip and knee) and small joints (e.g. finger and toe joints).

Each type of arthritis has particular characteristics such as the number and pattern of joint involvement, pathophysiology, aetiology, clinical findings, radiographic, biochemical and immunological features that correspond to a specific diagnosis. The most common type of arthritis is osteoarthritis (OA), which is characterised by premature degeneration of articular cartilage and tends to affect weight-bearing joints of the lower limbs and spine.

It is also important to recognise that other organ systems of the body can be affected, particularly in the context of inflammatory arthritis, e.g. eyes and lungs, and these are often termed *extra-articular complications*. There can be other disease associations, such as psoriasis and inflammatory bowel disease (IBD), which increase the risk of joint problems.

Recognising and treating inflammatory arthritis at an early stage is crucial to prevent permanent joint damage and deformity, impairment of function and quality of life, and disability. The introduction of new therapies and management strategies has significantly improved short- and long-term prognosis and outcomes for all patients with arthritis.

A general characteristic distinction between degenerative and inflammatory arthritis is the duration of early morning joint stiffness:

■ lasting <30 minutes: degenerative arthritis
■ lasting >30 minutes: inflammatory arthritis

Case 3.1 Pain and swelling in the knuckles

Presentation

Mrs Aimee Knowles, a 34-year-old school teacher, attends her GP surgery with persistent pain and swelling in her knuckles and wrists for the past 2 months. It initially started in her dominant hand but has progressed into her non-dominant hand within a week.

Initial interpretation

This is a patient who is rarely seen at the surgery. She has symptoms that are progressing in severity and the swelling in particular is affecting multiple joints, suggesting the possibility of inflammatory arthritis. It is important to find out more specific detail about her symptoms: has she had this before, and was there a trigger event (e.g. infection) that may suggest a reactive arthritis, which is more common in a younger patient? She is young and female, which may increase the likelihood of an inflammatory or autoimmune problem. Strong consideration should be given to referring her urgently to the specialist early

arthritis clinic in the Rheumatology department at the local hospital.

History

Mrs Knowles has noticed that she has slowed down in the mornings, with difficulties gripping and opening milk cartons; she also has stiffness in her feet. She has noticed she gets tired easily and has taken naps in the evening, which is unusual for her. She is finding it difficult to cope at work, particularly with writing on the whiteboard and standing still for long periods. She has noticed pins and needles in her fingers which wake her up early in the morning and tend to be relieved by shaking her hands.

Interpretation of history

Mrs Knowles' symptoms of prolonged early morning joint stiffness and systemic symptoms of tiredness suggest local and systemic effects of inflammation. This is clearly impacting on her levels of function at home and at work, so symptoms are no doubt significant. She also

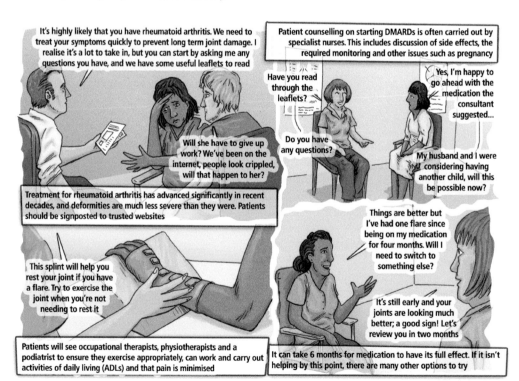

describes symptoms of carpal tunnel syndrome, most likely due to median nerve entrapment from joint and flexor tendon sheath swelling around the wrists, probably related to her inflammatory arthritis.

Further history

Mrs Knowles is married with two children. She is otherwise healthy with no significant past medical history or regular medications. She has bought ibuprofen from her local pharmacy and has been taking it for the past week; she finds that this helps with her joint pain and stiffness. She has not had any recent illness or symptoms of infection, skin rash or any other new symptoms. She is a smoker but does not drink alcohol. She has no family history of arthritis. There is no history of sexually transmitted infections.

Examination

On examination both wrists and the metacarpophalangeal (MCP) and proximal interphalangeal (PIP) joints of most fingers are tender with warm soft boggy swelling. She has positive Tinel's and Phalen's signs. She has tenderness across her metatarsophalangeal (MTP) joints in both feet when squeezed. All of her other joints are normal. There are no visible skin or nail changes, and general physical examination is normal.

Interpretation of findings

The nature of the swelling in Mrs Knowles' finger and wrist joints indicates synovial inflammation (synovitis). The distribution of symptoms across multiple small joints in the hands, wrists and feet in a symmetrical pattern also suggests an inflammatory cause. Tenderness on squeezing across the finger and toe joints can be a good screening examination for joint inflammation (**Figure 2.7**). Her symptoms of tingling in the fingers, relieved by shaking her hands, together with positive Phalen's and Tinel's tests (see *Section 9.8* and **Figures 2.22** and **2.23**) confirm a diagnosis of carpal tunnel syndrome which is likely to be related to synovial and tenosynovial

swelling causing compression of the median nerve. There are no nail changes or skin rash which makes psoriatic arthritis, connective tissue disease or vasculitis less likely. It is always important to consider systemic manifestations of inflammation, but in this case general physical examination is normal. Her response to ibuprofen (an anti-inflammatory treatment) supports an inflammatory cause.

All these clinical findings are strongly suggestive of an inflammatory polyarthritis. There is enough information to be confident to make this diagnosis and start appropriate treatment to suppress the joint inflammation. This should be facilitated by an urgent referral to the rheumatology specialist early inflammatory arthritis clinic at the local hospital.

Further investigation may allow a more exact diagnosis to be made, i.e. what specific type of inflammatory arthritis. For example, does she have specific antibodies for RA – RF and ACPA?; are there any systemic manifestations of inflammation such as anaemia or raised acute phase markers (e.g. ESR or CRP)?; is there any impairment of renal or liver function that may make you more cautious with certain treatments?; is there any joint damage on X-rays consistent with a specific type of arthritis? (permanent joint damage at diagnosis can also suggest a worse prognosis). Other tests such as a chest X-ray can help exclude other differential diagnoses such as infection or sarcoidosis, and ANA may be useful to help exclude other associated autoimmune disease.

Investigations

Blood tests show mild anaemia (Hb 11.1g/dl) with a normochromic, normocytic picture (mean corpuscular volume (MCV) 85, mean cell haemoglobin (MCH) 30), and raised acute phase markers (CRP 15, ESR 42). She has a normal renal and liver function tests. She has positive antibodies (RF 134, ACPA 88) but ANA is negative.

X-rays of her affected joints show soft tissue swelling around the wrists, MCP and PIP joints, with reduced bone density adjacent to these

Case 3.1 *continued*

joints (periarticular osteopenia), but no definite bone erosions. She has a normal chest X-ray.

Diagnosis

The persistent joint pain, swelling and stiffness after rest (especially first thing in the morning), in a symmetrical distribution favouring the small peripheral joints, raised acute phase markers, positive RF and ACPA, and characteristic hand X-ray features all point strongly towards a diagnosis of rheumatoid arthritis (RA).

Management

Following referral by her GP, the Rheumatologist at local hospital early arthritis clinic confirms the diagnosis of RA and after appropriate discussion, Mrs Knowles is given a single intramuscular injection of corticosteroid (Depo-Medrone) (see *Section 2.8.3*) to reduce the joint inflammation quickly. She is also started on the DMARD methotrexate (see *Section 2.8.4*) to control the inflammation. These drugs work by altering the

immune process of the disease. She is likely to need to take this treatment for a period of years. Her disease activity score is calculated using DAS28 (**Table 3.1**). This score assesses 28 joints (in the shoulder, elbow, wrist, MCPs, PIPs and knee) as well as CRP and the patient's assessment of activity on a Likert scale. Mrs Knowles is invited to attend regular follow-up visits to the rheumatology clinic to closely monitor her condition and ensure that the joint inflammation is controlled. She may require increased doses of her medication or the addition of further drug therapies to achieve this.

Table 3.1 *DAS28 definitions of disease activity*

DAS score	Disease activity
>5.1	High
3.2–5.1	Moderate
<3.2	Low
<2.6	Remission

Case 3.2 Loss of mobility and painful knee

Presentation

Mrs Dora Crediton, a 65-year-old retired police officer, attends her GP surgery. Her family have noticed a gradual decline in her mobility in the last year and she often complains of a painful knee that is slightly swollen. The pain is constant and her knee feels stiff in the morning; however, the stiffness usually lasts only for a few minutes. Her daughter says her knee looks swollen and 'creaks' a lot when moved. Mrs Crediton has had to move her bed downstairs as her knee occasionally 'gives way' when she climbs the stairs.

Initial interpretation

Symptoms are relatively long-standing and are mechanical in nature, i.e. worsening with exercise,

relatively short-lived stiffness after resting and in the morning, audible crepitus and minimal swelling. A single weight-bearing joint is less likely to have an inflammatory aetiology and her age and previous occupation may increase the likelihood of a degenerative problem. Function and mobility are impaired and she has had to modify her home circumstances, implying symptoms are significant and are affecting function and quality of life.

History

Mrs Crediton is usually independent and lives alone in a two-storey house. She takes aspirin and atenolol for ischaemic heart disease and has now started to take paracetamol for pain. She normally plays lawn bowls with her friends over the weekend but has had to miss this recently due to her symptoms. She is a non-smoker and does not drink alcohol. Her mother and sister have arthritis.

Examination

On examination, Mrs Crediton's left knee has a small cool effusion with a negative patellar tap. There is tenderness, particularly over the medial and lateral joint lines. She has near full range of movement but this is painful and there is marked crepitus felt around her patella on flexing her knee. She has some hard knobbly changes in her finger distal interphalangeal (DIP) joints but they are not tender and the swelling feels bony. Her general examination is otherwise normal, apart from some muscle wasting over her left quadriceps muscles.

Interpretation of findings

There are pathological changes in the symptomatic knee joint, confirming a likely degenerative problem with a small cool effusion, joint line tenderness, pain and crepitus on movement. The bilateral joint line tenderness indicates likely cartilage loss in the medial and lateral joint compartments and the crepitus on flexion indicates that the patellofemoral joint is likely to be similarly affected. The muscle wasting of the quadriceps muscles is generally due to relative disuse. Bony swellings of the finger DIP joints are known as Heberden's nodes and are a feature of OA. There are no conclusive features suggesting joint inflammation such as prolonged joint stiffness that improves with activity, or warm boggy joint swelling. The most likely diagnosis is OA affecting the knee and finger joints.

Investigations

The clinical diagnosis of osteoarthritis is fairly clear but an X-ray of the knee is performed to confirm this. Her knee X-ray demonstrates generalised reduction in the medial joint space, with osteophytes and subchondral sclerosis.

Diagnosis

Clinical and radiographic findings support the diagnosis of osteoarthritis of the left knee.

Management

Analgesia is increased to co-codamol 8/500 two tablets 4–6 hourly. A corticosteroid injection (40mg methylprednisolone) is given into the knee joint to provide temporary symptom relief. She is referred for physiotherapy to strengthen her quadriceps muscles and improve her range of movement and mobility. Unfortunately, she fails to improve and so is referred to the orthopaedic team for consideration of total knee replacement surgery.

3.1 Osteoarthritis

Osteoarthritis (OA) is a slowly progressing degenerative joint disorder that causes chronic pain and loss of mobility. It is the most common type of arthritis and is the most common indication for knee and hip replacement surgery.

Osteoarthritis is defined radiologically by joint space narrowing which reflects cartilage loss and osteophyte formation, with reparatory new bone formation as an attempted repair response (**Figure 2.34b**). Clinically it is defined by joint pain, reduced range of movement and crepitus.

3.1.1 Epidemiology

The prevalence of OA is increasing due to the ageing population and increasing levels of obesity. OA is more common in women and the elderly, with symptoms affecting over half of the population who are 60 years or older. In the UK, for example, about 2 million people consult their GP for OA every year.

3.1.2 Aetiology

Contributory factors causing increased biomechanical loading across a joint can precipitate OA; for example, occupation, traumatic injury, obesity or systemic conditions which may predispose to cartilage problems, e.g. diabetes and acromegaly. Family history and twin studies indicate a genetic link and a number of candidate genes have been proposed. This is a complex area and is the subject of ongoing research. At present the relative contribution and interactions of these multiple genes are not fully understood.

3.1.3 Pathogenesis

In OA there is progressive damage and thinning of articular hyaline cartilage over several years. The loss of cartilage leads to remodelling of surrounding bone, with sclerosis and cyst formation in the subchondral bone and bony proliferation producing osteophytes at the joint margins. It is increasingly recognised that inflammation plays an important role in this pathophysiology. The phrase "wear, tear and repair" is often applied to describe the disease process.

3.1.4 Clinical features

Patients complain of a deep aching pain ("toothache") in their joints which may feel stiff and difficult to move, and which worsens with activity. The most common joints to be affected are load-bearing joints such as the hip, knee, lower back, neck, great toe and thumb bases (**Figure 3.1**). The onset is usually gradual over years. Patients experience stiffness after resting, which usually lasts less than 30 minutes. In the finger joints three deformities are seen (**Figure 3.2**):

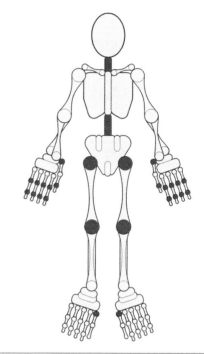

Figure 3.1 The pattern and distribution of joint involvement in osteoarthritis.

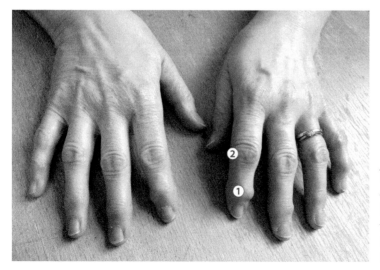

Figure 3.2 Osteoarthritis of the hands: note the Heberden's nodes at the DIP joints ① and Bouchard's nodes at the PIP joints ②.

- bony swelling of the proximal interphalangeal (PIP) joints, known as Bouchard's nodes
- bony swelling of the distal interphalangeal (DIP) joints, known as Heberden's nodes
- squaring deformity at the thumb carpometacarpal (CMC) joints.

There is reduced range of movement and audible or palpable crepitus when joints are moved. Muscle wasting occurs as a result of pain and disuse. Often a cool effusion is palpable, particularly around knee joints. The natural history is very variable between patients. OA can be confined to a single joint (e.g. following a previous injury) or progress to involve multiple joints (e.g. women with a positive family history of OA and an inflammatory component). Some joints can be relatively mildly affected, whereas other joints can be more severely affected and require surgical intervention. Patients have varied symptoms and functional impairment.

3.1.5 Diagnostic approach

Diagnosis relies on:
- thorough history taking to identify the characteristic symptoms
- clinical examination that notes the pattern of joint involvement and any pathological signs affecting the joints or soft tissues
- radiographs of the affected joints to visualise specific changes to cartilage and bone.

OA is usually formally defined by the degree of radiographic change. This may not necessarily correlate with symptoms, as a patient can have relatively mild changes on their X-rays but considerable symptoms or, conversely, severe X-ray changes but reasonable levels of pain and function. Both need to be carefully evaluated, particularly when considering treatment, especially surgery.

3.1.6 Investigations

OA is usually a clinical diagnosis, confirmed by X-ray findings. The characteristic radiographic features are (**Figure 3.3**):

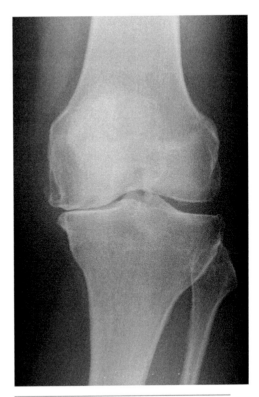

Figure 3.3 Radiograph demonstrating medial compartment osteoarthritis of the knee with reduced medial joint space, marginal osteophytes and subchondral sclerosis.

- joint space narrowing, representing cartilage damage and thinning
- subchondral sclerosis as a consequence of increased load bearing, causing the underlying bone to become hard
- subchondral cysts, as a result of bone damage and synovial fluid becoming trapped within damaged areas
- osteophytes at the joint margins, representing new bone formation as a result of joint instability.

Blood tests are characteristically normal and should only be performed if symptoms, signs or X-ray features are not typical of OA, or the patient does not respond as expected to treatment, suggesting an alternative diagnosis.

> **Radiographic joint space narrowing** is usually asymmetrical in osteoarthritis, reflecting localised damage to cartilage; but symmetrical in rheumatoid arthritis, as inflammation affects the whole joint, resulting in more diffuse cartilage loss.

If there is a discrepancy between clinical features and X-ray findings, e.g. severe pain but relatively normal X-ray, further imaging of the joint may be helpful to obtain an accurate diagnosis and exclude other pathology. MRI is the preferred imaging modality to visualise cartilage and surrounding soft tissue structures. MRI can detect early cartilage damage and associated inflammation which may respond to anti-inflammatory treatment. MRI can also detect other intra-articular pathology such as a labral or meniscal tear which can be the cause of joint symptoms and may increase the likelihood for later development of OA.

3.1.7 Management

Management of OA is aimed towards relief of symptoms and improving physical function, as patients usually present with established cartilage damage which cannot be reversed.

Self-management
Health professionals, including doctors and physiotherapists, should provide patients with education and information in order to advise and guide treatment. All patients should be advised to take regular aerobic exercise (e.g. walking or swimming), perform more specific local muscle strengthening (e.g. quadriceps exercises for knee OA) and maintain a healthy body weight. Employing these strategies generally helps relieve symptoms and reduces the risk of progression.

Physical and other therapies
Patients diagnosed with OA should be assessed by a multidisciplinary team (MDT) to assess their needs for treatment, which may include a physiotherapist, occupational therapist or podiatrist (**Table 3.2**). Other members of the MDT such as specialist nurses and clinical psychologists help patients cope with other

Table 3.2 *Physical therapies and support provided by the multidisciplinary rheumatology team*

Therapist	Therapy
Occupational therapist	Functional assessment; ergonomics; provision of splints; aids and appliances for home and work use
Physiotherapist	Exercise and physical therapies to improve mobility, function, muscular strength and core stability; joint protection; eccentric exercises for tendon inflammation; walking aids
Podiatrist	Assessment of biomechanical function; provision of orthotics and footwear; management and prevention of foot deformity
Specialist nurse	Drug counselling, pre-screening and monitoring; telephone clinics; patient helpline; review response to treatment; support and counselling
Clinical psychologist	Psychological support for adjusting to and managing a chronic illness, particularly if it has effects on function, quality of life, relationships and work

aspects of having a chronic disorder. Physical therapies such as a transcutaneous electrical nerve stimulation (TENS) machine or walking aids may be useful following assessment by a specialist physiotherapist. Hand function can be maintained by muscle-strengthening exercises and provision of splints to support the joints, as directed by an occupational therapist. Foot biomechanics and orthotic interventions can be provided by a podiatrist.

Medication
Paracetamol and topical NSAIDs should be first-line analgesic medications (see *Section 2.8.1*). Additional options include oral NSAIDs, topical capsaicin, opiates or intra-articular corticosteroid.

If there is significant inflammation, DMARDs may be trialled, e.g. systemic corticosteroid or hydroxychloroquine. However, unlike in RA, the results of trials of DMARDs in OA have been disappointing. There are a number of drugs in development and in active clinical trials that are directed at specific tissue targets in bone (e.g. osteoclasts) and cartilage (e.g. cell signalling pathways), that offer the opportunity to modify the disease process and reduce disease progression. Further drug trials are targeting specific inflammatory processes, e.g. antagonism of granulocyte colony-stimulating factor and mediators of pain, e.g. inhibition of nerve growth factor.

Surgery

Surgery is offered to patients with pain secondary to OA that cannot be controlled by analgesics, who have functional limitation and for whom other conservative measures such as weight management and physiotherapy have failed. Hip and knee replacements (arthroplasty) are commonly performed and generally have highly successful outcomes; reducing pain, restoring function and improving quality of life. The heterogeneous nature of symptoms and variability of radiographic signs can make surgical selection challenging, and careful balancing of risks and benefits and discussion between the patient and orthopaedic surgeon are required. Other surgical procedures for OA include removal of the trapezoid bone for CMC joint OA and fusion (arthrodesis) for the small finger joints.

Prognosis

Predicting prognosis is difficult because OA has a variable natural history. Modifying lifestyle factors such as weight and exercise helps considerably. Hand OA probably has the best prognosis, as knee and hip OA usually progress over time. However, only in rare cases does OA cause severe disability and, in most cases, progression is relatively slow over many years. It is common for symptoms to reach a peak in the first few years and then remain stable or even improve over time. However, some patients with hip or knee OA will inevitably progress and require joint replacement surgery.

3.2 Rheumatoid arthritis

Rheumatoid arthritis (RA) is an autoimmune disease that results in persistent joint inflammation. It is characteristically a chronic (persists over time), symmetrical (affects similar joints on both sides of the body), deforming (persistent joint inflammation will lead to permanent joint damage and deformity) polyarthritis (many joints affected), which mainly affects the small joints of hands, wrists and feet.

The development of new targeted immunomodulating therapies, modern strategies of early diagnosis and prompt commencement of treatment, often using combinations of drugs, have significantly improved outcomes for patients. The 'watch and wait' approach of earlier decades, reserving drug treatments for the most affected patients, is long gone. Prompt treatment increases the likelihood of disease remission, prevents joint damage and deformity, and restores normal function and quality of life.

3.2.1 Epidemiology

It is reasonable to assume that one in 100 of the general population will have RA. Prevalence data is reasonably consistent across populations, at less than 2% in women and less than 0.5% in men. The highest prevalence rates for RA have been recorded in certain Native American populations, in which prevalence is up to four times higher than it is in Europeans. There is no consistent evidence that any other ethnic group is at unusually high or low risk for RA. The most common age of onset is 40–60 years, but it can occur at any age. As with other autoimmune disease, it is more common in women than men.

3.2.2 Aetiology

Despite extensive research, the cause of RA remains unknown. It is likely to be multifactorial, involving an interaction between a number of genetic, host and environmental factors.

Genetic factors

Siblings of patients with RA have a two- to four-fold increased risk of developing RA when compared with those without an affected family member. There is an increased genetic susceptibility for RA associated with certain human leucocyte antigen (HLA) class II genes HLA DR1, DR4, DR10 and certain DRB1 'shared epitope' alleles HLA-DRB1*0401, *0404, *0405, *0101 and *1001. This is in contrast to other conditions associated with HLA class I genes, particularly HLA-B27, including psoriatic arthritis, axial spondyloarthritis, inflammatory bowel disease (IBD) and eye inflammation (e.g. anterior uveitis).

Host factors

The higher incidence of RA in pre-menopausal women has led to the suggestion that sex hormones and reproductive factors may influence susceptibility. Pregnancy seems to be relatively protective but in the postpartum period, particularly after a first pregnancy, there is an increased risk of development of the disease or a flare of existing RA.

There may be factors specific to the host which alter immune function and response. For example, there may be coexistence of autoimmune disease such as RA and thyroid disease in the same patient, and certain individuals may be predisposed to produce increased autoantibodies such as RF following immunisation.

Environmental factors

A number of environmental factors have been implicated. In particular, smoking is significantly associated with risk of developing RA, but only in the appropriate genetic or immune environment. For example, possession of the 'shared epitope' or presence of RA-associated autoantibodies such as RF or ACPA and smoking significantly increase the risk of RA. Prior infection is frequently associated with development of RA. Occupational factors such as heavy silica exposure in mining communities increase risk. Dietary factors such as red meat consumption and overeating and becoming obese may contribute.

3.2.3 Clinical features

Patients have joint pain, swelling and stiffness, usually of gradual onset, persisting over a period of weeks or months. Prolonged early morning stiffness improving with activity is common, and duration of at least 30 minutes indicates inflammatory arthritis (patients with degenerative arthritis can also have morning stiffness but this is usually less than 30 minutes). Other symptoms such as tiredness or fever are often present due to systemic inflammation.

Patients usually present with a symmetrical, polyarticular pattern of joint involvement affecting the metacarpophalangeal (MCP), proximal interphalangeal (PIP), metatarsophalangeal (MTP) and wrist joints (**Figures 3.4** and **3.5**). Other larger joints such as knees and cervical spine joints may also be affected. Less commonly, patients present with inflammation in a single joint (monoarthritis), in less than five joints (oligoarthritis), or symptoms moving from joint to joint (migratory or palindromic RA). In elderly patients there may also be proximal

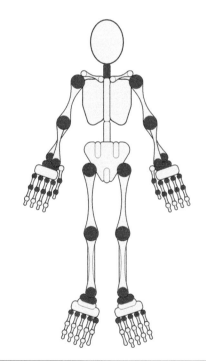

Figure 3.4 The pattern and distribution of joint involvement in RA.

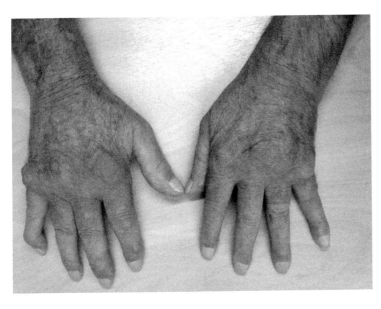

Figure 3.5 Rheumatoid arthritis of the hands – there is swelling of symmetrical MCP joints and left wrist with a swan-neck deformity of the right 5th finger DIP joint.

muscle pain and stiffness (polymyalgic-onset). Other extra-articular features such as Raynaud's phenomenon, skin rashes, nodules and carpal tunnel syndrome can occur, and other organs may be affected such as the eyes and lungs:

- rheumatoid nodules (**Figure 3.6**)
- carpal tunnel syndrome; peripheral neuropathy; mononeuritis multiplex; atlanto-axial subluxation
- palmar erythema; nailfold infarcts; ulceration
- pleural effusion; pleuritis
- pericardial effusion (**Figure 3.7**); pericarditis; nodules

- interstitial lung disease and fibrosis (N.B. Caplan's syndrome = RA + pneumoconiosis with intrapulmonary nodule formation)
- vasculitis
- lymphadenopathy
- splenomegaly
- Felty's syndrome (RA + splenomegaly + neutropenia)
- sicca syndrome (dry eyes and mouth)
- episcleritis; scleritis; scleromalacia perforans ('corneal melt')
- normochromic normocytic anaemia; leucopenia; pancytopenia
- amyloidosis
- fatigue, low-grade fever; weight loss.

With uncontrolled inflammation over time chronic joint damage and deformity will develop. Characteristic joint deformities are (**Figure 3.8**):

- ulnar deviation at MCPJs
- Z deformity of the thumb
- muscle wasting of dorsal interossei and thenar eminence
- boutonnière deformity
- swan-neck deformity
- thinning and bruising of the skin
- fixed flexion deformity

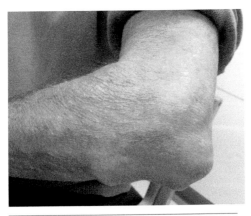

Figure 3.6 Rheumatoid nodules are shown over the extensor surface of the elbow.

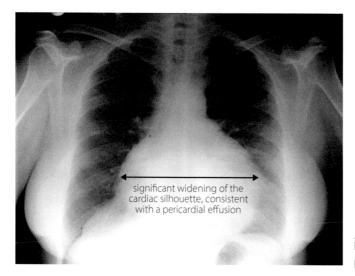

significant widening of the cardiac silhouette, consistent with a pericardial effusion

Figure 3.7 RA-related pericardial effusion.

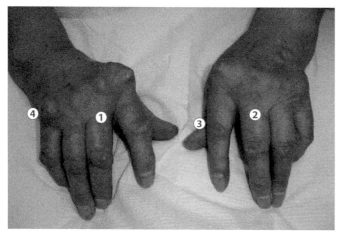

Figure 3.8 There is ulnar deviation at the MCP joints ①, flexion deformities of the fingers ② and a Z deformity of thumbs ③. Rheumatoid nodules are visible in the right hand ④.

3.2.4 Diagnostic approach

The diagnosis of RA requires a combination of characteristic inflammatory joint symptoms (pain, stiffness and swelling) and a typical pattern and number of tender and swollen joints (symmetrical, polyarticular small joints of hands and feet) that persists over time. Often the initial diagnosis of early inflammatory arthritis is made purely on these clinical grounds. The presence of autoantibodies (RF and ACPA), acute phase reactants (raised CRP) and imaging features (radiographic periarticular osteopenia and periarticular erosions) can help confirm the diagnosis but may not always be present, especially in the early stages.

The history should establish the duration and inflammatory nature of the symptoms, and examination should confirm tender soft synovial thickening and the pattern and number of joints involved. This may be enough to make a diagnosis. It is essential to perform a general physical examination to look for extra-articular manifestations of RA and rule out other disease processes (e.g. a polyarthritis can sometimes be a paraneoplastic presentation of malignancy; see **Table 2.4**).

Investigations are always carried out to exclude other causes and to gain additional information to corroborate the diagnosis and assess prognosis. Blood samples are taken to detect additional evidence of inflammation (e.g.

raised acute phase reactants, particularly CRP or ESR, anaemia) and to identify autoantibodies (e.g. RF and ACPA); X-rays are used to assess any reduction in bone density or joint damage (e.g. periarticular osteopenia, erosions or joint space narrowing). The presence of autoantibodies, raised inflammatory markers and radiographic damage at diagnosis confers a worse prognosis.

3.2.5 Investigations

Blood tests

Blood tests used in the diagnosis of RA are shown in **Table 3.3**.

Blood test markers of inflammation may be only mildly raised (and may even be normal), particularly when inflammation is confined to small joints.

RA-specific antibodies can also be negative at presentation.

> RA with positive antibodies is referred to as 'seropositive RA'. If antibodies are negative then it is known as 'seronegative RA'.

Imaging

Radiographs are usually performed of the affected joints, usually the hands and feet, and may show soft tissue swelling, periarticular osteopenia, erosions and joint space narrowing, particularly with ongoing disease activity

Table 3.3 *Blood tests used in the diagnosis of RA*

Test	Result if RA is present
Full blood count	Normocytic anaemia
Renal profile	Usually normal
Liver function test	Slight elevation in ALP (acute phase reactant)
Inflammatory markers	Raised CRP, ESR and PV
Autoimmune serology	Positive RF and ACPA
	Possible ANA positive, especially if overlap with associated connective tissue or other autoimmune disease

(**Figure 3.9**). Periarticular osteopenia is often the first radiographic sign of joint inflammation but radiographs are often normal at presentation. They are performed at diagnosis and usually periodically to assess any cumulative joint damage over time.

Ultrasound or MRI of the joints are more sensitive at detecting inflammation and joint damage than clinical or laboratory tests or radiographs, and may be performed particularly in equivocal cases (**Figure 3.10**).

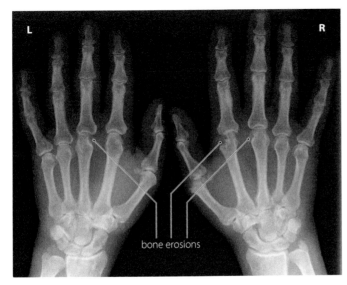

bone erosions

Figure 3.9 X-ray of rheumatoid arthritis.

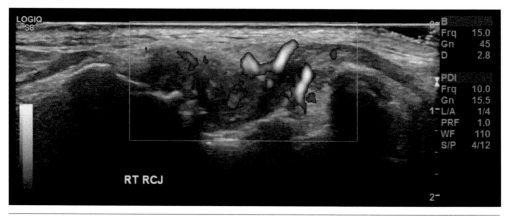

Figure 3.10 This patient with RA has active synovitis of the radiocarpal compartment of the wrist; there is grey scale synovial thickening and positive power Doppler activity.

A chest X-ray is often performed to exclude any other pathology, such as sarcoidosis or lung cancer. Chest radiographs are also requested prior to starting methotrexate (MTX) to rule out interstitial lung disease or other lung pathology which may increase the risk of MTX-associated lung complications.

Disease activity assessment

In RA, disease activity is measured objectively using the disease activity score (DAS). This is a number derived from a mathematical formula which combines:

- the number of tender and swollen joints, out of 28, hence the name DAS28
- the CRP
- the patient's own assessment of disease activity using a 0 to 100 Likert scale.

Often a commercially available calculator or a web-based application is used to calculate the score. This result is a value between 0 and 10 which is used to record disease activity (**Table 3.1**).

The goal of treatment should always be remission, and using the DAS28 score as a guide for increasing therapy ('treat to target') helps optimise treatment and improve outcomes.

3.2.6 Management

The aim of treatment is to stop inflammation as early as possible to prevent any permanent joint damage, functional impairment or disability.

This requires prompt initial assessment and identification of inflammation and an urgent referral to the local rheumatology department's early arthritis clinic, for review and treatment planning by a multidisciplinary team (MDT) of specialist doctors and allied health professionals.

Medication

Medication for RA falls into two classes: control of acute inflammation and modification of disease (see *Section 2.8*).

Control of acute inflammation

NSAIDs reduce inflammatory prostaglandins, which can help to reduce symptoms, but have little effect on disease progression, so should not be used alone.

Corticosteroids are used typically at disease onset or flare to rapidly reduce inflammation. They should be used sparingly, usually by intramuscular or intra-articular injection, to reduce the risk of side-effects (e.g. weight gain, osteoporosis, skin thinning and infection).

Modification of disease

Early commencement of disease-modifying antirheumatic drugs (DMARDs) is essential (see *Section 2.8.4*). Almost all patients should be prescribed traditional DMARDs and/or newer biologic DMARDs which are designed to stop the pathological process at the primary site of inflammation and so are much better at controlling symptoms and preventing progression. The key to a good outcome is prompt *early* commencement of treatment and rapid and continued suppression of inflammation.

> Research suggests that there is a 'window of opportunity' for intervention early in disease, when inflammation may be completely reversible and even curable with prompt treatment. This would render the patient asymptomatic, with undamaged joints and normal function. Using biomarkers such as genetics, autoantibodies and imaging, it may even be possible to identify patients either at risk or with very early subclinical disease.

Patients are usually started on a traditional DMARD at their first visit to the rheumatologist, as there is good evidence that starting treatment as early as possible improves outcome. Usually a single drug is used (most commonly MTX) but combination drug therapy (e.g. MTX +/− sulfasalazine +/− hydroxychloroquine) may be commenced in very active, poor prognosis disease.

If patients fail to respond to combination traditional DMARDs and have persistently active inflammation, they may be eligible for biologic DMARDs, which are usually monoclonal antibodies directed against specific pro-inflammatory cytokines (see *Section 2.8.5*). Usually an anti-TNF-α drug is tried first (e.g. adalimumab or etanercept) but if patients fail to respond, therapy may be switched to alternative mode of action drugs such as anti-B-cell therapy (e.g. rituximab), anti-IL-6 agents (e.g. tocilizumab), inhibition of T-cell activation (e.g. abatacept) or JAK inhibition (e.g. tofacitinib or baracitinib). Many more biologic DMARDs are in development.

Use of drugs that suppress the immune system requires careful balancing of risks and benefits in individual patients. This involves careful history taking and examination for other medical problems and screening for particular risk factors such as infection and malignancy. Baseline blood tests should also be performed to check FBC, renal profile and liver function, as these can be affected by DMARD therapy, and inflammatory markers as part of disease activity assessment. Check immunoglobulins before rituximab as these can reduce with repeated courses (**Table 3.4**).

It is important that patients with RA remain under regular specialist review and are assessed by a rheumatologist at regular intervals to ensure that inflammation remains controlled over time. It is often necessary to titrate the dose or change treatment to ensure good control and maintain

Table 3.4 *Screening before initiating traditional and biologic DMARDs*

Condition	Screening method
Active infection, including fungal infection, active herpes zoster infection, and non-healing infected skin ulcers	History and examination
Exposure, risk and contact with TB	Pre-biologic DMARD – all patients require screening to rule out active or latent TB by clinical assessment and chest X-ray in all patients and blood test (interferon-gamma release assays) in higher risk patients
Hepatitis B and C infection	History, examination and blood test
HIV infection	History, examination and blood test
Herpes zoster infection	In patients who have not had chickenpox, a blood test should be checked to detect zoster antibodies – if negative, vaccination or treatment with immunoglobulin in the event of exposure should be considered
Prior history of malignancy	History and examination

good outcome. It is also important to monitor for side-effects related to long-term drug therapy or any complications of chronic disease.

Surgery

Joint replacement or surgery to fuse joints is performed in patients with severe joint damage or deformity, in particular when it is accompanied by persistent pain. Soft tissue surgery such as tendon transfer is also performed to help restore function.

Physical and other therapies

All patients diagnosed with RA should be assessed by the multidisciplinary rheumatology team to assess their needs for treatment by a physiotherapist, occupational therapist and podiatrist (see **Table 3.2**). Other members of the MDT such as specialist nurses and clinical psychologists help patients cope with other aspects of having a chronic disorder.

3.2.7 Prognosis

With modern management strategies of early recognition and prompt initiation of treatment, the goal is to quickly return patients to normal with cessation of symptoms, no joint damage and normal function and quality of life. However, in the presence of persistent joint inflammation, the likelihood of ongoing symptoms and development of joint damage and functional impairment is increased. Other factors that may confer a worse prognosis include female sex, smoking, shared epitope genetics, presence of antibodies (RF and ACPA), elevated inflammatory markers and radiographic erosions.

3.3 Psoriatic arthritis

Psoriatic arthritis (PsA) is a diverse group of chronic inflammatory arthropathies which affect approximately one in five patients who have skin or nail psoriasis. A variety of joint and soft tissue structures can be affected, including single or multiple large and small joints; the spine; tendons, ligaments and their bony insertions (enthesitis). It may be referred to as a type of seronegative arthritis (negative for RA antibodies) or spondyloarthritis (if inflammation affects the spine) (**Figure 3.11**). The condition can range from relatively mild to a severe destructive arthropathy (arthritis mutilans).

> Psoriasis is an inflammatory skin condition characterised by red scaly plaques, usually affecting the extensor surfaces of elbows and knees, the hair line, the natal cleft and the umbilicus, but with potential to appear on any area of the skin.

3.3.1 Epidemiology

PsA affects between 0.3 and 1% of the population; 2–3% of patients with arthritis have psoriasis.

Approximately one in five patients with psoriasis will have inflammatory arthritis. Sex distribution is equal. Skin psoriasis may precede arthritis and vice versa by a number of years.

3.3.2 Aetiology

The aetiology of PsA is not known. Some patients may not have skin psoriasis themselves but have a family history of psoriasis or PsA. The development of psoriasis and PsA is associated with certain HLA class I genes, particularly HLA-B27, in contrast to RA which is associated with HLA class II genes. The genetic link to HLA-B27 means that other conditions associated with this gene, such as IBD or eye inflammation (e.g. anterior uveitis), may also be present.

> **HLA-B27 is an important test.** It is a common gene (present in 1 in 7 of the general population) but if present in the appropriate clinical circumstances it increases diagnostic certainty of PsA or axial spondyloarthritis and confers a worse prognosis.

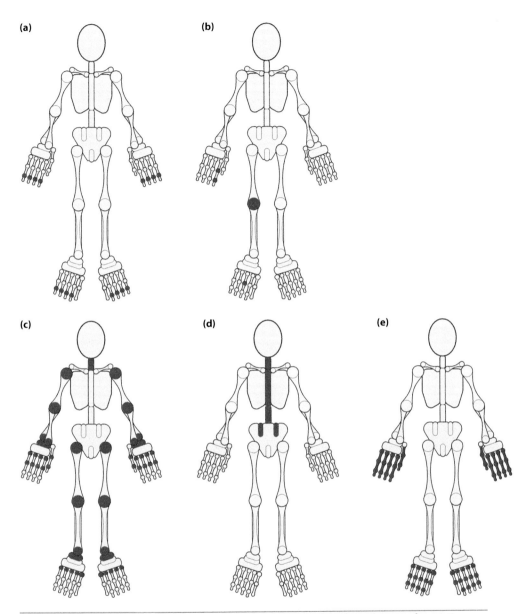

Figure 3.11 The pattern and distribution of joint involvement of the five subtypes of psoriatic arthritis: (a) arthritis with DIP joint involvement predominant; (b) asymmetrical mono-/oligo-articular; (c) symmetrical 'RA-like' polyarthritis; (d) spondyloarthropathy; (e) arthritis mutilans association with destruction, osteolysis and telescoping of fingers.

3.3.3 Clinical features

There is considerable variety in the pattern of joint involvement but asymmetry is common. Disease is traditionally classified into one of five subtypes:

1. Predominant distal finger and toe joint involvement, usually DIP joints (**Figure 3.12**)
2. Asymmetrical monoarthritis (single joint) or oligoarthritis (less than 5 joints), usually affecting the knees and small peripheral joints; this is the most common form

3. Symmetrical polyarthritis, which can mimic RA
4. Spondyloarthritis, i.e. affecting the spine and sacroiliac joints (SIJs), often more extensive and asymmetrical than in axial spondyloarthritis (ankylosing spondylitis)
5. Arthritis mutilans, with destruction, osteolysis and telescoping deformity of the fingers.

Symptoms are typical of inflammation with pain, stiffness and swelling. They are worse after resting, with a diurnal pattern with early morning stiffness >30 minutes. Swelling may be due to joint or soft tissue inflammation (e.g. dactylitis) and proliferative new bone formation may also be palpable, particularly in the DIP finger joints. Sites of tendon and ligament insertion may be inflamed and tender (enthesitis), e.g. Achilles tendon, plantar fascia, elbow epicondyles.

Nail involvement is classical of PsA. Common nail changes include pitting, discolouration, hyperkeratosis and onycholysis (**Figure 3.12** and **Figure 3.13**).

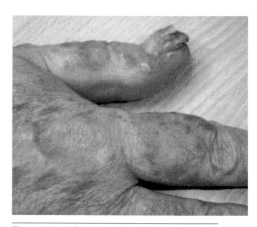

Figure 3.13 Psoriatic skin and nail changes.

Dactylitis or 'sausage digit' is a classical feature of PsA, characterised by diffuse swelling of a finger or toe, caused by inflammation of tendons (tenosynovitis), soft tissues and the synovium lining the joint (**Figure 3.14**).

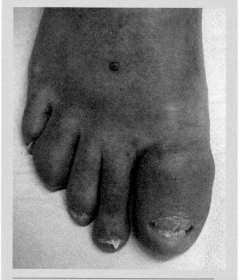

Figure 3.14 Dactylitis of the great and 4th toes and nail changes of psoriasis.

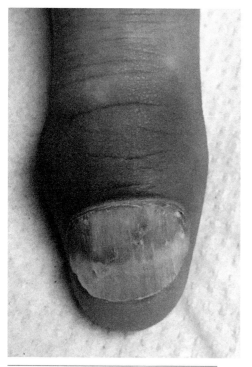

Figure 3.12 DIP finger joint arthropathy and psoriatic nail changes in psoriatic arthritis.

3.3.4 Diagnostic approach

The criteria for the diagnosis of PsA are a combination of inflammatory symptoms and signs affecting the joints, spine or entheses, with a personal or family history of psoriasis and/or other related symptoms such as psoriatic nail changes and dactylitis.

The ClASsification of Psoriatic ARthritis (CASPAR) group developed a set of validated diagnostic/classification criteria with high specificity and good sensitivity for PsA (**Table 3.5**). To meet the CASPAR criteria for PsA, a patient must have inflammatory articular disease (joint, spine or entheseal) and score 3 or more points based on these categories.

Blood tests can be useful to confirm a negative RF and demonstrate inflammation, and radiographs can demonstrate characteristic bony changes.

If a patient presents with an inflammatory polyarthritis in the hands and feet, as well as considering RA look for skin or nail psoriasis, especially if RF and ACPA are negative; this could be an RA-like presentation of PsA.

3.3.5 Investigations

Blood tests
There is no specific blood test for PsA. Tests are most commonly used to exclude other types of arthritis, or to help monitor inflammation (e.g. CRP) or drug therapy. Inflammatory markers (e.g. CRP) are elevated in the presence of inflammation in a large joint, e.g. knee effusion, but may be normal, particularly in the presence of enthesitis or small joint involvement.

Antibodies such as RF and ACPA are typically negative, although up to 13% of patients may have a modest elevation in RF, so clinical context is important to ensure accurate interpretation.

Imaging
Characteristic radiographic changes include proliferative new bone formation and erosions which may progress to produce a 'pencil in cup' appearance in the distal finger joints, which is characteristic of severe PsA (**Figure 3.15**). Periostitis, sacroiliitis and spondylitis may be present, as well as bony proliferation at entheseal attachments, e.g. Achilles tendon and pelvis.

Ultrasound and MRI are more sensitive than radiographs at detecting inflammation within joints as well as in soft tissues, tendons and entheses.

3.3.6 Management
Similar to RA, early diagnosis and prompt suppression of inflammation are key to controlling symptoms and optimising long-term outcomes.

Involvement of the multidisciplinary rheumatology team is important to assess and treat the various manifestations of the condition, e.g. physiotherapist, occupational therapist, podiatrist, specialist nurses and clinical psychologist. A dermatologist may also be useful to help manage skin psoriasis.

Table 3.5 *The CASPAR diagnostic/classification criteria for PsA*

Category	Description	Points
1. Psoriasis	Current psoriasis	2
	Previous history of psoriasis	1
	Family history of psoriasis	1
2. Psoriatic nail changes	Pitting, onycholysis, hyperkeratosis	1
3. Negative for RF		1
4. Dactylitis	Current dactylitis	1
	Previous history of dactylitis	1
5. Radiographic changes	Juxta-articular new bone formation	1

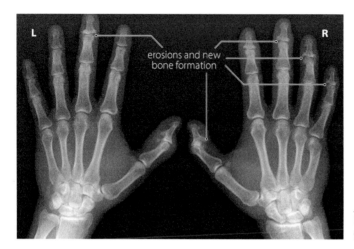

erosions and new
bone formation

Figure 3.15 Radiographic
findings in psoriatic arthritis.

Medication

Analgesics and NSAIDs can help symptoms
and corticosteroids control acute flares of
inflammation (but may flare skin psoriasis),
but DMARD therapy is often required, e.g.
methotrexate or sulfasalazine. Biologic
DMARDs are used for persistent uncontrolled
inflammation, e.g. anti-TNF-α inhibitors (e.g.
adalimumab or etanercept) or drugs targeting
IL-23 (e.g. ustekinumab), IL-17 (e.g. secukinumab,
ixekizumab) or JAK (e.g. tofacitinib).

Surgery

Surgery is reserved for particularly damaged
or deformed joints to improve pain or correct
deformity, and usually involves joint replacement
or fusion.

3.3.7 Prognosis

PsA prognosis is variable and less predictable than
RA. Many patients have relatively mild disease
but up to 20% may have a severe destructive
progressive arthropathy. Prompt recognition,
diagnosis and prolonged suppression of
inflammation improve the likelihood of remission.

3.4 Spondyloarthritis

In common with PsA, spondyloarthritis (SpA) is
strongly associated with the HLA-B27 gene and
so shares several similar clinical features, familial
predominance and other disease associations,
such as inflammatory eye and bowel disease.

The diagnostic and classification criteria for this
group of conditions have evolved over time and
most authors often now refer to this spectrum of
diseases as SpA (although spondyloarthropathy
is still sometimes used), with subtypes to reflect
which joints are affected and severity as judged
by radiographic changes:

■ Axial spondyloarthritis (aSpA) is inflammation
in the spine and/or SIJs

□ radiographic aSpA, with changes seen on
X-ray (ankylosing spondylitis is the classical
phenotype)

□ non-radiographic aSpA (nr-aSpA), without
changes on X-ray

■ Peripheral spondyloarthritis (pSpA) is
inflammation of joints in the peripheral
skeleton (i.e. non spine or SIJs).

The older, more traditional criteria make
distinctions between different types of
spondyloarthritis (or spondyloarthropathy):

■ ankylosing spondylitis – the classical
phenotype causing inflammation of the spine
and SIJs

- psoriatic arthritis (see *Section 3.3*)
- reactive arthritis (see *Section 3.5*)
- arthritis associated with IBD (enteropathic arthritis; see *Section 3.6*).

The clinical reality is that there is much overlap between these conditions and many share similar features, and often patients will not fit into a specific category (often termed undifferentiated spondyloarthritis), which is where the newer criteria describing the pattern of joint involvement and severity can be more useful. For example, PsA is usually a pSpA initially but can become an aSpA; ankylosing spondylitis is almost always a radiographic aSpA; and reactive arthritis may be either an aSpA, nr-aSpA or pSpA. Often a combination of terms are applied to each patient's case.

3.4.1 Epidemiology

Axial spondyloarthritis is the commonest type of arthritis within the SpA group, with a prevalence of between 0.2 and 0.5% in northern Europe. It is most common in Caucasian males, reflecting the prevalence of HLA-B27, although there are tribal communities in North America with an even higher frequency. Onset is typically in young adult life, before age 40. Ankylosing spondylitis is three times more common in men but nr-aSpA has an equal sex distribution.

HLA-B27 is present in up to 90% of patients with aSpA and this can be a marker of more severe and persistent disease. However, this gene is also common in the general population, present in approximately 8 out of 100 Caucasians. It is not a good screening test in itself as only 1 in 4 of these people will develop aSpA, and should only be tested in patients with appropriate symptoms.

3.4.2 Aetiology

The cause is unknown but the association of HLA-B27 confirms the importance of genetic susceptibility. Immunological factors, e.g. IL-23, and various environmental factors have been associated. Reactive arthritis usually has a clear infective trigger, e.g. group A *Streptococcus*, chlamydia, campylobacter, salmonella or others.

3.4.3 Clinical features

aSpA is characterised by inflammation affecting the spine and SIJs. pSpA is most commonly a mono- or oligoarthritis involving asymmetric large joints, e.g. hips and shoulders (**Figure 3.16**). In both types, enthesitis may occur, e.g. at elbow epicondyles, hip greater trochanters, Achilles tendon and plantar fascia.

Insidious onset of persistent lower back pain and stiffness is the commonest presentation of aSpA. The patient will describe typical features of inflammatory back pain which include:

- stiffness worse after rest or inactivity
- night pain and stiffness, disturbing sleep
- early morning stiffness of more than 30 minutes
- improvement with mobility and exercise.

Buttock pain may also be a common symptom which suggests sacroiliitis; this may be poorly localised in the buttock or lower back or upper hamstring region and can be bilateral.

In pSpA, pain, stiffness and swelling of other joints occur. Enthesitis is common in both subtypes. Dactylitis may be present.

Examination findings may include deformity such as hunched posture, exaggerated cervical flexion, loss of lumbar lordosis, reduced cervical

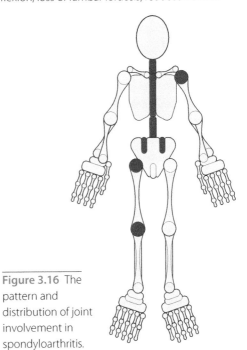

Figure 3.16 The pattern and distribution of joint involvement in spondyloarthritis.

rotation, reduced thoracic chest expansion and decreased lumbar spine forward and lateral flexion.

Other extra-articular manifestations may occur (**Figure 3.17**) such as psoriasis, anterior uveitis, IBD and, rarely, apical lung fibrosis, aortic valve regurgitation, osteoporosis and spinal fracture.

3.4.4 Diagnostic approach

Back pain is common in the general population, but only approximately 5% will have aSpA, so a careful history is needed to establish features of inflammatory back pain. This is usually supported by a blood test to check markers of inflammation and HLA-B27, and imaging to confirm evidence of inflammation or characteristic bone changes.

3.4.5 Investigations

Blood tests

Inflammatory markers such as ESR and CRP are most useful to confirm inflammation at diagnosis and to evaluate response to treatment. However, normal inflammatory markers do not exclude the diagnosis.

FBC may show anaemia of chronic disease if inflammation has been prolonged.

HLA-B27 is present in up to 90% of patients with aSpA.

> **Diagnosis is often delayed, sometimes by as much as 6 to 8 years.** This is because back pain is common, patients may tolerate symptoms, aSpA may not be recognised by some health professionals, and investigations – particularly inflammatory markers and X-rays – are often normal in the early stages.

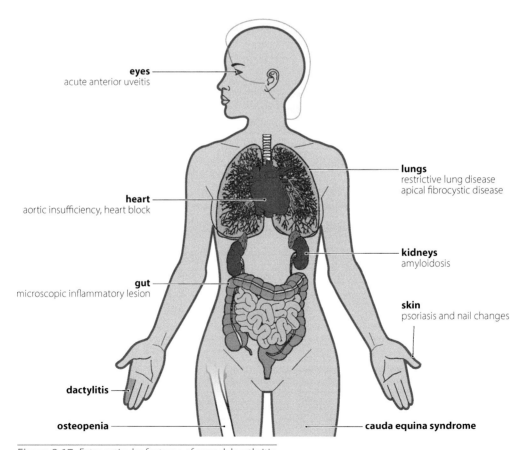

eyes
acute anterior uveitis

lungs
restrictive lung disease
apical fibrocystic disease

heart
aortic insufficiency, heart block

kidneys
amyloidosis

gut
microscopic inflammatory lesion

skin
psoriasis and nail changes

dactylitis

osteopenia

cauda equina syndrome

Figure 3.17 Extra-articular features of spondyloarthritis.

Radiology

The first radiographic signs are usually symmetrical sacroiliitis which is highly specific for aSpA. This usually starts in the lower synovial part of the joint on the iliac side, with loss of clarity of joint margins, erosions, followed by bony proliferation, sclerosis and eventually ankylosis and fusion. Changes of spondylitis may also be visible with erosion and new bone formation at the corners of vertebral bones, vertebral squaring as a result of new bone formation; calcification of intervertebral discs and spinal ligaments (syndesmophytes) may produce the characteristic 'bamboo spine' appearance (**Figure 3.18**).

MRI is much more sensitive than radiographs at detecting the early signs of aSpA, as it can detect inflammation (bone marrow oedema), enthesitis and structural changes (erosions) (**Figure 3.19**). If radiographs are normal then MRI is often performed, and some experts now perform MRI as a first-line investigation as it can detect both inflammation and structural damage.

(a) **(b)**

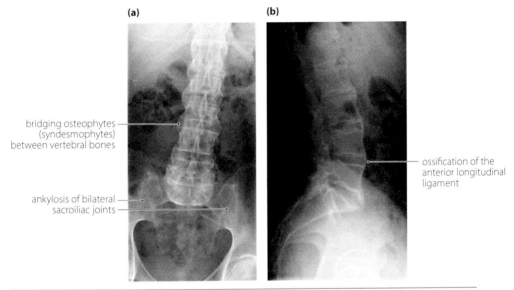

bridging osteophytes (syndesmophytes) between vertebral bones

ankylosis of bilateral sacroiliac joints

ossification of the anterior longitudinal ligament

Figure 3.18 Radiographic features of aSpA spine and SIJs: (a) antero–posterior view; (b) lateral view.

ankylosis of bilateral sacroiliac joints

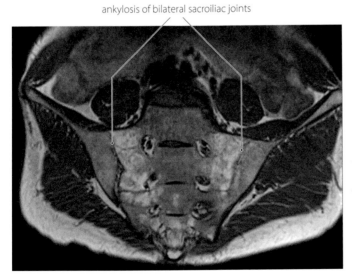

Figure 3.19 MRI of sacroiliac joints in aSpA, confirming ankylosis. There is no bone marrow oedema present to suggest currently active inflammation (same patient as in **Figure 3.18**).

3.4.6 Management

Management of SpA aims to control pain and stiffness, maintain spinal movement and restore normal function.

Medication

NSAIDs remain the mainstay of treatment for axial inflammation and are most effective if taken regularly. Corticosteroid tablets or injections can treat joint, entheseal or tendon inflammation. DMARDs such as MTX and sulfasalazine are helpful in treating peripheral joint and soft tissue inflammation but do not work as well for axial disease. Biologic DMARDs, e.g. TNF-α inhibitors (e.g. infliximab or adalimumab) or targeting IL-17 (e.g. secukinumab) are effective at treating axial and peripheral joint and soft tissue inflammation in SpA.

Physiotherapy

Physical therapy is a crucial part of effective management, particularly for axial disease, but also for enthesitis and tendon manifestations. A physiotherapy assessment of all patients should be undertaken, and specific regular daily exercises should be provided for each patient. It is essential that patients commit to performing these activities in order to improve stiffness and maintain range of movement and function. Periodic review and re-education are useful, and often there will be a physiotherapist present in specialist SpA clinics for this purpose.

Surgery

Surgery is rarely used as a treatment for SpA. Joint replacement or fusion may be considered in damaged joints from previous inflammation if patients have considerable pain or disability.

3.4.7 Prognosis

With earlier diagnosis, helped by the sensitivity of MRI, and more effective biological DMARD therapies, prognosis has improved. Good control of inflammation and regular exercise will prevent complications such as ankylosis and deformity. Many patients have relatively mild disease and continue to function normally. Some patients develop progressive deformity and postural changes over time.

3.5 Reactive arthritis

Reactive arthritis is an acute inflammatory arthritis that occurs within a few days or weeks following an infection such as a sore throat, food poisoning or sexually transmitted infection (STI) (**Table 3.6**). It is an immune system reaction to the infection and not a septic arthritis, as the trigger organism doesn't directly infiltrate the joint. It is more common in HLA-B27-positive individuals. The most common presentation is a monoarthritis or asymmetric oligoarthritis affecting the lower limb joints. Dactylitis and enthesitis can also occur, similar to other types of SpA.

Reiter's disease is a specific subtype characterised by arthritis, urethritis and conjunctivitis. The diagnosis is usually made on clinical grounds. The condition is often self-limiting but can persist and require anti-inflammatory treatment with NSAIDs, corticosteroid or DMARDs. The prognosis is usually good, but in a small number of patients the arthritis can persist and require long-term DMARD treatment and may reoccur.

Table 3.6 *Common infectious agents precipitating reactive arthritis*

Infection	Organism
STI	*Chlamydia trachomatis*
	Neisseria gonorrhoeae
Gastroenteritis	*Campylobacter jejuni* and *coli*
	Salmonella enteritidis
	Shigella flexneri
	Yersinia enterocolitica and *pseudotuberculosis*
Respiratory tract infection	Group A streptococci
	Mycoplasma pneumoniae
	Mycobacterium tuberculosis

3.6 Enteropathic arthritis

This is arthritis arising in the context of IBD. It can also be referred to as IBD-associated arthropathy. There are a range of musculoskeletal manifestations of Crohn's disease and ulcerative colitis which include arthralgia, spondylitis, sacroiliitis, enthesitis and peripheral joint arthritis.

HLA-B27 is prevalent in this group of patients. Bowel and peripheral joint disease activity are often linked but spondylitis may be independent; however, controlling colitis will often lead to an improvement in musculoskeletal symptoms. Management is similar to other types of SpA.

3.7 Crystal arthropathies

The most common types of crystal arthritis are gout and calcium pyrophosphate disease. They are characterised by deposition of crystals in the joints and surrounding tissue – monosodium urate (MSU) in gout and calcium pyrophosphate dihydrate (CPPD) – which leads to acute self-limiting episodes of inflammation and may progress to chronic tissue damage.

3.8 Gout

Gout is the most common type of inflammatory arthritis in men. It is characterised by recurrent, acute and very painful attacks of joint inflammation, most commonly affecting the great toe MTP joint. Joint pain, redness and swelling often develop over a period of only a few hours or overnight. It is caused by hyperuricaemia, an excess of serum uric acid which then crystallises in tissues around joints, causing the acute inflammatory reaction.

3.8.1 Aetiology and pathogenesis

The serum uric acid level depends on the balance of dietary intake, purine synthesis (e.g. increased cell turnover and metabolism) and excretion. An imbalance produces hyperuricaemia, for example as a result of:

- under-excretion of urate due to kidney impairment
- increased protein turnover in haematological diseases such as leukaemia or lymphoma.

Hyperuricaemia can be asymptomatic but increases the risk of developing the symptoms of gout. Risk factors for gout are listed in **Table 3.7**.

3.8.2 Clinical features

During a typical attack of gout there is sudden onset of severe pain, swelling and erythema of the affected joint (and soft tissues). Usually it is monoarticular – classically affecting the MTP joint of the great toe – but it may be oligo- or polyarticular, most commonly involving lower limb joints (**Figure 3.20**). Acute episodes usually settle after a few days but further events are likely to occur if risk factors are not addressed or prophylactic treatment not prescribed. With recurrent acute attacks over time, subcutaneous deposits of MSU crystals – called tophi – may be visible under the skin (**Figure 3.21**) and a destructive arthropathy of chronic gout may

Table 3.7 Risk factors for gout

Non-modifiable	Modifiable
Age	Hyperuricaemia
Male sex	High purine diet (e.g. red meat and seafood)
Race, e.g. African Americans, Pacific islanders and Maori races	Consumption of purine-rich alcoholic beverages (particularly beer)
Genetic factors, e.g. genes contributing to hyperuricaemia	Obesity
Chronic kidney disease	Certain medications, especially diuretics

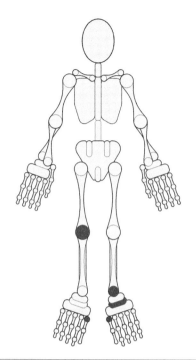

Figure 3.20 The pattern and distribution of joint involvement in gout.

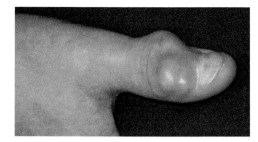

Figure 3.21 Tophaceous gout affecting the thumb IPJ.

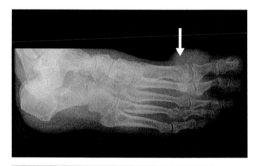

Figure 3.22 Radiographic features of gout affecting the first MTP joint.

develop, which is visible on radiographs (**Figure 3.22**).

> Gout is often described as 'the worst pain ever', so painful that it can suddenly wake patients from sleep in the middle of the night. They may be unable to tolerate even the weight of bedclothes on the affected region.

3.8.3 Diagnostic approach

In patients with a classical clinical presentation, i.e. an acute inflammatory arthritis of the great toe MTP joint, the diagnosis can be made without the need for further investigations. The gold standard for diagnosis is demonstration of uric acid crystals in a sample of synovial fluid. It is important to consider other possible causes of an acutely inflamed joint, particularly septic arthritis if it is a single joint.

Synovial fluid analysis

When the diagnosis is unclear, a sample of synovial fluid should be obtained from the affected joint and examined under polarised light microscopy by an experienced operator. This should be done quickly to maximise yield, because changes in temperature and pH affect the solubility of the crystals and therefore their visibility. MSU crystals are needle-shaped and negatively birefringent (the direction of refraction when the crystal is exposed to polarised light). The sample should be cultured to exclude septic arthritis.

Blood tests

Hyperuricaemia (raised levels of uric acid in the blood) is characteristic of gout. But hyperuricaemia is common and not everyone with hyperuricaemia will necessarily develop gout. Also, during an attack of acute gout, most uric acid will have moved to the affected joint, so there will be a falsely low reading on a blood test; thus a convalescent sample is important to obtain a true reading.

Inflammatory markers (e.g. ESR and CRP) and white blood cell count can be very high during an acute attack of gout.

Imaging

Radiographs of affected joints are often normal during initial acute inflammatory episodes; however, recurrent attacks can produce a destructive erosive arthropathy (**Figure 3.22**).

Acute inflammation and joint destruction can be seen on ultrasound and MRI; ultrasound and dual energy CT can be used to visualise tophaceous crystal deposits.

3.8.4 Management

Management of gout is divided into the acute episode and prophylaxis.

Acute management

The aim is to quickly settle the acute joint inflammation. Local measures such as 'RICE' can be used (rest, ice and elevation – compression is likely to be painful). Anti-inflammatory drugs, e.g. NSAIDs, corticosteroid or colchicine, are usually required. NSAIDs, e.g. ibuprofen, naproxen or etoricoxib, work well, but should not be used in renal impairment or if there is a risk of GI bleeding. Colchicine is effective but can cause diarrhoea as a side-effect. Corticosteroids can be injected into the affected joint or given as an intramuscular injection or as a short course of tablets, particularly if multiple joints are affected.

Prophylaxis

Any modifiable risk factors for hyperuricaemia should be addressed (**Table 3.7**), particularly diet, alcohol and any medication, e.g. diuretics.

The risk of recurrence after a single acute attack is high and is related to the level of serum uric acid. Two-thirds of patients will have another gout episode in the following year, increasing the likelihood of chronic gout with permanent joint damage and tophi. Hyperuricaemia itself is a risk factor for metabolic syndrome and cardiovascular disease; therefore most patients should be started on prophylactic urate-lowering therapy with dose titration aiming to reduce their uric acid level to a target of 300µmol/L. Reducing uric acid to <300µmol/L has been shown to significantly reduce the risk of further acute attacks of gout and dissolves uric acid crystals, promoting their excretion.

Xanthine oxidase inhibitors, usually allopurinol as first-line or febuxostat as second-line, are the most commonly used drugs. Uricosuric agents to promote excretion of uric acid by the kidneys are occasionally used (e.g. benzbromarone, probenecid or sulfinpyrazone) but should not be used if there is a history of renal stones as this can precipitate an exacerbation.

Prophylactic medications can precipitate an acute attack of gout as they mobilise uric acid in the body, so co-prescription with an anti-inflammatory drug such as NSAID or colchicine is recommended. If a patient develops an episode of acute gout during this period, they should be counselled not to stop their prophylactic therapy (they often blame this and stop the medication) and should receive treatment for the acute episode, as above.

3.9 Calcium pyrophosphate disease

Calcium pyrophosphate disease is increasingly common with age and may coexist with OA. It is caused by deposition of calcium pyrophosphate dihydrate (CPPD) crystals in the joint and surrounding tissues. It can manifest as asymptomatic chondrocalcinosis, an acute inflammatory arthritis ('pseudogout') or a chronic destructive arthritis ('chronic pyrophosphate arthropathy').

3.9.1 Aetiology and pathogenesis

In contrast to gout, calcium pyrophosphate disease is slightly more common in women than men. Prevalence increases with age. Chondrocalcinosis may be present in up to one-third of healthy people aged 65–75. It is usually sporadic but if it occurs in a younger person then consider a genetic association or a metabolic cause. Some metabolic conditions, e.g.

hyperparathyroidism and haemochromatosis, are associated with chondrocalcinosis.

3.9.2 Clinical features

CPPD crystals may deposit in articular hyaline cartilage and fibrocartilage, producing chondrocalcinosis. This is usually asymptomatic and can be found incidentally on radiographs (**Figure 3.23**). Common sites are the hyaline and fibrocartilage in the knees and triangular fibrocartilage in the wrist.

In a similar way to gout, CPPD crystals can provoke an acute inflammatory reaction in and around a joint, resulting in an acute inflammatory arthritis known as 'pseudogout'. Acute pseudogout usually presents as an inflammatory monoarthritis, with sudden onset of severe pain, stiffness, swelling, with signs of synovitis including joint effusion, tenderness, redness, warmth and restricted movement. Fever is common and

elderly patients may become generally unwell and confused. It may be indistinguishable clinically from gout or septic arthritis. The knee or wrist are the most commonly affected joints (**Figure 3.24**). It is the most common cause of an inflammatory monoarthritis in the elderly and can be a common occurrence if an elderly patient is admitted to hospital with an acute illness.

Chronic pyrophosphate arthropathy is usually an oligoarticular asymmetric pattern and overlaps with OA, with more chronic joint symptoms including pain, early morning and inactivity stiffness, reduced movement and functional impairment, superimposed by acute pseudogout episodes. It is a chronic asymmetric destructive arthritis with radiographic features of OA and chondrocalcinosis.

3.9.3 Diagnostic approach

The diagnosis is usually made in the presence of a characteristic clinical presentation supported by identification of CPPD crystals from a sample of synovial fluid. It is important to consider other

chondrocalcinosis affecting the hyaline and fibrocartilage in lateral and medial compartments of the knee

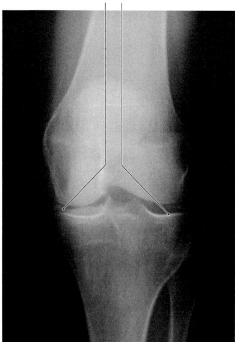

Figure 3.23 X-ray of chondrocalcinosis affecting the knee.

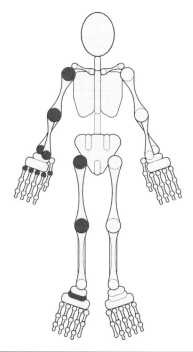

Figure 3.24 The pattern and distribution of joint involvement in calcium pyrophosphate disease.

differential diagnoses such as septic arthritis and gout.

Synovial fluid analysis

Confirmation of the diagnosis is obtained by examining a sample of synovial fluid from the affected joint under polarised light microscopy and demonstration of rod- or rhomboid-shaped non-birefringent or weakly positively birefringent CPPD crystals. The sample should be cultured to exclude septic arthritis.

Blood tests

Inflammatory markers (e.g. ESR and CRP) and white blood cell count can be very high during an acute attack of pseudogout. Other blood tests should be performed if a metabolic cause is suspected.

Imaging

Radiographs can be useful to demonstrate cartilage and soft tissue calcification and any bone and cartilage destruction that may develop over time, and often help in making the diagnosis (**Figure 3.23**). Changes of OA are usually present, e.g. cartilage loss, subchondral sclerosis and cysts, and osteophytes.

Ultrasound can demonstrate joint inflammation and chondrocalcinosis and dual energy CT can detect deposition of CPPD crystals and bone damage.

3.9.4 Management

Management of acute pseudogout is similar to gout, with anti-inflammatory drugs, e.g. NSAIDs, corticosteroid or colchicine. Unfortunately, there is no specific long-term or prophylactic treatment. Chondrocalcinosis does not require specific treatment. Chronic pyrophosphate arthropathy is usually managed in a similar way to OA, with NSAIDs, corticosteroid or colchicine used to manage inflammatory exacerbations.

> A hot swollen joint should be promptly aspirated and a sample sent for urgent microscopic analysis and culture to exclude septic arthritis. At the same time crystals can be identified, distinguishing between calcium pyrophosphate disease and gout.

3.10 Answers to starter questions

1. Education is key: patients and health professionals need to be aware of the symptoms and signs of arthritis, particularly inflammatory arthritis. In patients with joint stiffness, swelling and tenderness on squeezing, prompt referral to local rheumatology specialist services early arthritis clinic is required, to ensure early diagnosis of inflammatory arthritis and prompt initiation of DMARD treatment.

2. There is much evidence to support the concept that early intervention and halting inflammation in a joint with timely commencement of DMARD therapy will prevent joint damage and resultant deformity, loss of function and disability. Modern imaging techniques are able to demonstrate the rapidly adverse effects of even relatively small amounts of persistent synovial inflammation on adjacent cartilage surfaces.

3. RA is 2–3 times more common in women. This is similar in many other autoimmune diseases. It is

not exactly known why this should be the case, but hormonal and genetic factors seem important. Female sex hormones are involved in immune system regulation and the development of RA is uncommon during pregnancy but more common in the postpartum and perimenopausal phases.

4. This relies on aspirating synovial fluid from an affected joint and examination under a polarised light microscope. CPPD crystals are rhomboid-shaped and positively birefringent, whereas MSU crystals are needle-shaped and negatively birefringent.

5. Hip and knee replacement surgery are extremely effective operations in most patients and are most commonly performed for advanced OA. Data suggests an annual failure rate of 0.5–1% per year, with a 90–95% chance of 10-year survival. Between 80% and 85% of the joint replacements last 20 years. In more active patients they may wear out and require attention and revision earlier.

Chapter 4
Connective tissue disorders and vasculitis

Starter questions

1. Why does hypermobility lead to joint pain?
2. Why is systemic lupus erythematosus named after wolves?
3. Why can cancer be associated with muscle inflammation?

Answers to questions are to be found in *Section 4.22*.

Connective tissue connects the framework and organs of the body, providing support both structurally and metabolically whilst allowing inter-cellular communication. It comprises:

■ cells
■ extracellular matrix
■ protein fibres (elastic, collagenous, reticular)
■ ground substance (gelatinous material composed of glycoprotein and proteoglycan).

Connective tissue is not uniform throughout the body and different compositions of cells and extracellular matrix (ECM) confer particular properties. For example, the ECM is calcified in bone and teeth. Other specialised connective tissues are:

■ cartilage
■ bone marrow
■ lymphoid tissue
■ tendons and ligaments
■ cornea of the eye.

Inherited connective tissue disorders affect various components of connective tissue, e.g. skin, blood vessels, joints and bones. Recognising the patterns of affected sites and accompanying symptoms and signs, aided by genetic testing, helps diagnose a specific condition.

Autoimmune connective tissue disorders (also called inflammatory systemic connective tissue disorders) are caused by the immune system erroneously recognising elements of the connective tissue as foreign. These disorders can be life-limiting and cause significant morbidity. Often, they are not diagnosed immediately because their symptoms are non-specific, and their onset insidious. Diagnosis generally relies on a combination of symptoms, clinical signs and autoantibody tests.

Vasculitis is a general term describing inflammation of the wall of any blood vessel. This pathological process can compromise blood flow and lead to tissue ischaemia and infarction. Vascular disorders can also be caused by inherited or acquired disorders of the vascular connective tissue. Vasculitis is often classified by the size of blood vessel affected, e.g. large vessel or small vessel. Alternatively it can be classified by the cause, e.g. primary autoimmune disease, or secondary, e.g. to infection or another autoimmune disease, or specific antibody associations such as ANCA positive. There may be overlap with other connective tissue disorders.

Case 4.1 Pain in the shoulders and hips

Presentation

Miriam Dawes is 72 years old. She attends her general practice with a 3-week history of an aching pain in both of her hips and shoulders.

Initial interpretation

Musculoskeletal pain like this has many common causes including trauma, physical exertion, viral illnesses and adhesive capsulitis (frozen shoulder). If the patient has systemic symptoms such as fever or weight loss then polymyalgia rheumatica, polymyositis, underactive thyroid disease or cancer should be considered.

History

Mrs Dawes is normally fit and well, apart from high blood pressure which is controlled adequately by her medication. She reports aching and particularly stiffness around both shoulders and hips which is especially bad in the mornings or if she has sat down for a long period of time. She hasn't experienced any injury or trauma or changed her activity levels. She had a bad cold

last month and thought that had been the reason for feeling unwell, but now her cold has gone but still her pain and stiffness is not getting any better. She must wait for about an hour to 'loosen up' before she can walk her dog in the morning and does not feel as active as she was. It is becoming a struggle to get out of a chair on her own or brush her hair. She feels very tired all the time and has lost her appetite, but her clothes don't feel particularly loose. Sometimes she feels very hot and sweaty. She has taken paracetamol, but this hasn't helped her symptoms.

Interpretation of history

The predominant symptom is stiffness with some pain but no weakness. It is affecting symmetrical proximal muscular sites around shoulders and hips, rather than being confined to specific joints. The prolonged stiffness first thing in the morning and after resting indicates an inflammatory cause. Persistent symptoms lasting for a few weeks suggest an underlying disease process. A recent cold could be a trigger for her symptoms of musculoskeletal inflammation. She does have some other symptoms, i.e. fatigue, appetite loss and sweats, that need

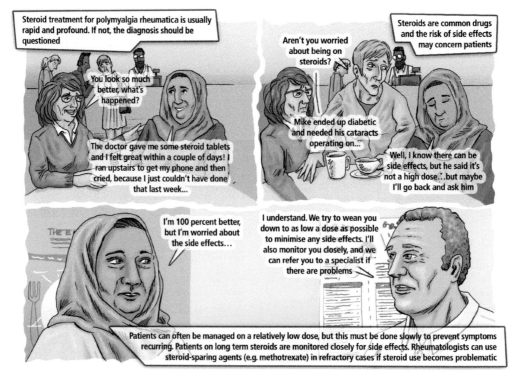

Steroid treatment for polymyalgia rheumatica is usually rapid and profound. If not, the diagnosis should be questioned

You look so much better, what's happened?

The doctor gave me some steroid tablets and I felt great within a couple of days! I ran upstairs to get my phone and then cried, because I just couldn't have done that last week...

Aren't you worried about being on steroids?

Steroids are common drugs and the risk of side effects may concern patients

Mike ended up diabetic and needed his cataracts operating on...

Well, I know there can be side effects, but he said it's not a high dose...but maybe I'll go back and ask him

I'm 100 percent better, but I'm worried about the side effects…

I understand. We try to wean you down to as low a dose as possible to minimise any side effects. I'll also monitor you closely, and we can refer you to a specialist if there are problems

Patients can often be managed on a relatively low dose, but this must be done slowly to prevent symptoms recurring. Patients on long term steroids are monitored closely for side effects. Rheumatologists can use steroid-sparing agents (e.g. methotrexate) in refractory cases if steroid use becomes problematic

further interrogation. At this stage, polymyalgia rheumatica (PMR) is the most likely diagnosis. The following features are typical of PMR:

- symmetrical generalised stiffness around the shoulders and hips
- prolonged morning stiffness
- persistent symptoms lasting over 2 weeks
- patient is always over 50 years old (usually over 70)
- systemic symptoms such as fatigue and loss of appetite are common.

However, inflammatory arthritis, myositis, malignancy or infection should also be considered as they can cause similar symptoms and signs, so careful history taking and physical examination are essential. Temporal arteritis may coexist with PMR, so it is important to assess for this specifically, e.g. headache, jaw claudication, scalp tenderness, visual symptoms.

Further history

Mrs Dawes does not report any symptoms of temporal arteritis. Her shoulders, lower back and hips feel stiff and sore but she has not noticed any pain in other joints and there is no joint swelling. She feels hot from time to time but has not recorded her temperature. She doesn't think she has lost weight. She has never smoked. She has not noticed any rash, cough or change in bowel habit. There have been no previous similar episodes.

Examination

Mrs Dawes is comfortable at rest; her observations are normal and her BMI is 27kg/m². There is no rash. She is uncomfortable standing up from a seated position and raising her hands above her head. There is no specific joint line tenderness or swelling but there is tenderness of the proximal muscles of both the upper and lower limbs. Power in these proximal muscles is 4+/5. Neurological examination is otherwise normal. Cardiovascular, respiratory and abdominal examinations are normal.

Interpretation of findings

The further history and examination findings support the diagnosis of PMR. Mrs Dawes describes characteristic proximal muscle aching and stiffness that is worse in the morning or after resting. She fits the age and sex profile for PMR. She does not report any 'red flag' symptoms suggestive of malignancy, such as weight loss, cough, or change in bowel habit. There are no signs of inflammatory arthritis or any definite indicators of persistent infection. While myositis can present with muscle aches, you would normally find muscle weakness and wasting. Mrs Dawes did have some mild reduced muscle power, but patients who have a great deal of stiffness and pain will often have a mild reduction in muscle strength so this can be a non-specific finding. Mrs Dawes should be investigated to confirm the presence of an inflammatory response and to help exclude other differential diagnoses.

Investigations

Blood tests show a normal FBC but raised inflammatory markers; CRP is 47mg/L and ESR is 74mm/hour. ALP is elevated slightly at 165IU/L. Thyroid function and CK are normal, which rule out thyroid disease and inflammatory myositis. A mild anaemia may be present, reflecting a systemic inflammatory response. If the inflammatory markers are normal then further investigations would be warranted to exclude alternative diagnoses, particularly malignancy.

Diagnosis

The characteristic clinical presentation, associated with raised inflammatory markers, means that the most likely diagnosis is PMR. The raised ALP is also an acute phase reactant and, like CRP and ESR, is raised in inflammatory states. Mrs Dawes is started on prednisolone at a dose of 15mg daily. It is expected that her symptoms will dramatically improve in around 48 hours. If they do not, the diagnosis should be reconsidered. Patients usually require corticosteroid treatment for two years; the prednisolone dose is gradually weaned, according to symptoms and CRP levels. To prevent steroid-induced side-effects on bones and gut, Mrs Dawes is also given vitamin D and calcium supplementation, a weekly bisphosphonate tablet and a PPI.

INHERITED CONNECTIVE TISSUE DISORDERS

There are more than 200 heritable connective tissue disorders. Any alteration in genetic code that leads to a defective protein being produced in connective tissue may result in abnormalities in these structures. Due to the variety of errors that are possible, there is a wide spectrum of effects involving different elements of connective tissue, but clinical manifestations are variable, ranging from no apparent consequence to organ-threatening disease. Fortunately, life-threatening inherited connective tissue disorders are rare.

Hypermobility ('bendy joints') is the most common symptom, as the connective tissue structures stretch and are less able to hold the joints in place. It can be the first sign of a potentially serious connective tissue disease such as Ehlers–Danlos syndrome (EDS) or Marfan syndrome. However, joint hypermobility is common, particularly in young females, and is not a specific sign, being most often a benign isolated finding. A simple screening questionnaire, devised by A.J. Hakim, can be used to assess for joint hypermobility (**Table 4.1**) and a screening physical examination is used to calculate the Beighton Score (**Figure 4.1**), where one point is scored for each joint up to a maximum of nine.

Table 4.1 *Hypermobility questionnaire: if a patient answers 'yes' to two or more questions, they should be fully evaluated for joint hypermobility*
Can you place your hands flat on the floor without bending your knees?
Can you bend your thumb to touch your forearm?
As a child could you do the splits OR did you amuse your friends by contorting your body into strange shapes?
As a child or teenager did your shoulder or kneecap dislocate on more than one occasion?
Do you consider yourself double-jointed?

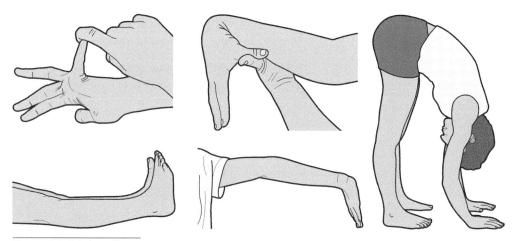

Figure 4.1 Beighton Score.

Connective tissue disorders and vasculitis are multisystem disorders, so a good way to think about them is to break them down into their effects on each body system, e.g. respiratory, renal, musculoskeletal, skin, etc. You can also apply this when you gather information from patients by conducting a 'systems review'. This involves asking about a range of symptoms in each body system. The patient may think not all their symptoms are relevant or may be reluctant to discuss them, but this approach will ensure all information is captured to inform a correct diagnosis and identify potential complications.

4.1 Marfan syndrome

Marfan syndrome is caused by a defect in the fibrillin 1 gene which encodes a glycoprotein. Usually this is inherited in an autosomal dominant pattern, but it can also be caused by a spontaneous mutation in the gene within a gamete. It affects males and females equally around the world with an estimated prevalence of 6 in 100 000. The leading cause of death in patients with Marfan syndrome is aortic root dissection (a tear in the innermost lining, the intimal layer of the vessel).

4.1.1 Clinical features

Marfan syndrome doesn't tend to be diagnosed until adolescence, as symptoms are rarely present until then. Whilst it can be life-threatening, most patients can expect a relatively normal life expectancy, particularly with screening for potential complications. Clinical features of Marfan syndrome are listed in **Table 4.2**. Patients will not present with all features but the more features they have, the more likely the diagnosis. Cardiac, ophthalmic and musculoskeletal manifestations are characteristic of Marfan syndrome but the nervous system, skin and lung are also affected (**Figure 4.2**).

4.1.2 Management

Management should involve the following disciplines:

■ Cardiology: annual echocardiography and regular cardiac CT/MRI scanning to assess the heart valves and thoracic aorta. Elective repair of the aortic root is preferred to emergency repair. Beta blockers are prescribed to help prevent dilatation.

Table 4.2 *Clinical features of Marfan syndrome*

System/area	Key features
Cardiovascular	Thoracic aorta dilatation (leading to dissection/rupture) Aortic regurgitation Mitral regurgitation Abdominal aortic aneurysm
Musculoskeletal	Arachnodactyly (fingers and toes are abnormally thin and long) Arthralgia Hypermobility Long thin limbs (arm span greater than height) Pectus excavatum (sunken chest) or carinatum (chest pushed out) Scoliosis
Ophthalmic	Myopia Glaucoma Cataracts Lens dislocation
Respiratory	Apical blebs and bullae causing pneumothoraces
Nervous system	Dural ectasia (enlargement of the dura in the spinal column, leading to back pain, headache, numbness)
Skin	Striae
Facial	Long face, high arched palate, enophthalmos (eyes appear sunken), small and recessed jaw (micrognathia and retrognathia)

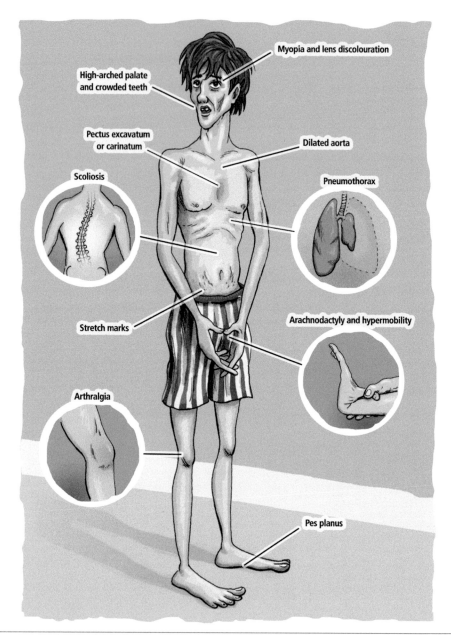

Figure 4.2 Marfan syndrome is characterised by long tall stature with arm span wider than height and long slender arms, legs, fingers and toes.

- Ophthalmology: regular screening for complications; treatment options include eye drops, laser treatment or surgery.
- Orthopaedic surgery: for correction of scoliosis and chest abnormalities if causing significant problems, e.g. respiratory compromise.
- Physiotherapy: regular exercise and joint protection activities.

Prognosis is usually good if complications are carefully monitored and treated. Patients may require genetic counselling if they are planning a family of their own.

4.2 Ehlers–Danlos syndrome

The Ehlers–Danlos syndromes (EDS) are a group of inherited connective tissue disorders with different inheritance patterns. In 2017, their classification was updated and now includes thirteen subtypes. They are rare conditions with an overall prevalence of around 1 in 5000. The gene defects either affect collagen itself or proteins which support collagen within the extracellular matrix. Hypermobility and stretchy skin are the characteristic features but there may be a wide variety of other manifestations, depending on the subtype and severity. Those of African origin are affected more than other ethnic groups and women are affected up to eight times more than men.

> Patients with EDS are at increased risk of complications when undergoing surgery, due to skin and blood vessel fragility.

4.2.1 Clinical features

The skin and joints are the most commonly affected systems. Hypermobility is common. Depending on the subtype, other systems and organs can be affected. Hypermobile EDS is the most common; others are rare. Vascular EDS is the most dangerous, as arterial and organ rupture can occur. The key features of three of the most important subtypes are outlined in **Table 4.3**. Diagnosis is made based on clinical manifestations and genetic testing.

4.2.2 Management

Management centres around joint and skin protection, with physiotherapy to strengthen muscles, tendons and ligaments, orthoses to provide stability, and taking appropriate precautions, e.g. avoiding high impact sports. Occasionally, orthopaedic surgery is required for joint stabilisation or correction of scoliosis.

Patients need extra support around the time of pregnancy (increased oestrogen) and childbirth due to increased musculoskeletal symptoms including symphysis pubis dysfunction and back pain. Because of the fragility of connective tissue in EDS, preterm rupture of membranes can occur, and vaginal births can lead to extensive perineal tissue damage unless managed carefully.

Patients with vascular EDS are managed by an expert MDT. Counselling is offered due to the burden of ongoing risk. Beta blockers have reduced the risk of arterial rupture.

Prognosis is variable. Lifespan is normal except for vascular EDS. Patients may have chronic pain, functional impairment and disability.

Table 4.3 *Common and important features of Ehlers–Danlos syndrome*

Hypermobile	Classical (type 1)	Vascular
Joint hypermobility	Joint hypermobility	Joint hypermobility (tends to be restricted to small joints)
Increased skin elasticity (not as fragile as in classical type)	Increased skin elasticity and fragility	Spontaneous hollow organ or arterial rupture, e.g. colon, uterus
Musculoskeletal pain (can be widespread)	Widespread atrophic scars	Characteristic facial features: lobeless ears, thin lips, prominent eyes
Hernias, genitourinary prolapse	Hernias, genitourinary prolapse	Thin skin and easy bruising
	Cardiovascular complications (aortic root dilatation, mitral valve prolapse)	Early varicose veins

4.3 Osteogenesis imperfecta

Osteogenesis imperfecta (OI) is a group of genetic disorders that affect type 1 collagen and most commonly result in fragile bones which break easily. They are rare conditions with a prevalence of between 1 in 10 000 and 1 in 20 000. Inheritance can be both autosomal dominant (least severe) or autosomal recessive (most severe), or the condition can result from a new spontaneous mutation.

OI is caused by mutations in type 1 collagen genes (*COL1A1*, *COL1A2*) which lead to increased bone fragility, fractures and deformity. Connective tissue in the sclerae, heart valves, blood vessels and skin can also be affected.

4.3.1 Clinical features

There are at least eight subtypes. The main clinical features are:
■ fractures – more common in children
■ blue sclerae
■ hearing difficulties
■ joint hypermobility
■ deformity – which occurs in more severe types affecting the spine, chest, skull and long bones – and short stature

■ cardiac complications, including aortic root dilatation and valvular dysfunction.

Diagnosis is usually suspected if there is a family history or recurrent fractures, and is confirmed with genetic testing.

> The sclera is so thin in patients with osteogenesis imperfecta that veins in the underlying tissue can be seen, giving the sclera a blue hue.

4.3.2 Management

There is no cure, but strategies to maintain good bone health and prevent fractures are key. Physiotherapy to build muscle and bone mass is important; medical management includes bisphosphonates to reduce pain and increase bone density; orthopaedic surgery to stabilise fractures and correct skeletal deformities. Patients should be screened and monitored for cardiac abnormalities.

Prognosis ranges from a normal life expectancy to death in early infancy, depending on the subtype.

AUTOIMMUNE CONNECTIVE TISSUE DISORDERS

Autoimmune connective tissue disorders vary significantly in their presentation and response

to treatment. The most common are discussed below.

4.4 Systemic lupus erythematosus

Systemic lupus erythematosus (SLE) is a chronic autoimmune disease characterised by the formation of autoantibodies to host cell nuclear material. The resulting inflammation leads to unpredictable patterns and severity of disease from patient to patient, but often multiple body systems are affected. The different types of lupus erythematosus (often just referred to as lupus) are outlined in **Table 4.4**.

4.4.1 Epidemiology

SLE is six to nine times more common in women and the peak age range of presentation is in child-bearing years. It has a predilection for those of Afro-Caribbean, Chinese and south-east Asian descent.

4.4.2 Aetiology

The cause of SLE is unknown. Genetic factors may predispose patients and the HLA alleles B8,

Table 4.4 *Types of lupus erythematosus*

Type of lupus	Features
SLE	A systemic inflammatory disease causing widespread symptoms including fatigue, joint pain, rash
	Serious complications involving the brain, heart and kidney can occur
Discoid lupus	Characterised by a chronic, scaly rash causing scarring and pigmentation; the face, scalp, lips, V-neck area and other parts of skin typically exposed to sunlight are affected
	Symptoms are restricted to the skin
Neonatal lupus	Maternal autoantibodies are passed to the developing foetus, causing a characteristic rash on the scalp and eyelids; this is transitory but complete heart block is a serious complication
Drug-induced lupus	Drug-induced lupus is rare and caused by medication such as hydralazine (antihypertensive), procainamide (anti-arrhythmic) and the oral contraceptive pill; symptoms tend to be mild and cease when the drug is stopped
Subacute cutaneous lupus erythematosus	Rare and the symptoms are restricted to the skin; a photosensitive rash occurs in the summer months over the sun-exposed upper body

DR2 and DR3 are associated with SLE. Other risk factors include a family history and complement deficiency. Environmental factors are thought to be triggers, via an epigenetic effect, and include ultraviolet light, drugs and viruses. **Figure 4.3** illustrates how autoantibodies may develop in SLE. During development and maintenance of tissues, apoptosis (programmed cell death) is a necessary process. This results in the release of nuclear material that is rapidly phagocytosed by self-tolerant macrophages. In SLE, this material is inappropriately presented to the immune system by antigen-presenting cells. An inflammatory response is then triggered. Autoreactive T and B cells that have not been quiesced are activated.

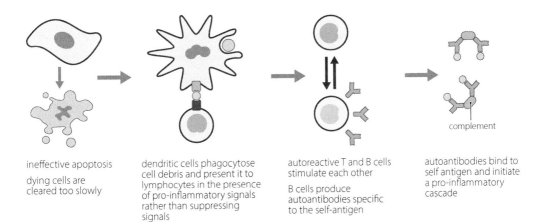

ineffective apoptosis
dying cells are cleared too slowly

dendritic cells phagocytose cell debris and present it to lymphocytes in the presence of pro-inflammatory signals rather than suppressing signals

autoreactive T and B cells stimulate each other

B cells produce autoantibodies specific to the self-antigen

complement

autoantibodies bind to self antigen and initiate a pro-inflammatory cascade

Figure 4.3 Development of autoantibodies in SLE.

4.4.3 Prevention

SLE cannot be prevented. However, there is some evidence that the risk of neonatal lupus is reduced if the mother's SLE is adequately treated during pregnancy.

4.4.4 Pathogenesis

The pathogenesis of SLE is not fully understood but is likely to involve a series of breaks in immune tolerance to nuclear material that becomes extracellular during the process of host cell death. The exact pathogenicity of each autoantibody involved in SLE is not known. The antibody anti-dsDNA is thought to bind directly to autoantigens, activating the complement cascade and causing inflammation.

4.4.5 Clinical features

The clinical features of SLE can be non-specific and vary from patient to patient, which can make diagnosis difficult (**Figure 4.4**). The most common symptoms are:
- joint pain (most commonly aches and stiffness affecting multiple joints – 'polyarthralgia')
- skin rash (classically raised, red or purplish, in a butterfly shape over the nose and cheeks – 'butterfly rash')
- fatigue (of variable intensity, but can be disabling).

Always ask about effects on other body systems, and specifically assess for any organ-threatening complications (**Table 4.5**).

There is a wide spectrum of disease intensity:
- Mild, usually involving musculoskeletal and skin symptoms, and fatigue
- Moderate, where one or more organ system becomes involved
- Severe, where multiple organs (e.g. kidney, heart and lungs) are involved, with life-limiting effects.

Table 4.5 *The multisystem clinical features of SLE*

System	Manifestation
General	Constitutional symptoms including: ■ fever ■ malaise ■ fatigue
Musculoskeletal	Polyarthralgia Myalgia Arthritis of the small joints
Skin	Photosensitivity Raynaud's phenomenon Butterfly rash Purpura Urticaria Vasculitic changes (fingertips, nail folds) Alopecia
Blood	Anaemia Lymphopenia Leucopenia Thrombocytopenia
Nervous system	Depression Psychosis Migraines Seizures Ataxia Polyneuropathy
Renal	Glomerulonephritis
Cardiac	Pericarditis Endocarditis
Other	Abdominal pain Mouth ulcers Episcleritis Pleurisy Antiphospholipid syndrome (leading to thrombosis, miscarriage)

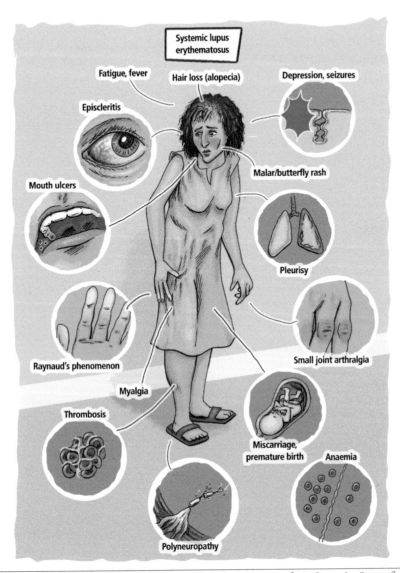

Figure 4.4 There are multiple features of SLE; however, the most specific is the malar (butterfly rash) over the cheeks.

4.4.6 Diagnostic approach

There is no single specific test for SLE; diagnosis is made from a combination of signs, symptoms and investigations.

4.4.7 Investigations

Investigations are used as part of diagnosis and monitoring of SLE (**Table 4.6**). Important investigations include:

- autoantibody tests (positive ANA and dsDNA)
- urine dipstick (if haematuria and proteinuria, consider renal involvement)
- FBC (cytopenias)
- inflammatory markers (usually raised ESR > CRP)
- complement levels (reduced C3 and C4 in active disease).

Table 4.6 *Investigations used in diagnosis of SLE*

Investigation	Results in SLE
FBC	Anaemia, leucopenia, lymphopenia or thrombocytopenia
Inflammatory markers	ESR or PV is generally raised more than CRP (N.B. if CRP>ESR/PV consider infection)
Autoantibodies	Antinuclear antibodies (ANA) almost always positive
	Double-stranded DNA (dsDNA) is more specific
	Antihistone antibodies in drug-induced lupus
	In secondary antiphospholipid syndrome, anticardiolipin antibodies may also be positive
Complement and immunoglobulins	Complement levels may be low
	IgG and IgM may be raised
Urine dipstick testing	Haematoproteinuria present if there is renal involvement
Biopsies (skin or renal)	Histological abnormalities
Imaging	Chest X-ray (pleural effusion or infiltrates)
	MRI brain (CNS lupus)
	Echocardiogram (pericarditis or endocarditis)

If the antinuclear antibody (ANA) is negative, the diagnosis of lupus should be reconsidered, as ANA-negative SLE is rare.

Subsequent investigations are dependent on the patient's presentation and affected organ systems. The antibody dsDNA is most specific for diagnosis and is associated with an increased risk of glomerulonephritis; it is also used as a marker of disease activity with ESR and complement.

Secondary antiphospholipid syndrome should be considered in SLE patients, as up to 40% will have antiphospholipid antibodies and half of these will have clinical manifestations of antiphospholipid syndrome (see *Section 4.11*).

4.4.8 Management

SLE is usually managed by rheumatologists but other specialists are likely to be involved, depending on the organ-specific manifestations, e.g. renal, neurology, etc. Pregnant patients with SLE are managed jointly with obstetricians in a high-risk pregnancy clinic.

Education and self-management are important, e.g. sun protection, exercise and healthy lifestyle. As with other inflammatory conditions, the risk of cardiovascular disease is increased, and patients should be screened and treated for other modifiable risk factors such as hypertension and hypercholesterolaemia.

Drug treatment (see *Section 2.8*) aims to suppress inflammation using immunosuppressive agents, including corticosteroids, hydroxy-chloroquine, azathioprine, mycophenolate and MTX. Intravenous cyclophosphamide and biologic targeted therapies (e.g. rituximab) are used in patients with persistent inflammation and organ-threatening disease.

Women of child-bearing age should be counselled about the risks of pregnancy in SLE, particularly if their disease is not well controlled. Risks are highest if they have antiphospholipid antibodies, and include miscarriage, thrombosis, preterm delivery and pre-eclampsia.

Prognosis

Patients with mild disease can expect to live a normal life if their condition is managed appropriately; there is now a 90% 10-year survival rate. Patients with serious multi-organ involvement have a worse prognosis and die due to infection, renal failure or cardiovascular disease.

4.5 Sjögren's syndrome

Sjögren's syndrome is an autoimmune condition characterised by lymphocytic infiltration of the exocrine glands, which consequently leads to reduced bodily secretions, most commonly saliva and tears, leading in turn to dry mouth and eyes. Women over 30 years of age are most likely to be affected.

4.5.1 Types

There are two types of Sjögren's syndrome, classified according to their aetiology:
- Primary Sjögren's syndrome is a stand-alone condition of unknown aetiology which classically causes dry eyes and dry mouth, joint pain and fatigue.
- Secondary Sjögren's syndrome occurs in patients who already have an autoimmune condition, such as rheumatoid arthritis.

4.5.2 Clinical features

The most common symptoms are dry eyes (xerophthalmia or keratoconjunctivitis sicca) and dry mouth (xerostomia). Fatigue and musculoskeletal pain are also common. Most symptoms relate to reduced glandular production of lubricant fluid. Some are related to a general autoimmune profile and others remain unexplained. An overview of clinical features is provided in **Table 4.7**.

4.5.3 Diagnostic approach

Diagnosis is usually made based on typical ocular and oral symptoms, a positive Schirmer's tear production test (**Figure 4.5**), and the presence of anti-Ro and anti-La autoantibodies. There are classification criteria for identifying Sjögren's syndrome, e.g. The American–European Consensus Criteria, but these are mainly used for research purposes. **Table 4.8** is a simplified version of these criteria and can be useful to target history taking and appropriate investigations. Patients seldom volunteer symptoms such as dyspareunia (pain on penetrative sex – often caused by vaginal dryness) or consider seemingly unconnected symptoms, e.g. cough. Salivary gland or lip biopsies can provide confirmatory histopathology but are seldom performed in clinical practice.

> When there are clinical grounds to suspect autoimmune disease, order autoantibody tests for only the suspected disease. Requesting blanket tests without the appropriate clinical context can complicate diagnosis if false positive results are found.

Table 4.7 *Symptoms of Sjögren's syndrome*

Frequent (>50%)	Less frequent (<50%)	Rare
Dry eyes	Cough	Peripheral neuropathy
Dry mouth	Raynaud's phenomenon	Vasculitis
Parotitis	Dyspepsia	Pulmonary fibrosis
Fatigue	Hoarse voice	Pleuritis
Arthralgia	Kidney involvement (glomerulonephritis, interstitial change)	Hearing loss
	Vaginal dryness and dyspareunia	Liver disease (primary biliary cirrhosis, autoimmune hepatitis)

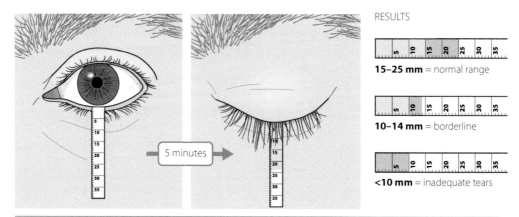

RESULTS

15–25 mm = normal range

10–14 mm = borderline

<10 mm = inadequate tears

Figure 4.5 Schirmer's test in Sjögren's syndrome. A sterile paper strip is placed under the lower eyelid of each eye for 5 minutes, and the amount of moisture on each strip is measured. A positive test is ≤5mm. ≤10mm is considered a moderately dry eye.

Table 4.8	Criteria for diagnosing Sjögren's syndrome: primary Sjögren's syndrome is diagnosed if a patient has four of the six criteria (must include a histopathology or serological component) or has three objective criteria (III, IV, V, VI)
I Ocular symptoms	Dry eyes for >3 months
	Foreign body sensation in eyes
	Use of artificial tears (>3 times a day)
II Oral symptoms	Dry mouth >3 months
	Recurrently or persistently swollen salivary glands
	Use of liquids to swallow dry food
III Objective ocular signs	Schirmer's test (≤5mm in 5 mins)
IV Histopathology	Salivary gland biopsy demonstrating focal lymphocytic sialadenitis
V Objective oral signs	Poor salivary flow (≤1.5ml in 15 mins)
	Abnormal parotid sialography (contrast medium is injected into salivary glands and the jaw is then X-rayed to observe flow)
	Abnormal salivary scintigraphy (nuclear medicine test whereby a radioactive tracer is injected and observed being secreted from salivary glands)
VI Serology	Antibodies to Ro (SSA) or La (SSB) antigens, or both

4.5.4 Management

Symptom relief is the mainstay of treatment, including:
■ artificial tears
■ saliva replacements
■ vaginal lubricants.

Regular dental review is advised due to the increased risks of dental decay (because of reduced neutralising saliva) and ophthalmology input is beneficial to reduce the risk of ocular complications from dry eyes, e.g. corneal ulcers. If symptoms do not respond to conservative measures, oral pilocarpine can be given to stimulate gland function. Hydroxychloroquine can help joint and skin inflammation. Additional immunosuppressant treatments are used in the presence of systemic or organ-threatening inflammation.

There is an increased risk of non-Hodgkin's lymphoma in Sjögren's syndrome, so any new lymphadenopathy should be investigated promptly.

4.6 Scleroderma

In Greek, 'sclero' means hard and 'derma' is skin. Localised scleroderma affects only the skin (e.g. morphea), and as this usually presents to the dermatology clinic it is not discussed here. Systemic scleroderma (sometimes also called 'systemic sclerosis') is an autoimmune condition characterised by fibrosis within the skin and internal organs, and vascular inflammation. Fibrosis leads to skin tightening and organ dysfunction. Vascular inflammation can lead to ischaemia and infarction. Scleroderma can cause significant morbidity and result in premature death.

4.6.1 Types

There are two types of systemic scleroderma, which are defined according to the extent of skin involvement:

- Limited cutaneous – skin involvement is usually confined to the face and extremities. It is the most common type; it is insidious, and has more vascular manifestations, e.g. digital ulceration and pulmonary artery hypertension. It was previously known as 'CREST' syndrome (this acronym can be helpful to remember the key clinical features: **C**alcinosis (**Figure 4.6**), **R**aynaud's phenomenon, o**E**sophageal dysmotility, **S**clerodactyly and **T**elangiectasia).
- Diffuse cutaneous – skin involvement extends beyond extremities. It has more rapid disease progression, with earlier and more widespread internal organ involvement, e.g. of the lungs and kidneys. It is usually more severe.

The features of both types are presented in **Table 4.9**.

4.6.2 Epidemiology

Although there can be geographical differences in the incidence of scleroderma, there is no predilection for a specific racial group. As with most autoimmune conditions, women are more likely to be affected than men.

4.6.3 Aetiology

The cause of scleroderma is unknown. It is suspected that environmental triggers in genetically susceptible individuals cause the immune system to be activated, leading to vascular damage and the deposition of excess normal collagen.

4.6.4 Clinical features

Raynaud's phenomenon is often the first symptom and is present in almost all patients. Skin changes usually start in the fingers with generalised puffiness, swelling or thickening (**Figure 4.7**). Other features vary with subtype (**Table 4.9**). Digital ulceration and pulmonary hypertension are more common, with pulmonary arterial hypertension being the principal cause

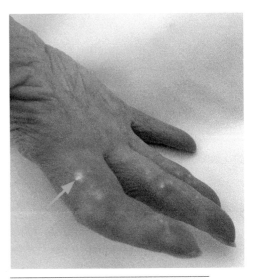

Figure 4.6 Calcinosis in limited cutaneous scleroderma – chalky white deposits (arrowed) beneath the skin.

Table 4.9 *Clinical features of scleroderma divided by subtype*

	Limited cutaneous scleroderma	Diffuse cutaneous scleroderma
Typical areas for thick/tight skin	Arms (below elbow only)	Arms (above and below the elbow)
	Legs (below knees only)	Legs (above and below knees)
	+/− face (e.g. mouth appears small)	Torso
		+/− face
	Thickening progresses slowly	Thickening progresses rapidly for 2–3 years, then can stabilise and regress
GI manifestations	Dysphagia, dyspepsia	Dysphagia, dyspepsia, constipation
Pulmonary manifestations	Pulmonary hypertension	Interstitial lung disease, pulmonary hypertension and fibrosis
Renal manifestations	Less common	Acute hypertensive renal crisis
Cardiac manifestations	Less common	Myocardial fibrosis leading to arrhythmia
Other skin changes	Digital ulcers, telangiectasia, dilated nail fold capillary loops	
Raynaud's phenomenon	Common	
Fatigue	Common	
Musculoskeletal manifestations	Arthralgia and myalgia	

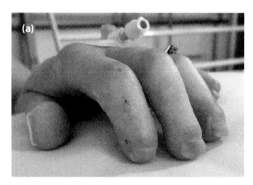

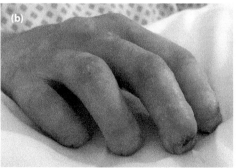

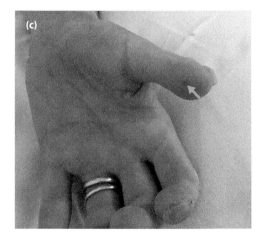

Figure 4.7 Skin and vascular changes in scleroderma include sclerodactyly (localised thickening and tightening of skin) causing contractures; ulcers also develop due to vascular insufficiency: (a) global sclerodactyly of the hands with finger contractures; (b) healing ulcer on nail bed (arrowed); (c) new ulcer forming (arrowed).

of death in limited cutaneous scleroderma. Internal organ involvement with interstitial lung disease and acute renal crisis are more common in diffuse cutaneous scleroderma. Complications usually occur in a progressive fashion; however, on rare occasions a 'renal crisis' can occur. Patients present with headache or visual disturbance with hypertension and acute kidney injury. Careful stabilisation of blood pressure and dialysis are required. This complication is now rare as patients are prophylactically treated with angiotensin-converting enzyme (ACE) inhibitor drugs.

> A renal crisis can occur when patients with scleroderma and renal involvement are commenced on corticosteroids, therefore these patients should be monitored closely.

4.6.5 Diagnostic approach

As with most autoimmune connective tissue diseases, diagnosis is made using a combination of clinical features and immunological markers. Skin changes are usually specific, especially in established disease. The presence of specific symptoms and signs may trigger additional tests (e.g. dry cough and chest crackles may suggest interstitial lung disease which should be further evaluated by pulmonary function tests and imaging such as chest X-ray or high resolution CT (HRCT) scan).

4.6.6 Investigations

A number of additional tests are usually performed, as part of both the diagnostic workup, assessment and ongoing monitoring of scleroderma.

Blood tests

Blood tests are usually normal but normochromic anaemia, raised ESR and renal impairment may be present.

Autoantibodies:
- ANA is generally positive, but is not specific to scleroderma.
- Anti-topoisomerase (Scl70) is associated with diffuse skin involvement, pulmonary fibrosis and renal disease.
- Anti-centromere antibody is more common in limited cutaneous systemic sclerosis.

- Anti-RNA polymerase III is associated with more severe skin and internal organ involvement.

Imaging

Hand X-rays may demonstrate calcinosis.

Echocardiogram is used in screening and monitoring of pulmonary arterial hypertension.

Barium swallow assesses oesophageal dysmotility.

Chest X-ray and HRCT can be carried out if interstitial lung disease or pulmonary fibrosis are suspected (**Figure 4.8**).

Urinalysis

Carry out urine dipstick analysis for haematuria and proteinuria (a sign of glomerular disease). If positive, then consider further renal assessment and investigation, e.g. protein: creatinine ratio, blood pressure, renal function and urine culture.

Other tests

Pulmonary function tests are used for the assessment and monitoring of interstitial lung disease and pulmonary artery hypertension.

Nail fold capillaroscopy can identify patients who are at risk of developing internal organ complications and digital ulcers (**Figure 4.9**).

Blood pressure should be assessed and monitored.

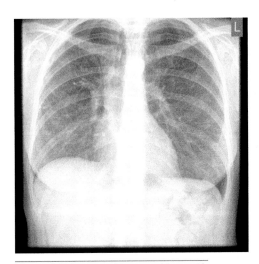

Figure 4.8 Increased lung markings with reticular-nodular showing most obviously in the lower zones of both lungs, consistent with interstitial lung disease and pulmonary fibrosis.

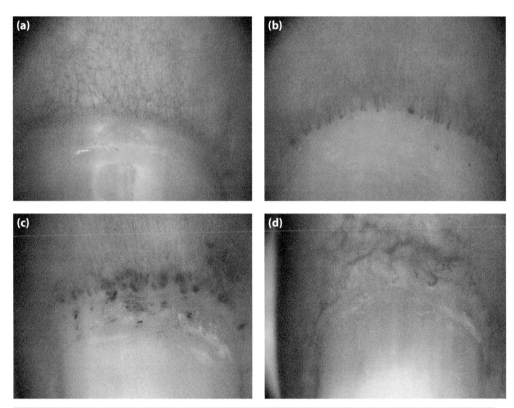

Figure 4.9 Nail fold capillaroscopy: (a) normal: uniform 'hairpin-shaped' arrangement of capillaries, at least 9 capillaries per mm; (b) early: few giant capillaries, few capillary haemorrhages, relatively well-preserved capillary distribution and no evident loss of capillaries; (c) active: frequent giant capillaries, frequent capillary haemorrhages, moderate loss of capillaries, mild disorganisation of the capillary architecture, absent/mild ramified capillaries; (d) late: irregular enlargement of capillaries, few or absent giant capillaries and haemorrhages, severe loss of capillaries with avascular areas, disorganisation of the normal capillary array, ramified/bushy capillaries.

4.6.7 Management

Treatment is tailored according to individual patient symptoms and to the body systems involved. The condition is chronic and may worsen acutely or over time, so ongoing regular assessment and monitoring is important in order that any new or worsening symptoms are acted upon quickly. This involves patient education and recognition of important new symptoms. Regular exercise and good nutrition help to minimise symptoms. Annual or biennial echocardiogram and pulmonary function tests are recommended to identify and monitor interstitial lung disease and pulmonary arterial hypertension.

Medication

Medications used include the following:

- Raynaud's syndrome is managed conservatively in the first instance, e.g. hand protection or warmers. An oral calcium channel blocker, e.g. nifedipine, is used when required. An intravenous vasodilator (iloprost) is used if symptoms are particularly severe.
- If there is kidney involvement, then ACE inhibitors are the preferred treatment. These are also used in cases of renal crisis and as prophylaxis in patients with diffuse cutaneous scleroderma.
- Cyclophosphamide can help reduce the progression of skin and interstitial lung disease.

- PPIs and H2 receptor antagonists are used for dyspepsia secondary to dysmotility.
- Pulmonary hypertension can be treated with vasodilators (e.g. sildenafil, iloprost) and endothelin receptor antagonists, e.g. bosentan.

Surgery

Surgery is rarely performed unless there are debilitating contractures requiring release, or oesophageal strictures requiring dilatation.

Prognosis

In diffuse scleroderma the prognosis is poor but improving due to advances in management, including treatment and prophylaxis of renal crisis. In limited scleroderma the 10-year survival rate is somewhat better at 70%.

4.7 Adult onset Still's disease

Adult onset Still's disease (AOSD) is a rare inflammatory disease with an incidence of less than 1 in 100 000. Its aetiology is poorly understood, but the condition is thought to be an over-zealous reaction of the immune system to a foreign microbe. Patients tend to present with a pyrexia of unknown origin and are investigated for infection before the diagnosis is made.

4.7.1 Clinical features

Classically there is a triad of:
- a salmon pink rash (**Figure 4.10**)
- symmetrical arthralgia
- high spiking fever.

Patients may also complain of a sore throat or myalgia. Haematology and biochemistry results will be consistent with an acute phase response, but RF and ANA will be negative. Serum ferritin is usually significantly elevated, in the thousands.

> Highest temperatures and rash tend to occur in the evening, so this needs to be taken into consideration when assessing any potential patient with AOSD. Temperature charts will frequently show acute spikes and troughs and the rash is often referred to as 'the rash that the physician never sees' due to its timing.

4.7.2 Management

As AOSD is rare, there are no formal guidelines for its management. Generally, it is treated symptomatically, with immunosuppressive drugs used in refractory cases.

Medication

NSAIDs are used initially, followed by oral prednisolone. If there is no improvement, then drugs such as MTX or hydroxychloroquine may be used.

Prognosis

Most commonly AOSD is a 'one-hit' condition that resolves, but chronic refractory disease requiring ongoing immunosuppression may occur.

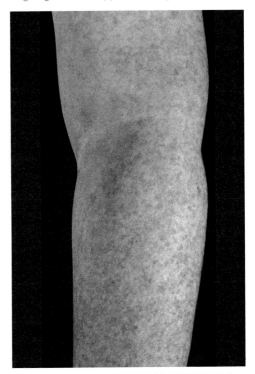

Figure 4.10 Characteristic salmon pink rash of Still's disease.

4.8 Sarcoidosis

Sarcoidosis is a systemic inflammatory condition. Usually seen in young adults (<50 years old), it is most common in African-American and European populations. It has a predilection for the respiratory system, with 9 out of 10 patients reported to have lung involvement. Non-caseating granulomas and inflammatory cells aggregate in affected tissues.

4.8.1 Clinical features

Sarcoidosis can present differently in individuals, depending on which system(s) are affected. Common symptoms or features include:

- systemic: fever, sweats, malaise, lymphadenopathy, hypercalcaemia
- respiratory: dyspnoea, cough

- cutaneous: erythema nodosum, maculopapular rash
- neurological: headache, Bell's palsy
- ocular: uveitis
- musculoskeletal: inflammatory arthritis.

Löfgren's syndrome is an acute presentation of sarcoidosis with fever, hilar lymphadenopathy, erythema nodosum and an inflammatory arthritis (most commonly in the ankles).

4.8.2 Management

Oral corticosteroids are the mainstay of treatment. If a patient's condition takes a chronic course, other immunosuppressive agents, e.g. MTX or azathioprine, are used.

4.9 Myositis

Myositis means muscle inflammation and has many causes including viral infection, or it can be drug-induced. The two common types, which are autoimmune in origin, are:

- polymyositis: there is inflammation of skeletal muscle leading to progressive proximal muscle weakness and muscle wasting
- dermatomyositis: symptoms are similar to those of polymyositis, accompanied by a distinctive rash.

4.9.1 Clinical features

Polymyositis

In polymyositis, the patient reports slowly progressive symptoms of symmetrical proximal muscle weakness; for example, difficulty in rising from a chair or raising their arms above their head. However, distal muscles are unaffected initially so fine motor skills are intact. Unlike PMR, there is little in the way of muscular pain or stiffness, although muscles may be tender.

Constitutional symptoms such as fatigue and night sweats may also be present. Muscle

wasting may be seen on examination and CK will be elevated. Symptoms of dysphagia, dysphonia, breathlessness and aspiration indicate involvement of the respiratory and pharyngeal muscles and severe disease with poor prognosis.

Diagnosis relies on characteristic symptoms associated with elevated CK and inflammatory markers. The autoantibodies ANA and anti-Jo-1 tend to be positive. Additional confirmatory investigations include MRI demonstration of muscle inflammation, electromyography changes and muscle biopsy with identification of characteristic histopathological changes.

Dermatomyositis

In dermatomyositis the features of polymyositis are accompanied by characteristic skin changes including:

- heliotrope rash: lilac discolouration of the eyelids, often associated with periorbital oedema (**Figure 4.11**)
- Gottron's papules: lumpy red scaly eruptions over the extensor aspects of the fingers and hands (**Figure 4.12**)

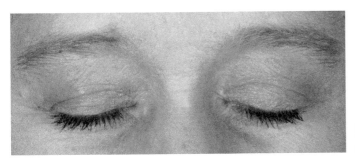

Figure 4.11 Heliotrope rash of dermatomyositis.

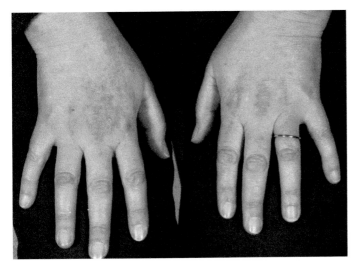

Figure 4.12 Gottron's papules of dermatomyositis.

- anti-Mi-2 antibodies: these are specific for dermatomyositis but only present in approximately 25% of patients.

> Malignancy should always be considered in the initial assessment of polymyositis and dermatomyositis, as both conditions can be a 'paraneoplastic presentation' of an underlying malignancy.

4.9.2 Management

Management centres on excluding malignancy and treating with immunosuppression. Steroids are the treatment of choice. Other immunosuppressive agents are used in resistant cases, e.g. azathioprine and MTX. Patients should also be advised to keep active to improve and maintain muscle strength. Sunblock is particularly important in dermatomyositis as UV light exacerbates the rash.

It is wise to screen for malignancy in the initial presentation of myositis and to reconsider a paraneoplastic process if there is unsatisfactory response to treatment.

Prognosis

Patients without an underlying malignancy will often do well and can gradually come off steroids, although a proportion will require ongoing immunosuppressive therapy.

4.10 Polymyalgia rheumatica

Polymyalgia rheumatica (PMR) is the most common inflammatory musculoskeletal condition in the elderly population and a common reason for corticosteroid prescriptions in this age group.

It is associated with temporal arteritis / giant cell arteritis (GCA; see *Section 4.13*). Up to half of patients with temporal arteritis will develop PMR at some stage and around 10% of patients with PMR may have temporal arteritis.

4.10.1 Epidemiology

The incidence of PMR is 1 in 1000 in the general population. Those living in northern Europe are most likely to be affected. Women are three times more likely to be affected than men. The condition affects those over 50 years old and prevalence increases with age; the typical patient is over 70.

4.10.2 Pathogenesis

The cause of PMR is unknown. There is an increase in pro-inflammatory cells and a reduction in immune-modulating signalling, which indicate disruption of the normal balance within the patient's immune system. This also occurs in temporal arteritis. The pro-inflammatory cytokine IL-6 is increased in PMR, which may explain some of the systemic features of the condition, e.g. fever, fatigue, anaemia and raised CRP.

4.10.3 Clinical features

There is symmetrical persistent aching and stiffness involving the shoulders, hips and surrounding muscles and soft tissues; the neck and torso may also be involved. Morning stiffness lasting at least 30 minutes, and often longer, is characteristic, relieved with movement and worsened by inactivity. Patients often complain of disturbed sleep with difficulty in rolling over in bed at night and getting up in the morning. Shoulder movements are reduced, noticeably abduction, and patients will have difficulty raising their arms above their head. Associated symptoms are common and include malaise, anorexia, fatigue, low-grade fever and depression. There may be peripheral joint inflammation and, if present, this raises the possibility of polymyalgic-onset rheumatoid arthritis. Not all patients present in the same way: some will have just shoulder involvement; others will have more widespread musculoskeletal symptoms; some may not have many systemic symptoms, whilst others may be

overwhelmed by them. Any patient who presents with features of PMR must be assessed for features of temporal arteritis (see *Section 4.13*), due to the overlap between these conditions and risk of visual loss with undiagnosed temporal arteritis.

4.10.4 Diagnostic approach

The following characteristics make a diagnosis of PMR more likely:

- The patient is >50 years old (usually >70).
- There is a new onset (>2 weeks) of persistent symmetrical aching and stiffness affecting the shoulders and/or pelvic girdle with morning stiffness >30 minutes.
- Systemic symptoms such as fatigue and loss of appetite are common.
- ESR and CRP are elevated.
- There is a rapid and profound clinical and biochemical response to corticosteroids.

4.10.5 Investigations

Laboratory investigations are important in the diagnosis and to exclude other causes and should include:

- ESR and CRP – these are key as they are invariably raised; if they are both normal, PMR is far less likely and alternative diagnoses should be considered
- FBC, U&Es and liver function tests (LFTs) – there may be anaemia of chronic disease (normochromic, normocytic)
- CK – normal and helpful to exclude myositis.

Other investigations depend on the clinical picture, diagnostic certainty and response to treatment. Malignancy should be considered as part of the differential diagnosis, particularly in this age group as PMR may be a paraneoplastic presentation. Imaging (ultrasound, MRI) may detect joint and soft tissue inflammation, and subacromial/subdeltoid bursitis appears to be the most helpful ultrasound feature for PMR diagnosis.

4.10.6 Management

Oral prednisolone should be commenced, usually in primary care, at a dose of 15–20mg once daily. Clinical response is usually rapid, e.g. 70% improvement in clinical symptoms within

1 week and normalisation of inflammatory markers within 4 weeks. Once symptoms are consistently under control, there should be a very gradual reduction in the prednisolone. The dose is titrated according to symptom control and reduction in CRP. If steroids are reduced too quickly, symptoms can flare, requiring an increase in steroid dose and a slower wean. Patients who do not report an improvement in their symptoms, or those who cannot reduce their prednisolone because of exacerbations of symptoms, should be reassessed and other diagnoses considered, e.g. polymyalgic-onset RA, temporal arteritis and malignancy. Bone prophylaxis with vitamin D and calcium supplementation and an oral bisphosphonate should be used to prevent steroid-related osteoporosis. A gastroprotective agent (e.g. PPI) should also be used to counteract the gastric irritation side-effects of steroids. In patients who become steroid-dependent and whose dose cannot be weaned or who develop significant steroid-related side-effects, other immunosuppressants, e.g. MTX or azathioprine are used, under the guidance of a rheumatologist. If temporal arteritis occurs, then the prednisolone dose must be increased to 40–60mg daily to prevent sight-threatening complications (see *Section 4.13* and *Case 11.1*).

Prognosis

Prognosis is excellent if treatment is initiated rapidly with regular monitoring of clinical symptoms and CRP, and appropriate titration of treatment. Most patients should expect to receive prednisolone for about 2 years, but some may stop sooner, and others may require a longer treatment course. Patients should be monitored for clinical features of temporal arteritis or inflammatory arthritis.

4.11 Antiphospholipid syndrome

Antiphospholipid syndrome (APLS) can occur as a stand-alone condition (primary APLS) or as a condition associated with other autoimmune conditions, most commonly SLE (secondary APLS). It is characterised by recurrent thrombosis, obstetric complications and the presence of antiphospholipid autoantibodies.

4.11.1 Clinical features and diagnosis

APLS causes recurrent arterial and venous thromboses and pregnancy-related complications such as miscarriage, unexplained foetal loss, premature birth and pre-eclampsia. There may be skin rashes, characteristically mottled net-like erythematous discolouration of the skin called livedo reticularis, splinter haemorrhages (**Figure 4.13**), coagulation defects and thrombocytopenia.

Autoantibodies should be positive on two occasions at least 12 weeks apart:
- anti-cardiolipin antibodies
- lupus anticoagulant
- anti-beta2-glycoprotein 1.

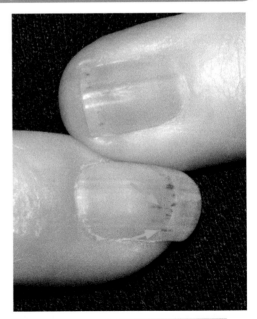

Figure 4.13 Splinter haemorrhages in APLS – small capillaries under the nail are damaged, resulting in small blood streaks seen under the nail (arrowed).

The diagnosis of APLS requires the presence of at least one clinical event and persistently positive antibodies.

> Transient production of antibodies can occur in response to, for example, infection, but persistent antibody production is more likely to be associated with autoimmune disease.

4.11.2 Management

Patients should be advised to reduce their risk of thrombosis by modifying risk factors, including not smoking, exercising regularly and maintaining a healthy weight. Diabetes mellitus, hypertension and hypercholesterolaemia should be tightly controlled and patients are usually commenced on low dose aspirin. Once a thrombosis has occurred, patients should be treated with lifelong anticoagulation, usually with warfarin. Preconception expert advice and planning, and care in a high-risk pregnancy clinic is needed for women with known APLS considering pregnancy; low molecular weight heparin and low dose aspirin are usually prescribed during pregnancy (warfarin is teratogenic) to reduce the risk of miscarriage and other complications.

Prognosis

Prognosis varies according to the site, frequency and extent of thrombosis. Lifelong anticoagulation can improve morbidity and mortality but events such as stroke, pulmonary haemorrhage, myocardial infarction and eclampsia can be fatal.

4.12 Raynaud's phenomenon

Raynaud's phenomenon is abnormal paroxysmal vasoconstriction of the peripheral blood vessels, leading to temporarily reduced blood flow. It can be a primary condition or secondary, where it is associated with another illness, e.g. scleroderma or SLE. Primary Raynaud's is most common, especially in young women. If ANA is positive, secondary Raynaud's is more likely and symptoms are more severe, with increased risk of digital ulceration and ischaemia. Pathophysiology is uncertain, but abnormalities of the vessel wall and mechanisms for controlling appropriate vasodilatation and constriction are likely to be involved.

4.12.1 Clinical features and diagnosis

Symptoms and signs include colour change, pain and numbness in the fingers or toes. The nose, lips and ear lobes can also be affected. Common triggers include cold weather and stress; smoking, vibrating tools and the oral contraceptive pill may be implicated.

Diagnosis is based on typical triphasic symptoms:

■ pallor and numbness of the digits associated with cold-induced vasospasm (**Figure 4.14**)

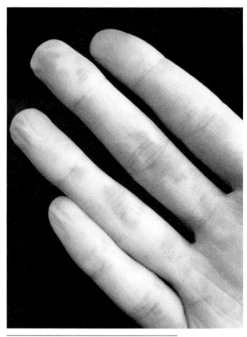

Figure 4.14 First stage of Raynaud's phenomenon, in which the digits turn white due to abnormal peripheral vasoconstriction.

- digits turn blue, associated with pain
- digits then become red and warm with burning discomfort following vasodilatation and hyperaemia.

Patients may not exhibit all three classical stages in all episodes, especially in milder cases.

4.12.2 Management

Education and lifestyle advice are important, e.g. stop smoking, avoid temperature changes and maintain core temperature. Medications include vasodilators, e.g. calcium channel blockers such as nifedipine.

VASCULITIS

Vasculitis is pathological inflammation of the blood vessels. Arteries and veins of all sizes may be affected, from large vessels such as the aorta, to small vessels and capillaries. Symptoms depend on the location and type of blood vessel affected; they can be localised to a single organ or may be vague and non-specific (**Table 4.10**). Such non-specific symptoms can mimic other conditions, which typically leads to a delay in diagnosis. A skin rash is often the first sign of small vessel inflammation (**Figure 4.15b**).

Vasculitis can be classified according to the

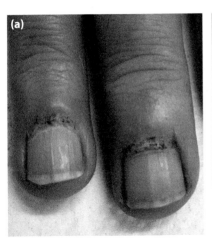
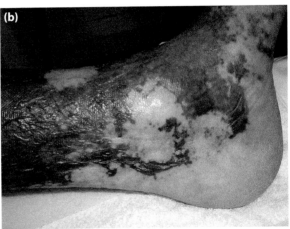
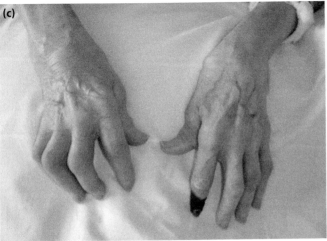

Figure 4.15 The cutaneous presentation of vasculitis can vary from (a) small nailfold infarcts; (b) purpuric skin rash; to (c) significant tissue ischaemia and necrosis.

Table 4.10 *Symptoms of vasculitis*

System	Symptoms
General	Fatigue, fever, weight loss, malaise
Respiratory	Dyspnoea, cough, haemoptysis
Ear/nose/throat	Deafness, nasal crusting, nose bleeds, sinus pain, hoarse voice
Dermatological	Rash, ulcers
Ocular	Eye pain, visual loss, dry eyes
Neurological	Paraesthesia, weakness
Musculoskeletal	Arthralgia, joint swelling
GI	Diarrhoea, abdominal pain, bleeding

aetiology, type or size of blood vessel (**Table 4.11**). The epidemiology, clinical features and management vary according to the type of vasculitis. They are rare conditions which require specialist assessment and management, with potential for significant morbidity and mortality.

Classification

Vasculitis can be classified according to aetiology:
- Primary vasculitis: these are autoimmune disorders of unknown aetiology which target the endothelium of the blood vessel wall.
- Secondary vasculitis: causes include drugs (e.g. hydralazine, cocaine), infection (e.g. hepatitis B and C), malignancy, or coexisting connective tissue disease, e.g. RA and SLE.

> **When vasculitis presents, take a careful drug history.** Certain drugs can cause vasculitis even when the patient has been taking them for some time.

Vasculitis can be classified according to the size of vessel affected, i.e. large vessel, medium vessel or small vessel (**Table 4.11**).

> **In patients with vasculitis always check the urine for blood and protein.** Renal involvement is common, often has minimal symptoms, and can progress rapidly.

Table 4.11 *Vasculitis classification by predominant size of vessel affected*

Class	Types of vasculitis	
Large vessel	Giant cell arteritis	
	Takayasu's arteritis	
Medium vessel	Polyarteritis nodosa	
	Kawasaki's disease	
Small vessel	ANCA-associated	Granulomatosis with polyangiitis (Wegener's granulomatosis)
		Eosinophilic granulomatosis with polyangiitis (Churg–Strauss syndrome)
		Microscopic polyangiitis
	Immune complex associated (ANCA negative)	Henoch–Schönlein purpura
		Cryoglobulinaemic vasculitis
Venules/veins	Behçet's disease (which also affects small and medium arteries)	

4.13 Giant cell arteritis

Giant cell arteritis (GCA) is the most common type of vasculitis and the most common type of large vessel vasculitis. It typically affects the temporal artery (so it is also called temporal arteritis) but can affect any branch of the aorta. Untreated involvement of the ophthalmic artery causes irreversible visual loss, so prompt diagnosis and treatment are needed. The cause is unknown. Characteristic histopathological features visible on biopsy of an affected temporal artery include inflammatory infiltrates, granuloma and multinucleated giant cells (hence 'giant cell arteritis'). Caucasian women over 50 years of age are most commonly affected.

4.13.1 Clinical features

GCA typically presents with acute onset of unilateral temporal headache or scalp tenderness (see *Case 11.1*). Occipital headache may also be a feature. Visual symptoms such as blurring, visual loss or amaurosis fugax suggest potentially serious sight-threatening ischaemic complications and require urgent treatment. Jaw claudication and features of PMR may also be present. The temporal artery may feel tender, enlarged or pulseless on examination. Laboratory findings are similar to those in PMR, with the hallmark being a raised inflammatory response. A temporal artery biopsy is the gold standard test for GCA and will confirm vessel wall inflammation. 'Skip lesions' can occur where only certain sections of the vessel are affected and can lead to a false negative biopsy if the diseased portion of the vessel is missed on biopsy. Vascular ultrasound can also be used in specialist centres to detect vessel wall inflammation.

4.13.2 Management

Immediate treatment with high dose corticosteroids (prednisolone 40–60mg) is required as soon as a clinical diagnosis of GCA is suspected, to prevent irreversible visual loss, whilst waiting for any blood or temporal artery biopsy results. In the presence of visual symptoms, intravenous (IV) methylprednisolone should be considered and the patient seen by Ophthalmology the same day. Due to this regime, gastroprotection with a PPI and prophylaxis against osteoporosis with calcium, vitamin D and a bisphosphonate is required.

Prognosis

Visual loss occurs early and is usually irreversible. A high clinical index of suspicion of the diagnosis is important, with prompt initiation of steroid treatment, and this significantly improves morbidity. Prompt recovery is the usual outcome. Patients can expect to be on oral steroids for at least two years, with gradual tapering of the dose balanced against symptoms and CRP measurement. Relapses may occur. Some patients require additional immunosuppression, e.g. MTX or azathioprine. Aortic dissection or aneurysms are rare complications of persistent large vessel inflammation.

4.14 Takayasu's arteritis

Takayasu's arteritis is a rare vasculitis affecting large vessels of the aorta and its branches. It is most common in Japanese and Asian women <40 years old. It usually presents with ischaemic symptoms such as claudication of an arm or leg with loss of pulsation and reduced blood pressure in the affected limb (measure and compare blood pressure in both arms). Vascular bruits may be present. Vascular imaging (e.g. CT or MR angiography) and inflammatory markers (CRP and ESR) are useful in the diagnosis and monitoring of disease. Treatment is suppression of inflammation with corticosteroids and other immunosuppressant drugs.

4.15 Polyarteritis nodosa

Polyarteritis nodosa (PAN) is a necrotising vasculitis affecting medium-sized vessels. It is more common in men and may be precipitated by hepatitis B infection. Kidneys are most often affected but multiple systems can be involved, and symptoms depend on the location of the disease. It may cause ischaemia, infarction, thrombosis and aneurysm formation. GI features include abdominal pain, bleeding or even perforation. Cardiovascular involvement may result in angina or myocardial infarction. Kidney involvement may present with hypertension or acute kidney injury. Other clinical presentations may include mononeuritis multiplex or constitutional symptoms. Treatment involves immunosuppression with corticosteroids, cyclophosphamide, azathioprine or rituximab.

4.16 Kawasaki's disease

Kawasaki's disease is vasculitis of medium-sized blood vessels and usually affects children under 5 years of age; it is particularly prevalent in Japan, although does have a worldwide distribution. Coronary aneurysms are a particularly significant complication and can occur in 20% of untreated patients. Specific clinical features include persistent fever, conjunctival congestion, inflammation of the mouth (e.g. cracked lips, strawberry tongue – red, bumpy lesions on tongue surface), cervical lymphadenopathy, skin rashes, red and swollen palms and soles of feet. Treatment includes IV immunoglobulin, aspirin and corticosteroids.

4.17 Granulomatosis with polyangiitis

Granulomatosis with polyangiitis (GPA; formerly known as Wegener's granulomatosis) is a chronic necrotising granulomatous inflammation of the small arteries, which affects mainly the nasal and oral cavity, lungs and kidneys. The presence of c-ANCA and anti-proteinase 3 (anti-pr3) antibodies is very specific for GPA.

4.17.1 Clinical features

Some patients have disease limited to the ear, nose and throat (ENT) whilst others have multisystem involvement. Upper airway disease may produce symptoms including nasal crusting, epistaxis (nosebleed), obstruction, recurrent otitis media (inflammation of the middle ear), and eventually complications such as nasal bridge or septal collapse and subglottic stenosis (narrowing of the windpipe). Lung involvement may produce cavitating nodules and pulmonary haemorrhage (**Figure 4.16**). Kidney disease may range from haematoproteinuria and hypertension to acute

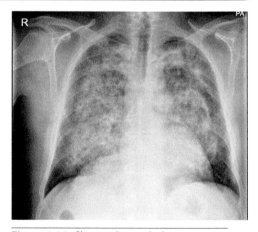

Figure 4.16 Chest radiograph demonstrating pulmonary haemorrhage in vasculitis. There are widespread patchy lesions caused by blood entering the lung tissue, which impairs the transfer of oxygen over the specialised surfaces of the alveoli, causing hypoxia.

kidney injury. Scleritis and episcleritis may occur. Constitutional symptoms such as fever, malaise, lethargy and weight loss are common.

4.17.2 Management

Remission induction with high dose IV corticosteroids combined with cyclophosphamide is the management for organ-threatening disease; oral corticosteroids for ENT-limited disease. Maintenance therapy is with MTX or azathioprine and tapering of corticosteroids. Additional therapies such as plasma exchange

(plasma is removed from the blood and replaced with donated blood plasma) or B-cell blockade with rituximab are used for resistant or relapsing disease. Co-trimoxazole is an antibiotic and can be useful in ENT-limited disease.

Prognosis

Prompt assessment and treatment has significantly improved prognosis such that following remission, around 80% of patients survive for 5 years. Half of patients will relapse, which is more common in the presence of c-ANCA pr3 antibodies.

4.18 Eosinophilic granulomatosis with polyangiitis

Eosinophilic granulomatosis with polyangiitis (EGPA; formerly known as Churg–Strauss syndrome) is a necrotising granulomatous vasculitis affecting small arteries associated with eosinophilia. It is most common in adults over 40 years of age, and often patients have a previous history of atopy or asthma. The presence of p-ANCA and anti-myeloperoxidase (anti-MPO) proteinase 3 antibodies is more specific for

EGPA. Skin lesions such as purpura (purple spot rash), nodules (raised lumps) or vesicles (small, fluid-filled sacs) are common. Patients may present with mononeuritis multiplex secondary to nerve vessel ischaemia, or abdominal pain secondary to reduced flow to the mesenteric artery causing bowel ischaemia. Corticosteroids are usually an effective treatment, but additional immunosuppression is often required.

4.19 Microscopic polyangiitis

Microscopic polyangiitis (MPA) is a necrotising vasculitis affecting small blood vessels. It commonly targets the kidneys, but skin, lungs, nerves and joints may be involved, and constitutional symptoms are common. p-ANCA

and anti-MPO proteinase 3 antibodies are most commonly present. Treatment is suppression of inflammation with corticosteroids and other immunosuppressant drugs.

4.20 Henoch–Schönlein purpura

Henoch–Schönlein purpura is an IgA-mediated small vessel vasculitis, characterised by a palpable purpuric rash. It is the most common vasculitis in children but can also occur in adults. It may occur following an upper respiratory tract infection and is often self-limiting.

4.20.1 Clinical features

Purpura of the skin over the back of the legs, buttocks and forearms is the characteristic presentation. An inflammatory arthritis, particularly in the knees and ankles, may occur.

GI involvement may produce abdominal pain, bloody diarrhoea and, rarely, intussusception (where the bowel folds in on itself, causing ischaemia). Glomerulonephritis leads to haematoproteinuria, hypertension and acute kidney injury.

4.20.2 Management

Henoch–Schönlein purpura is usually a self-limiting disease. Patients with renal or GI involvement may require corticosteroids or additional immunosuppressive therapy.

4.21 Behçet's disease

Behçet's disease is unusual among the vasculitides because it predominantly targets the venous system, as well as small and medium-sized arteries. Prevalence is highest in Middle-Eastern and Mediterranean populations. It presents with recurrent oral and genital ulcers, skin lesions and eye inflammation. Rarely, it presents with thromboembolism or meningoencephalitis (inflammation of the brain and its surrounding protective membranes). Treatment targets local symptoms. However, aggressive or persistent disease requires immunosuppression.

> Behçet's disease is sometimes known as the 'silk road disease' as high prevalence of the condition appears to track the old silk trading routes in the Middle East and Asia.

4.22 Answers to starter questions

1. In hypermobility, the range of motion of a joint becomes larger. Joints and associated tendons and ligaments stretch to accommodate the extended movement. This causes multiple 'sprain and strain'-type injuries to occur.

2. *Lupus* is Latin for wolf. There are differing opinions on whether the term lupus for the condition was because the rash resembles wolf markings, or the fact that some erosive lesions look like bite marks.

3. We don't yet know why cancer can sometimes be associated with muscle inflammation (myositis). It is possible that there is a crossover of antigen expression between cancer and muscle cells, so as the normal immune response targets cancer cells, it may also attack the muscles.

Chapter 5
Metabolic bone disease

Starter questions

1. Should everyone who takes corticosteroids be put on medication to prevent osteoporosis?
2. If PTH rises in response to low calcium levels in the blood, in what condition can both a raised PTH and raised calcium be seen, and why does this occur?

Answers to questions are to be found in *Section 5.5*.

Bone is not a static framework but a constantly regenerating matrix. Any disruption to cells or minerals available for this turnover can lead to bone pathology. Due to the number of pathways that can be affected, there are a large number of different bone diseases that can occur. This chapter will illustrate examples of conditions where the bone matrix becomes disrupted due to:

- failure of the kidneys to ensure adequate levels of calcium and phosphate (renal osteodystrophy, part of chronic kidney disease metabolic bone disorder)
- reduced bone mass (osteoporosis)
- insufficient mineralisation (osteomalacia/rickets)
- deregulated bone turnover (Paget's disease).

Case 5.1 Bone pain with a raised ALP

Presentation

Mr Green is a 73-year-old man who presents to his GP with left knee and thigh pain that has been becoming more troublesome over the past two months.

Initial interpretation

Knee pain is a common presentation and osteoarthritis becomes more common with advancing age. The thigh pain could be referred from the knee but any bone pain requires further detailed evaluation. Malignancy such as multiple myeloma needs to be excluded, particularly in this age group.

History

Mr Green reports a constant ache in his knee and thigh. The pain doesn't seem to vary according to the time of day. Weight-bearing exacerbates the pain, and painkillers help. No other joints are affected. He hasn't lost any weight but does complain of a persistent headache and some hearing loss.

Examination

Mr Green is overweight, with a BMI of 27. There is no specific bony tenderness on palpation of the knee, thigh or hip, and no obvious deformities but there is reduced range of movement of the knee with associated crepitus. Cranial nerve examination and fundoscopy are normal but hearing acuity is reduced. Cardio-respiratory and abdominal examinations are normal.

Interpretation of findings

Whilst the clinical findings suggest some features of knee OA, this does not necessarily explain his thigh pain, the unremitting nature of symptoms, or the headache. Other conditions in this age group, e.g. multiple myeloma, can have subtle symptoms in the initial stages. Polymyalgia rheumatica is unlikely given the localised unilateral symptoms. Overall, the diagnosis is not clear on clinical grounds, so further investigations are warranted.

Investigations

Routine blood tests demonstrate an elevated ALP (520IU/L). Bone biochemistry and liver function tests are otherwise normal. Plain radiograph demonstrates reduced joint space and marginal osteophytes, consistent with OA of the knee. However, the thigh bone is abnormal with bony expansion with a coarse trabecular pattern. On the report, the radiologist suggests Paget's disease as a possible explanation. Subsequently the GP rings Mr Green and enquires further about the headache. He is referred back to the local hospital radiology department for a skull X-ray which also demonstrates similar changes consistent with Paget's disease.

Diagnosis

Although the symptoms described by Mr Green were non-specific, they could not be completely explained by OA. Subsequent investigations suggest a diagnosis of Paget's disease, which would explain the thigh pain, headache, hearing loss and raised ALP, supported by characteristic radiographic appearances. Mr Green was prescribed a bisphosphonate drug (annual IV injection of zoledronic acid) and analgesia, to which he made a good response.

Paget's disease is a condition which is often not suspected on initial assessment. Frequently patients are completely asymptomatic and the diagnosis is only considered when ALP is elevated or an X-ray, sometimes taken for another reason, shows characteristic changes.

5.1 Renal osteodystrophy

Renal osteodystrophy is a collective term for a variety of abnormal bone morphologies caused by kidney disease. It is part of a systemic condition termed chronic kidney disease – mineral and bone disorder (CKD-MBD). Due to the kidneys' pivotal role in bone metabolism and mineral homeostasis, chronic kidney disease results in significant abnormalities affecting both skeletal and non-skeletal sites.

Long-term rises in serum calcium levels result in the deposition of calcium in blood vessels, increasing the risk of cardiovascular disease.

5.1.1 Epidemiology

Once patients reach stage 3 of chronic kidney disease (CKD), their kidneys are working at 50% of their normal function. Many patients will now have a mild degree of renal osteodystrophy. Once a patient is on dialysis (stage 5 CKD) they will almost certainly have bone disease.

5.1.2 Aetiology

Renal disease can affect the skeleton in different ways. **Figure 5.1** illustrates how declining renal function leads to disruption of the bone matrix.

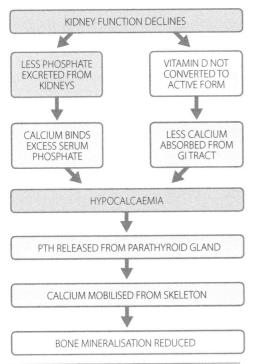

Figure 5.1 How chronic kidney disease results in reduced bone mineralisation.

Hypocalcaemia triggers PTH release and bone resorption. **Table 5.1** lists the different types of renal osteodystrophy. Hyperparathyroid bone disease is the most common.

5.1.3 Clinical features

Most patients are asymptomatic and abnormalities are detected on routine blood testing in patients known to have CKD. Symptoms include bone pain and/or muscle weakness (secondary to low calcium). Fractures may result from a weakened bone architecture.

5.1.4 Diagnostic approach

Patients with declining renal function typically have routine blood tests to monitor bone biochemistry and PTH levels. Once these become abnormal, treatment can be instigated. The typical changes seen on blood testing are:

- low (but sometimes high or normal) serum calcium
- high (but sometimes normal) serum phosphate
- high PTH
- high ALP
- low vitamin D.

The typical results from blood testing in different metabolic bone diseases are illustrated in **Table 5.2**. The gold standard for diagnosing renal osteodystrophy is a bone biopsy but this is seldom performed in clinical practice. Radiographs are not usually necessary but may demonstrate a wide variety of appearances depending on the stage, severity and duration of CKD and dominant pathological process.

Table 5.1 *Types and features of renal osteodystrophy*	
Type of renal osteodystrophy	**Main features**
Secondary hyperparathyroid bone disease	High turnover bone disease
	High PTH triggers increased osteoblast and osteoclast activity
Adynamic bone disease	Low turnover bone disease
	Low levels of PTH
	Low numbers of osteoblasts and osteoclasts
	Can be triggered by overtreatment of hyperparathyroid bone disease
Osteitis fibrosa	Seen in advanced primary hyperparathyroidism; very rare
	Excessive bone resorption and marrow fibrosis with cyst formation

Table 5.2 *Typical blood test results in metabolic bone disease*

Osteomalacia	Osteoporosis	Paget's disease	Primary hyperpara-thyroidism	Secondary hyperpara-thyroidism	Adynamic bone disease
Low vitamin D	Normal	High ALP	High PTH	High PTH	Low PTH
Low Ca			High Ca	Low Ca	
Low Phos			Low Phos	High Phos	
High ALP					
High PTH					

5.1.5 Management

Renal and bone biochemistry is monitored by renal physicians. An important part of prevention and treatment of CKD-MBD is to preserve renal function. Regular monitoring of blood biochemistry should ensure early detection of abnormalities and intervention to prevent bone damage. Once calcium levels drop and/or PTH levels rise, the following strategies are employed:

- reduction of phosphate levels through avoiding certain foods in the diet (e.g. milk, beer, sardines, nuts, cereals) and use of phosphate-binding drugs, which bind phosphate in the stomach (e.g. calcium carbonate)
- vitamin D supplementation (e.g. alfacalcidol), to increase calcium absorption from the gut and subsequently reduce PTH secretion

- parathyroidectomy in patients with tertiary hyperparathyroidism or medical treatment with a calcimimetic drug that mimics calcium and tricks the parathyroid glands into thinking there is enough calcium and therefore reducing PTH secretion
- bisphosphonates are generally avoided in patients with CKD as they are primarily excreted by the kidneys.

Prognosis

Patients with renal bone disease are at increased risk of fracture. However, the overall morbidity and mortality is determined by the severity of renal disease, and the complications arising from this. Depending on an individual's comorbidities, once on dialysis life expectancy ranges from 5–20 years.

5.2 Osteoporosis

In osteoporosis, the bone microarchitecture (trabecular bone) becomes fragile and bone density is reduced, resulting in an increased risk of fracture. Postmenopausal women are most affected by osteoporosis and it becomes more common in the elderly where there can be a vicious cycle of falls, fractures and reduced confidence, which can strip patients of their independence.

5.2.1 Epidemiology

Osteoporosis is primarily an age-related disease and more women than men will suffer from

osteoporotic fractures due to the effects of sex hormones on bone remodelling. A third of women will suffer an osteoporotic fracture in their lifetime compared to a fifth of men. By the age of 60, one-tenth of women have osteoporosis, and by the age of 90, this increases to two-thirds.

> Osteoporosis causes nine million fractures worldwide every year.

5.2.2 Aetiology

Osteoporosis occurs when there is either excess osteoclast activity or reduced osteoblast activity. This leads to the balance of bone remodelling being in favour of resorption rather than formation. There are numerous risk factors for osteoporosis (**Table 5.3**). Peak bone mass is reached at 30 years of age, followed by a gradual decline; thus any risk factors prior to this will make premature osteoporosis more likely.

> Osteoporosis is a reduction of normal mineralised bone; however, the structure of the bone is unchanged. This is a disorder of bone quantity, not bone quality.

5.2.3 Prevention

The aim is to reduce the risk of fracture and two strategies should be employed to achieve this:

1. Prevention of osteoporosis by addressing known risk factors, e.g. lifestyle modification such as smoking cessation; prophylaxis with a bisphosphonate for patients on long-term corticosteroids.
2. Prevention of falls, i.e. the mechanical cause of fracture. The risk of falls is increased by conditions or medications that affect vision, balance or strength, so these risk factors need to be addressed.

5.2.4 Pathogenesis

The pathogenesis of osteoporosis in an individual varies according to their unique set of risk factors. There are multiple stages of bone remodelling which are affected by both local and systemic factors, e.g. hormones, cytokines and drugs.

Figure 5.2 demonstrates changes in bone structure and mineralisation in osteoporosis, osteopenia and osteomalacia. Osteopenia is a term for low bone mineral density (BMD) which is not as severe as osteoporosis. Patients with osteopenia are more likely to go on to develop osteoporosis, but not all will.

Table 5.3 *Risk factors for osteoporosis*

Increasing age (reduced activity, secondary hyperparathyroidism, low vitamin D levels)
Female gender
Early menopause
Hyperthyroidism
Glucocorticoid therapy
Chronic disease, e.g. rheumatoid arthritis, diabetes mellitus, Cushing's syndrome, CKD, liver disease, coeliac disease
Low BMI and anorexia nervosa
Family history of hip fracture
Personal past history of a fragility fracture
Smoking
Excess alcohol intake
Testosterone deficiency

5.2.5 Clinical features

There are usually no symptoms of osteoporosis. Generally, it is diagnosed after a low impact fracture affecting the wrist, spine or hip, or through routine bone density screening in a patient at risk, e.g. on long-term corticosteroids or with RA.

A patient may present with back pain due to a vertebral compression fracture (**Figure 5.3**).

Following a fracture there can be noticeable changes to the skeleton, e.g. loss of height due to vertebral collapse, spinal deformities such as kyphosis, or persistent bone pain.

5.2.6 Diagnostic approach

If a patient presents with a fracture, a plain X-ray can raise suspicion of osteoporosis if the bone density appears reduced; however, this is not a reliable radiographic sign. The diagnosis is made formally using a DEXA (dual energy X-ray

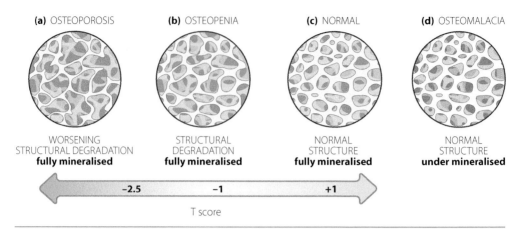

(a) OSTEOPOROSIS   **(b)** OSTEOPENIA   **(c)** NORMAL   **(d)** OSTEOMALACIA

WORSENING STRUCTURAL DEGRADATION **fully mineralised**   STRUCTURAL DEGRADATION **fully mineralised**   NORMAL STRUCTURE **fully mineralised**   NORMAL STRUCTURE **under mineralised**

−2.5   −1   +1

T score

Figure 5.2 Bone architecture in osteoporosis, osteopenia and osteomalacia: (a) osteoporosis (T score <−2.5); (b) osteopenia (T score −1 to −2.5); c) normal (T score −1 to +1); (d) osteomalacia – failure of mineralisation.

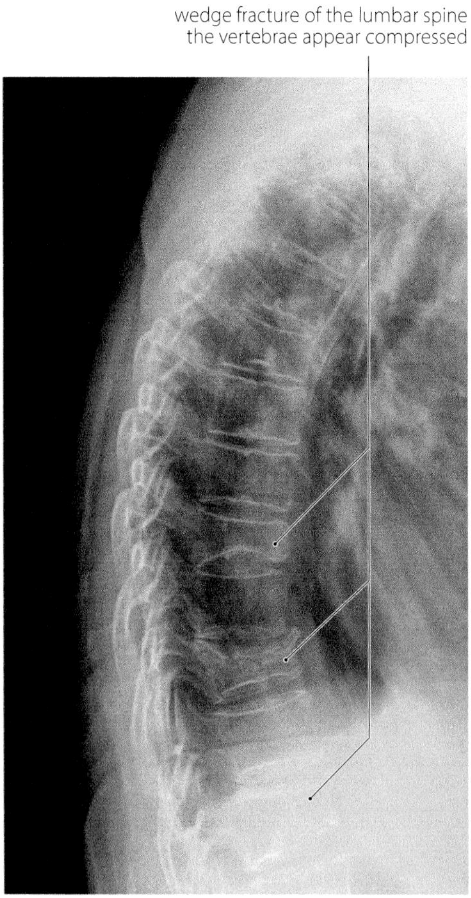

wedge fracture of the lumbar spine the vertebrae appear compressed

Figure 5.3 Osteoporotic vertebral fractures.

absorptiometry) scan (see *Section 2.7.5*). BMD is described using a T or Z score:

- ■ **T score** represents the number of standard deviations the patient's BMD sits above or below the average BMD of a young person of the same sex
  - ☐ T score of <−2.5 is diagnostic of osteoporosis
  - ☐ T score −1 to −2.5 is diagnostic of osteopenia
- ■ **Z score** represents the number of standard deviations above or below the average BMD in an age-matched population.

5.2.7 Investigations

A DEXA scan should be performed to formally diagnose osteoporosis and repeated at timely intervals to assess response to treatment. Patients who are diagnosed with osteoporosis should be screened for risk factors for an underlying cause for osteoporosis (**Table 5.3**) with a thorough clinical history and examination and appropriate laboratory tests.

5.2.8 Management

Risk factors should be minimised where possible. Those with borderline BMD values but at high risk of falls may also qualify for preventative treatment. Patients should be educated on fall prevention and avoidance, which may require referral to occupational therapy and physiotherapy. Advice on smoking cessation and alcohol intake is important. All patients should follow advice on diet and weight-bearing exercise, to optimise bone strength.

> **Weight-bearing exercise** includes low impact activities such as walking, but does not include swimming or cycling.

Medication

Calcium and vitamin D supplementation are prescribed to all patients.

Bisphosphonates are first-line treatment and include weekly oral alendronate, monthly oral or 3-monthly IV ibandronate or annual IV zoledronate. They inhibit osteoclastic bone resorption, so tip the homeostatic balance towards osteoblastic bone formation. GI side-effects are common and can affect compliance. Osteonecrosis and atypical fractures are uncommon but important complications.

> Patients receiving long-term bisphosphonates may be at risk of atypical fractures. After sustained treatment, bisphosphonates can conversely reduce the deposition of bone by osteoblasts, ultimately weakening the bone. A 'drug holiday' may be considered in stable patients but in patients at high risk of fracture, treatment may be continued or one with an alternative mode of action considered.

In patients intolerant of or unresponsive to bisphosphonates, other medications are considered. Usually an oral bisphosphonate is tried first-line, with IV bisphosphonates second-line. Other medications include:

- denosumab (blocks RANK ligand, inhibiting osteoclasts)
- teriparatide (synthetic parathyroid hormone)
- strontium ranelate (mineral salt)
- raloxifene (selective oestrogen receptor modulator)
- hormone replacement therapy in postmenopausal women.

Surgery

Surgery is reserved for fracture management.

Prognosis

Elderly patients presenting with hip fractures have high mortality and morbidity. This is usually related to poor physiological reserve and increased risk of perioperative complications such as chest infection or heart failure. Combined care from orthopaedic teams and elderly care physicians is having a positive effect on outcomes. Osteoporotic fractures cause pain and disability and are frequently associated with loss of both confidence and independence.

5.3 Osteomalacia and rickets

Activated vitamin D is essential for intestinal absorption of dietary calcium and helps to regulate its renal excretion and storage in bone. The term osteomalacia refers to vitamin D deficiency in adults, whereas the term rickets is used in children. In children, the insufficient mineralisation of the bone occurs before closure of the epiphyses, so bone growth and development are affected, resulting in deformity. In adults, osteomalacia may be asymptomatic or cause bone pain, but bone deformities are rare.

> Osteomalacia is a failure of bone mineralisation causing a structural change of the bone matrix. This is a disorder of bone quality, not quantity.

5.3.1 Epidemiology

Vitamin D insufficiency affects 50% of adults in the UK and 16% have severe deficiency during winter and spring. Children are becoming more frequently affected as outdoor play and exercise have reduced. The groups most at risk are young children, pregnant women, people who do not expose their skin to the sun, those who are dark-skinned and the elderly.

5.3.2 Aetiology

Vitamin D deficiency is caused by one or more of:
- inadequate diet
- lack of sunlight
- malabsorption
- liver or kidney disease
- certain drugs, e.g. the anticonvulsant phenytoin.

Other causes of osteomalacia or rickets include:
- significant deficiency of calcium, independent of vitamin D levels
- genetic conditions, e.g. hypophosphatemic rickets or hypophosphatemic osteomalacia.

5.3.3 Prevention

Measures to prevent osteomalacia include:
- increasing vitamin D through the diet, using supplements
- increasing exposure to sunlight, within safe levels accounting for skin type
- providing information on foods rich in vitamin D.

Public health education concerning vitamin D rich foods, e.g. oily fish and eggs, should be made available for the whole population. People at high risk of deficiency should be provided with supplements, e.g. pregnant or breastfeeding women and children aged between 6 months and 5 years.

> In northern Europe, sunlight is only at the correct wavelength for vitamin D synthesis from April to late September. During spring and summer it is advisable to expose a certain amount of skin to daylight, without sunscreen, for 10–15 minutes between 11am and 3pm; exposing the forearms is sufficient. Darker-skinned individuals need longer in the sun to get the same benefit.

5.3.4 Pathogenesis

Vitamin D goes through several processes of hydroxylation, via the liver and kidneys, to be converted into its active form, 1,25-dihydroxyvitamin D. A reduction in active vitamin D leads to reduced calcium absorption from the intestine and triggers the release of PTH which acts to retain calcium in the kidneys at the expense of loss of phosphate in the same process. PTH indirectly increases osteoclast activity to increase bone and calcium resorption. Demineralisation means new bone formation is inadequate (**Figure 5.2**).

5.3.5 Clinical features

In adults, osteomalacia may be asymptomatic if it is mild. However, severe deficiency can lead to:
- bone and muscle pain
- muscle weakness (secondary to hypocalcaemia)
- paraesthesia
- fractures and deformities.

Rickets leads to more devastating deformities due to the impact of vitamin D deficiency in growing bones. Affected areas tend to be wrists, knees and costochondral junctions. Features include:
- leg bowing (genu varum – most common)
- knock knees (genu valgum)
- soft malleable skull (craniotabes)
- prominent costochondral joints (rachitic rosary)
- dental deformities
- short stature.

5.3.6 Diagnostic approach

Osteomalacia should be considered in adults presenting with joint or muscle pain. A simple blood test to assess levels of vitamin D can be performed. Occasionally it is picked up when a radiograph demonstrates partial or complete fracture of a bone.

Rickets should be considered in any child who presents with any of the clinical features above, particularly if they are in an at-risk group, e.g. those who have been exclusively breastfed with no supplementation, or have little exposure to sunlight. Vitamin D levels can be easily tested but an underlying cause of rickets (e.g. hereditary rickets) may need to be considered if there are atypical features.

If replacement of vitamin D does not improve symptoms then the patient should be reassessed to exclude other pathology such as conditions causing GI malabsorption of vitamin D (e.g. coeliac disease) or a different disease process entirely, such as bony metastases in adults.

5.3.7 Investigations

Multiple investigations are usually not warranted. A low serum vitamin D is often sufficient to make the diagnosis and start treatment but there are other characteristic blood test findings (**Table 5.4**) and radiological changes that may be observed (**Figure 5.4**). Additional investigations depend on whether a specific underlying cause is suspected.

5.3.8 Management

Management for those who are vitamin D deficient with no underlying cause is vitamin D replacement with dietary supplements.
In children, concurrent calcium supplementation is often required due to the needs of growing bones. It is prudent to consider offering the family of an affected child supplementation as they are likely to share the same environmental and social risk factors. Education should be provided, e.g. dietary sources of vitamin D and avoiding prolonged exposure to sunlight.

Prognosis

All but the most severe cases of rickets and osteomalacia are reversible with treatment, but bone deformities are often permanent. Prolonged vitamin D deficiency has been associated with other medical problems, such as autoimmune conditions, cardiovascular disease and cognitive impairment.

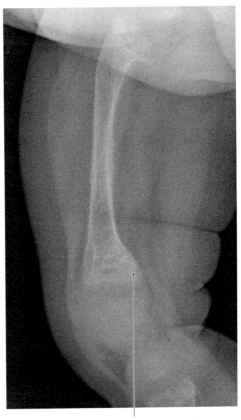

flared, widened metaphysis with diffuse demineralisation and bowing of the long bones

Figure 5.4 Plain radiograph of the right femur of an infant with features of rickets.

Table 5.4 *Investigations in osteomalacia and rickets*		
Blood test findings	**X-ray findings**	**Additional investigations**
Low vitamin D (<25nmol/L indicates deficiency, 25–50nmol/L indicates insufficiency)	Demineralisation	Kidney and liver function
	Loss of cortical bone	Coeliac antibodies
	Insufficiency fractures	Cystic fibrosis screening
PTH elevated	Looser's zones (pseudofractures, transverse cortical lucency with surrounding sclerosis, e.g. proximal femur, pubic rami, lateral scapula)	DEXA scan
ALP elevated		Isotope bone scan
Calcium and phosphate low		
Anaemia may be present (due to other dietary insufficiency)	Deformity	

As with any medication, vitamin supplements also have side-effects. Too much vitamin D can cause hypercalcaemia and, paradoxically, weaker bones, so it is important to stick to the recommended dose and duration.

5.4 Paget's disease

Paget's disease is a condition of disordered bone metabolism, with rapid unregulated turnover of bone resulting in abnormal bone remodelling. This causes bone enlargement and weaker bone matrix, with pain and increased risk of fracture.

Paget's disease presents with symptoms that are common in old age, e.g. musculoskeletal pain and hearing loss, so the diagnosis is easily overlooked. Unexplained bone pain or raised serum ALP should raise suspicion of the diagnosis.

5.4.1 Epidemiology

Patients over the age of 40 years are affected. It is more common in men than women and can affect up to 1% of people over the age of 50 years. Northern populations are most at risk but there are large geographical variations.

5.4.2 Aetiology

The aetiology is not fully understood. There is certainly genetic susceptibility because a third of patients will have a family history of the condition and specific genes have been identified in 25%. Viral infections, e.g. paramyxoviruses, have been implicated but not proven.

5.4.3 Pathogenesis

High osteoclastic activity is the predominant pathological finding; however, this is coupled with disorganised osteoblastic activity. The body tries to lay down bone quickly to counteract the bone resorption but in doing so the bone is disorganised and weak, leading to deformity and fractures.

5.4.4 Clinical features

Paget's disease can either lead to softer bones (lytic stage) or excessive bone growth (sclerotic stage) or a mixed pattern of both, depending on the stage of the disease. The sites most commonly affected are the femur, pelvis and lower back, leading to bone pain, pathological fractures, neuropathy and deformity. The cochlear bone within the inner ear and the skull can also be affected, leading to tinnitus, deafness and headaches. Sometimes the disease is asymptomatic at the time of diagnosis and is picked up as an incidental radiological finding or an isolated raised ALP. Rare complications include spinal cord compression and osteosarcoma.

5.4.5 Diagnostic approach

Paget's disease is diagnosed when there is raised ALP, usually in the presence of normal calcium and phosphorus levels, and typical radiographic findings, with or without symptoms.

Characteristic radiographic appearances include (**Figure 5.5**):
- coarse trabeculation, cortical thickening, bone expansion and sclerosis
- 'blade of grass' sign where there is a V-shaped area of radiolucency in a long bone
- 'cotton wool skull' with poorly defined or fluffy areas of sclerosis
- 'picture frame' vertebral body where the cortex is enhanced relative to the centre.

An isotope bone scan can be performed to visualise the whole skeleton, with Pagetic bone being easily identified due to its increased metabolic activity.

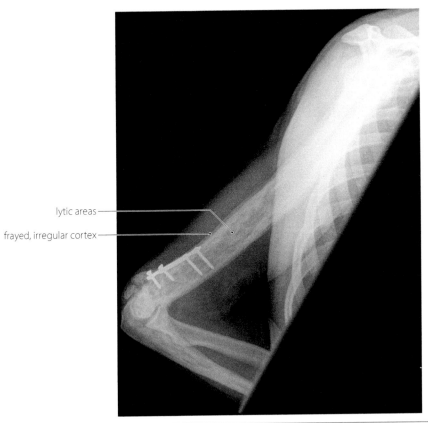

lytic areas
frayed, irregular cortex

Figure 5.5 Radiograph of the right humerus showing features of Paget's disease (note the disorganised pattern of bone); it also shows a plate used for fixation of a previous fracture.

5.4.6 Management

The main indication for pharmacological treatment is bone pain, and modern bisphosphonate drugs are highly effective. Early referral to physiotherapy and occupational therapy is helpful to provide patients with appropriate aids and strategies for coping with their individual symptoms or deformities, and improving mobility.

Medication

Bisphosphonate drugs, e.g. alendronate, risedronate and zoledronate, suppress osteoclast activity to regulate bone remodelling and ease bone pain. Re-treatment is based on symptoms rather than serial checking of ALP. Simple analgesia, including paracetamol and NSAIDs, is also helpful to treat bone pain.

Surgery

Surgery is indicated when there is a significant deformity, fracture or serious complication.

Prognosis

This is dependent on the extent of disease. Often the condition is mild, but recurrent bone pain may require repeat courses of treatment. Rare complications of Paget's disease include nerve compression, osteosarcoma (<1% malignant change) and hypercalcaemia. Heart failure is rare and is caused by hyperdynamic blood flow in Pagetic bone which requires an increased effort from the heart, which may precipitate high output heart failure.

5.5 Answers to starter questions

1. All patients on corticosteroids should be considered at risk of osteoporosis, particularly those on high doses or on long-term treatment. An osteoporosis risk assessment should be carried out in all patients using, for example, the FRAX Fracture Risk Assessment Tool algorithm (www.sheffield.ac.uk/FRAX/tool.aspx) to give the 10-year probability of fracture. This will help guide the need for specific treatment. Usually calcium and vitamin D, weight-bearing exercise and attention to any modifiable risk factors for osteoporosis is recommended for all, with the addition of a bisphosphonate, dependent on perceived fracture risk.

2. In tertiary hyperparathyroidism, the chronic overstimulation of the parathyroid glands causes them to become enlarged. The release of PTH becomes unregulated and it continues to be released, despite a rise in serum calcium.

Chapter 6
Skeletal injuries and disorders

Starter questions

1. Why are the elderly susceptible to hip fractures?
2. Why is it rare to manage a hip fracture non-operatively?
3. Why would you advise a patient with a fracture to stop smoking?

Answers to questions are to be found in *Section 6.18*.

Injury to the bony skeleton often results in a break in the bone known as a fracture. The type of fracture is dependent on the mechanism of the injury and bone density. Skeletal injuries in children act differently and they often injure through the growth plate (the weakest part), or the bone will deform and bend instead of fracture.

Case 6.1 Elderly woman with hip pain after a fall

Presentation

Doris James, a 75-year-old woman, presents to the Emergency Department complaining of a painful right hip following a fall and is not able to walk. She is accompanied by her daughter.

Initial interpretation

A fracture is suspected as Doris is unable to bear weight after a fall.

History

Mrs James was on her way to the kitchen when she fell. Due to the severe pain in her hip she was unable to get herself up or call for help. She doesn't remember losing consciousness or injuring her head but she is unclear how the fall happened; "*it all happened so fast*". Her daughter Gillian found her on the floor several hours later after returning from work.

Interpretation of history

Mrs James' fall does not sound like a simple trip and there may be other medical causes for her fall. Further history should enquire about similar events, her past medical history (including medications) and level of daily activities and independence. In the elderly, minor infections or medication can often cause confusion and falls. This is a good opportunity to obtain a collateral history from her daughter, as Mrs James may not be able to give a comprehensive history, especially if she is in pain or confused.

Case 6.1 *continued*

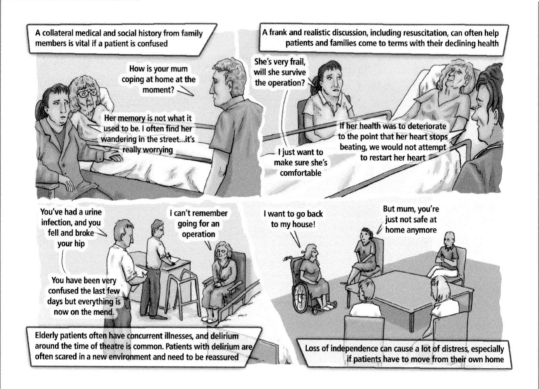

A collateral medical and social history from family members is vital if a patient is confused

How is your mum coping at home at the moment?

Her memory is not what it used to be. I often find her wandering in the street...it's really worrying

A frank and realistic discussion, including resuscitation, can often help patients and families come to terms with their declining health

She's very frail, will she survive the operation?

If her health was to deteriorate to the point that her heart stops beating, we would not attempt to restart her heart

I just want to make sure she's comfortable

You've had a urine infection, and you fell and broke your hip

I can't remember going for an operation

You have been very confused the last few days but everything is now on the mend.

I want to go back to my house!

But mum, you're just not safe at home anymore

Elderly patients often have concurrent illnesses, and delirium around the time of theatre is common. Patients with delirium are often scared in a new environment and need to be reassured

Loss of independence can cause a lot of distress, especially if patients have to move from their own home

Further history

Mrs James reports dizziness and lethargy but she denies any previous fall. She has been going to the toilet frequently over the last few days and noticed her urine had an unusual smell. She normally does her own shopping and cleaning. Gillian says it looks like her mum has not left the house and has not done her shopping in the last few days. She has had some concerns with her mother's memory over the last year.

Examination

Mrs James appears uncomfortable when she tries to move her right leg. Her right leg is shorter compared to the left and is in an externally rotated position (**Figure 6.1**). There is no visible bruising. Palpation reveals tenderness in the groin.

Interpretation of findings

Tenderness in the groin and severe pain when trying to move the hip strongly suggest a fracture. Shortening of right leg suggests that the fracture

is displaced. The absence of bruising does not exclude a hip fracture, as the hip joint is deep and covered by thick layers of soft tissue. Mrs

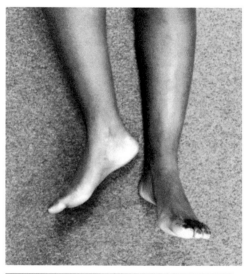

Figure 6.1 A shortened externally rotated leg is pathognomonic of a fractured hip.

James also appears to have some mild confusion coupled with lower urinary tract symptoms, including frequency of urine. It is likely she is suffering from a urine infection and mild delirium.

Investigations

Mrs James is referred for an X-ray of her pelvis and hip to confirm and establish the exact nature of the fracture. A urine dipstick is positive for nitrites and leucocytes, suggesting a urinary tract infection (UTI).

Diagnosis and management

The radiograph shows a displaced intracapsular neck of femur fracture (**Figure 6.2**). She is promptly provided with analgesia, IV hydration and antibiotics for her UTI. The next morning, she undergoes surgery to replace her fractured neck of femur, which enables her to mobilise soon after surgery. Early surgery helps prevent complications normally associated with prolonged bed rest, such

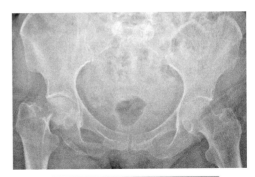

Figure 6.2 Mrs James' pelvic AP radiograph, showing a displaced intracapsular neck of femur fracture.

as pneumonia and pressure ulcers. Rehabilitation, with the help of physiotherapy and occupational therapy teams, allows her to return home sooner, but it is often the case that hip fracture patients will not return to their own home or will need care at home. She will be reviewed by the fragility fracture team before discharge, who will discuss options for osteoporosis treatment.

6.1 Fractures

Normal healthy adult bone requires significant force to fracture. Due to the shape of the skeleton and common mechanisms of injury, certain fracture patterns are common.

6.1.1 Types

Fractures are first described by the type of bone, where in the bone it is fractured, how many pieces it is in and how far away the pieces are from their normal position. The method for describing a radiograph is presented in **Table 2.15**.

6.1.2 Epidemiology

Fractures can happen in all ages. Postmenopausal women are more susceptible to fragility fractures due to lack of oestrogen resulting in osteoporosis (see *Section 5.2*).

6.1.3 Aetiology

Trauma is the most common cause of fractures. Sports such as long-distance running cause stress fractures due to repeated stress on the bone. Defects in bone such as cysts and cancers weaken the bone, making it prone to fracture (pathological fracture).

6.1.4 Prevention

Safety features such as seat belts, airbags and body armour for motorcyclists are some examples that have significantly reduced fracture morbidity. Screening and treating osteoporosis in those at risk reduces fractures.

6.1.5 Pathogenesis

Fracture patterns are determined by mechanism and force of the injury (**Table 6.1**). Fracture

Table 6.1 *Fracture patterns*

Type	Mechanism	Low/high energy	Picture
Transverse	Tension force	Low or high	
Spiral	Twisting force	Low or high	
Oblique	Compression and angulation force	Low or high	
Multifragmentary	Compression and angulation force	High	
Segmental	Compression and angulation force	High	
Avulsion	Tension force	Low or high	
Butterfly	Bending force	Low or high	

healing is discussed in *Section 1.9.3*. Infection and smoking prevent fractures from healing by reducing the blood flow to the fracture site.

6.1.6 Clinical features

Fractures are painful and cause deformity, swelling and bruising. Displaced fractures can pierce nerves, vessels and the skin. They can occur at the time of injury or during a reduction technique. It is therefore important to document an examination of the pulses, motor and sensory nerves and the overlying skin before and after any fracture reduction or cast application.

6.1.7 Investigations

Simple radiographs are enough to diagnose simple fracture patterns. CT scans are helpful to visualise and evaluate multifragmentary or intra-articular fractures as they can produce 3D reconstructive images which are useful to plan surgery (see *Section 2.7.4*).

6.1.8 Management

Fractures with significant deformity should be reduced (realigned) and temporarily held in a

plaster back slab before taking any radiographs. This reduces the pain for the patient and reduces any tension or further damage to the soft tissues, nerve and vessels. Pictures should be taken of any skin cuts, abrasions or lacerations before being dressed, to prevent multiple persons re-evaluating the wounds.

Medication

Oral and IV morphine are opiate medications and are effective for acute pain. Entonox (inhaled nitric oxide) and benzodiazepines are used to mildly sedate patients when manipulating fractures. Local anaesthetic can be injected into the fracture site (haematoma block) – this technique is useful when manipulating distal radius fractures.

Non-surgical

Fractures suitable for casting are well aligned and are unlikely to displace (stable fractures).

Surgery

Surgery is indicated when there is an inadequate reduction of the fracture or if the fracture can't be held reduced by casting. Intra-articular fractures need to be fixed quickly and accurately to restore movement to the joint and reduce the early OA that occurs if joints are not restored to their

Table 6.2 *Causes of non-union*

	Type	Mechanism
Patient factors	Smoking	Vasoconstriction
	Diabetes	Reduced blood supply
	Peripheral vascular disease	Reduced blood supply
	Hyperparathyroidism	Calcium resorption
Injury factors	Periosteal stripping	Reduced blood supply
	Comminuted or bone loss	Comminuted pieces become avascular
	Infection/contaminated wound/open fracture	Bacterial enzymes interfere with bone healing
Mechanical factors	Too much movement at fracture site	Unable to form bridging callus
	Too little movement at fracture site	Reduced osteoblast activity
	Gap too big	Osteoclast unable to cross fracture site as fracture ends are too far apart

normal anatomical alignment. Depending on the type of bone, fracture pattern and the overlying soft tissue injury, surgical fixation can include plates and screws (fixed to the bone under the skin), intramedullary fixation (inside the bone), K wires (piercing bone from outside the skin) and external fixation (outside the skin with a frame) – see *Section 2.9.1*.

Prognosis

Fractures almost always heal even without treatment, but the functional outcome is dependent on the adequacy of the reduction and the ability to rehabilitate early and restore range of movement. Most upper limb fractures heal within 6 weeks and lower limb fractures 12 weeks. Fractures that do not heal within these timescales are called delayed union and can go on to non-union if the underlying cause is not treated (**Table 6.2**). A malunion is when a bone has healed but is misaligned or deformed. The consequences of a non-union can be avascular necrosis, in which the blood supply to the bone is damaged and the bone begins to weaken and fracture.

UPPER LIMB FRACTURES

Bones of the upper limb encompass all bones from the clavicle to the distal phalanx of the finger. Fractures have a range of effects, from impairing ability to place the hand in a position to perform tasks to affecting fine finger movements directly. The most common mechanism of injury is a fall on an outstretched hand. The common injuries in each age group are shown in **Table 6.3** and the associated common nerve injuries in **Table 6.4**.

6.2 Scaphoid fracture

The scaphoid is the most commonly fractured wrist bone in the young. It is notoriously difficult to diagnose as it is poorly visualised on radiographs. Scaphoid fractures carry a risk of avascular necrosis (AVN) and non-union due to the bone's retrograde (distal to proximal flow) arterial blood supply.

Table 6.3 *The most common upper limb fractures in different age groups*

Age group	Type of fracture	Mechanism
Child	Supracondylar	During growth and maturation, supracondylar bone is the weakest part of upper limb
Adult	Scaphoid	Scaphoid is weakest bone as it is the most exposed when landing on extended hand (a child's scaphoid is covered in a dense layer of cartilage, giving it some protection)
Elderly	Distal radius Neck of humerus	Distal radius and proximal humerus are often affected by osteoporosis and are prone to fracture

Table 6.4 *Nerve injuries associated with upper limb fractures*

Fracture	Associated nerve
Proximal humerus	Axillary
Midshaft humeral	Radial
Supracondylar	Anterior interosseous (ulnar nerve during surgical medial wire placement)
Radial head/neck	Posterior interosseous
Midshaft forearm	Ulnar
Distal radius	Median (within the carpal tunnel)

6.2.1 Aetiology

The most common mechanism of injury is following a fall loading the wrist in dorsiflexion and radial deviation.

6.2.2 Clinical features

Scaphoid tenderness can be elicited on the dorsum of the wrist in the anatomical snuffbox (**Figure 6.3**), or palmar (scaphoid tubercle) aspects of the hand, but these are painful tests even in normal subjects and are therefore not very specific. Axial loading of the thumb also produces pain.

6.2.3 Investigations

Plain radiographs (AP, lateral, oblique and scaphoid views) often do not visualise the fracture due to the overlap of the other carpal bones. The treatment pathway for suspected scaphoid fractures is summarised in **Figure 6.4**. Scaphoid fractures are often not seen on radiographs and therefore an MRI may be required.

6.2.4 Management

Non-operative management of scaphoid fracture involves immobilising the wrist in a below elbow cast for 6 to 12 weeks. Surgery is indicated in displaced fractures and those with established non-union and includes stabilisation with a screw.

Complications
Non-union and AVN of the scaphoid have the highest incidence in proximal fractures, due to the break in the retrograde blood supply when fractured.

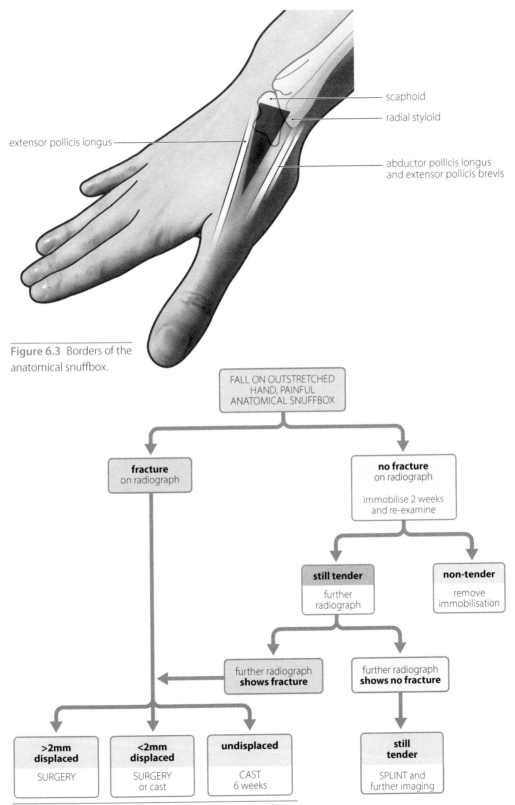

Figure 6.3 Borders of the anatomical snuffbox.

scaphoid

radial styloid

extensor pollicis longus

abductor pollicis longus and extensor pollicis brevis

FALL ON OUTSTRETCHED HAND, PAINFUL ANATOMICAL SNUFFBOX

fracture on radiograph

no fracture on radiograph

immobilise 2 weeks and re-examine

still tender further radiograph

non-tender remove immobilisation

further radiograph **shows fracture**

further radiograph **shows no fracture**

>2mm displaced SURGERY

<2mm displaced SURGERY or cast

undisplaced CAST 6 weeks

still tender SPLINT and further imaging

Figure 6.4 Suspected scaphoid fracture treatment pathway.

6.3 Distal radius fracture

6.3.1 Clinical features

Deformity, pain and swelling of the wrist occur following a fall. In the elderly, the most common fracture is the Colles' fracture which presents with a dinner fork deformity. Fractures are commonly referred to by their eponymous names instead of the more usual description of their fracture pattern. Several of the eponymously named fractures are shown in **Table 6.5**.

To orientate yourself on a lateral radiograph of the wrist, the thumb points to the palm.

6.3.2 Management

Non-displaced fractures are immobilised in a below elbow cast for 6 weeks. A consequence of immobilisation is joint stiffness; physiotherapy will help regain functional movement and strength more quickly. Displaced fractures require manipulation and if unlikely to displace, can also be treated in a cast (usually 6 weeks).

Surgery

Surgery is indicated in those fractures that cannot be reduced by closed reduction or are unstable. Extra-articular fractures with simple dorsal displacement are held by percutaneous (through the skin) K wires to restore the overall alignment. Intra-articular fractures often need an open reduction so the joint line can be visualised and reduced anatomically; most are fixed with a plate and screws.

Table 6.5 *Fractures of the distal radius*			
Fracture	**Mechanism of injury**	**Description**	**Fracture pattern**
Colles' fracture	Wrist extended Low energy	Extra-articular with dorsal displacement	DORSAL Lateral view
Smith's fracture	Wrist flexed Low energy	Extra-articular with volar displacement	VOLAR Lateral view

Table 6.5 *Fractures of the distal radius – continued*

Fracture	Mechanism of injury	Description	Fracture pattern
			VOLAR
Barton's fracture	Wrist flexed or extended High energy	Intra-articular fracture with subluxation of the radiocarpal joint	Lateral view
Chauffeur's fracture	Wrist extended	Fracture of radial styloid	PA view

6.4 Proximal humeral fracture

6.4.1 Clinical features

Proximal humerus fractures occur as a fragility fracture in the elderly after a fall on an outstretched hand. They can be very painful as the fracture cannot be immobilised in a plaster cast. Fractures occur around the surgical neck and the greater and lesser tuberosities. Fractures are described as parts if the fragment is displaced more than 1cm or more than 45° of angulation (**Figure 6.5**).

6.4.2 Management

Most proximal humerus fractures are treated in a collar and cuff, so the elbow weight is used as traction while the wrist is suspended up towards the chest. Even if the fracture does not heal it may not be painful and could have good function:

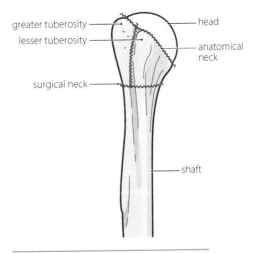

Figure 6.5 Locations of proximal humeral fractures.

this is termed a painless non-union and may be preferable in patients with low demand or who are not fit for surgery. Intra-articular fractures can be fixed in the young and those with good bone stock but are often replaced with joint arthroplasty in the elderly if they have ongoing pain.

LOWER LIMB FRACTURES

Lower limb fractures occur as a result of falls, sporting injuries and road traffic accidents. Ankle fractures are common in younger adults and hip fractures are common in the elderly. Long bone (tibia and femur) fractures are more common in sports and road accidents, due to the energy required to break these large bones.

6.5 Hip fracture

Fractures of the hip include the femoral neck, trochanteric region and up to 5cm distal to the lesser trochanter.

6.5.1 Epidemiology

The incidence of hip fractures is increasing globally, due to the growing ageing population. In the elderly, hip fracture affects women more commonly as their bone density reduces more quickly after the menopause than in men. Hip fractures in younger patients are usually caused by high energy trauma, e.g. a road traffic accident.

6.5.2 Pathogenesis

Hip fractures are classified according to the location of fracture:
- Intracapsular fractures involve the neck of femur within the hip capsule (**Figure 6.6**).
- Extracapsular fractures are in the trochanteric region outside the hip capsule (**Figure 6.2**).

The blood supply to the femoral head is dependent on the retrograde arterial supply (**Figure 6.7**). The capsule inserts onto the femoral neck at the intertrochanteric line. Fractures above this line are intracapsular and below this line are extracapsular.

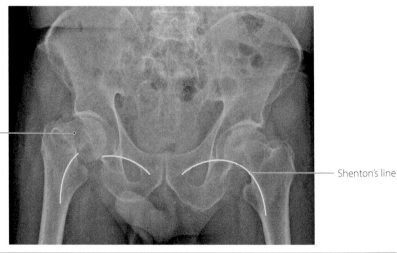

intracapsular neck of femur fracture

Shenton's line

Figure 6.6 The AP radiograph of the pelvis shows an intracapsular neck of femur fracture on the right side. Shenton's line is smooth on the left side but is disrupted on right.

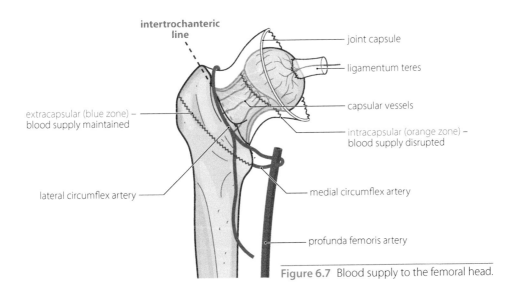

Figure 6.7 Blood supply to the femoral head.

Labels on figure:

intertrochanteric line

joint capsule

ligamentum teres

capsular vessels

extracapsular (blue zone) – blood supply maintained

intracapsular (orange zone) – blood supply disrupted

lateral circumflex artery

medial circumflex artery

profunda femoris artery

An intracapsular hip fracture with displacement severely compromises the vascular supply from the capsular arteries. This means that intracapsular fractures are at high risk of AVN and non-union due to the lack of blood supply causing collapse of the femoral head and therefore subsequent fixation failure.

6.5.3 Prevention

Patients who are at risk of falls should be offered walking sticks, frames and bannisters to help keep their independence and prevent falls. Osteoporosis treatment is discussed in *Section 5.2.8*.

6.5.4 Clinical features

Patients complain of pain in the affected hip, with an inability or difficulty in weight-bearing. If the hip fracture is displaced, the affected leg will be noticeably shorter and in an externally rotated position due to the pull of the external rotator muscles of the hip (**Figure 6.1**).

6.5.5 Investigations

Most hip fractures are easily seen on radiographs. However, if the history and clinical signs are suggestive of a hip fracture, CT and MRI can pick up undisplaced fractures that are not readily seen on simple radiographs.

6.5.6 Management

Patients with hip fractures should be admitted to the orthopaedic ward urgently and given analgesia to relieve pain. **Table 6.6** summarises the management of hip and pelvic trauma. Patients' medical conditions should be optimised for surgery to reduce the risk of surgical and anaesthetic complications. Hip fracture patients have a greater risk of deep vein thrombosis (DVT) due to their immobility, so mechanical and

Table 6.6 *Management of hip and pelvic trauma in the elderly*

Diagnoses	Management
Pubic ramus fracture	Analgesia, mobilisation and rehabilitation
Acetabular fracture	Immediate: skin traction
	Non-operative: mobilisation non-weight bearing
	Operative: internal fixation
Femoral shaft fracture	Immediate: Thomas splint, resuscitation (potential significant loss of blood into thigh compartments)
	Internal fixation using plate or intramedullary nail

pharmacological thromboprophylaxis agents are provided perioperatively.

Surgery

The type of surgery performed is dictated by the type of fracture and aims to allow a return to weight-bearing and mobility as soon as possible. The surgical options are either a hip arthroplasty or internal fixation (**Figure 6.8**).

Total hip replacement (replacement of the acetabulum and femoral head and neck) or hemiarthroplasty (replacement of only the femoral head and neck) are the standard operations for displaced intracapsular fractures where the risk of non-union or AVN would potentially subject a patient to a revision operation. There is a high risk of fracture displacement if an undisplaced intracapsular hip fracture is managed non-operatively. Internal

fixation is an option in undisplaced fractures or young patients in an attempt to preserve the femoral head. Total hip replacements are offered for more active, higher demand patients rather than hemiarthroplasty, as they last longer.

Internal fixation using a sliding hip screw or intramedullary nail is used to treat extracapsular fractures, as the blood supply is almost always preserved and the fracture is likely to heal.

Prognosis

There is a significant rate of morbidity and loss of independence following a hip fracture. Mortality is high, with a 30-day mortality rate of 10% and up to 60% at one year after hip fracture. This is an indication that hip fractures occur in patients who are already experiencing a decline in their general health.

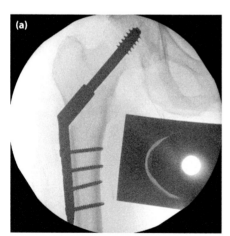 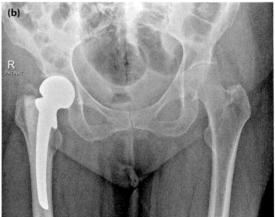

Figure 6.8 Anteroposterior radiograph of the pelvis depicting: (a) extracapsular fracture fixed with a dynamic hip screw; (b) intracapsular neck of femur fracture replaced with a hemiarthroplasty.

6.6 Ankle fracture

6.6.1 Clinical features

Ankle fractures are a result of a twisting injury: most commonly eversion or supination (see **Figure 1.39**). Pain, bruising and swelling are common in both sprains and fractures, so to help decide whether a patient needs an X-ray it is often helpful to use the Ottawa ankle rules (**Figure 6.9**).

A radiograph is needed if there is tenderness in the malleolar region and any one of the following:

- bone tenderness along the 6cm posterior edge of the tibia or tip of medial malleolus
- bone tenderness along 6cm posterior edge of fibula or tip of lateral malleolus
- inability to weight-bear more than four steps in the Emergency Department.

(a)   LATERAL

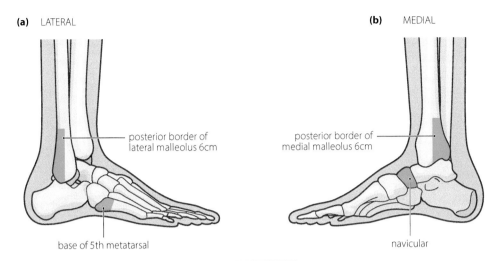

posterior border of
lateral malleolus 6cm

base of 5th metatarsal

(b)   MEDIAL

posterior border of
medial malleolus 6cm

navicular

Figure 6.9 Ottawa ankle rules: (a) lateral view; (b) medial view.

Fractures are classified (Weber A, B and C) in relation to the syndesmosis, which is a tough ligament complex made up of several ligaments that holds the distal tibia to the fibula and maintains the ankle joint shape (**Figure 6.10**).

6.6.2 Management

Fracture dislocations result in an obvious deformity and should be reduced and placed in a temporary back slab plaster prior to going for an X-ray, in order to reduce pain, prevent swelling and reduce damage to the skin and soft tissues. These are unstable injuries and require internal fixation with plates and screws, or temporary fixation in an external fixator.

Weber A fractures are stable as the syndesmotic ligaments are intact. Patients are able to walk on these injuries and a cast may be placed for comfort. Undisplaced Weber B fractures can be treated in a cast and if stable, can be allowed to weight-bear. Displaced Weber B and Weber C fractures are typically unstable and the fracture is likely to have disrupted the syndesmotic ligaments and requires fixation to restore the ankle joint.

Casting reduces movements in the ankle and the venous pump in the calf, so patients

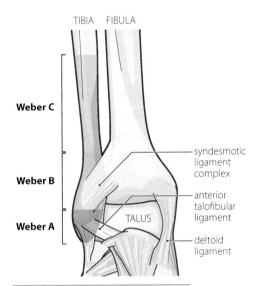

TIBIA   FIBULA

Weber C

Weber B

Weber A

syndesmotic
ligament
complex

anterior
talofibular
ligament

TALUS

deltoid
ligament

Figure 6.10 The Weber ankle fracture classification: a fracture below the syndesmosis ligament is a Weber A; at the level of the syndesmosis a Weber B; and above the syndesmosis a Weber C.

with ankle fractures are at increased risk of DVT. Therefore, thromboprophylaxis should be considered in all patients with an ankle fracture.

CHILDHOOD INJURIES AND DISORDERS

Skeletal injuries in children are different from those in adults. This is for two reasons: first, the more elastic bones in children often bend rather than break. Secondly, the physes are still open and, if injured, this could lead to growth arrest, causing deformity. Often young children are not able to say they have been injured and present to healthcare professionals with a limp or not using the injured limb.

6.7 Paediatric fractures and growth plate injury

Injuries of the growth plate include separation of the epiphysis through the growth plate, fractures crossing the growth plate and crush injuries.

6.7.1 Radiological features

Plain radiographs will not show the physis, as it is made of non-mineralised cartilage. This makes it more difficult to diagnose a child with a suspected growth plate injury. Assessing the alignment of the joint and looking for swelling in the soft tissues helps diagnose fractures, especially around the elbow and hip physis (**Figure 6.11**).

Growth plate injuries are assessed and described using the Salter–Harris classification (**Table 6.7**). The classification is also an indicator

Table 6.7 *Salter–Harris classification*		
Grade	**Fracture location and extent**	metaphysis / physis / epiphysis
I	Along width of physis	
II	Along physis with involvement of metaphysis (extra-articular)	
III	Along physis with involvement of epiphysis (intra-articular)	
IV	Across physis, involving metaphysis and epiphysis	
V	Crush injury	

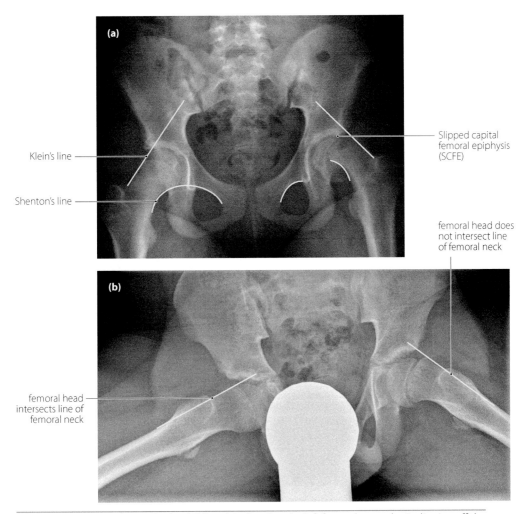

Figure 6.11 (a) AP radiograph of a child's pelvis showing the left femoral metaphysis slipping off the femoral epiphysis – the normal femoral head is intersected by Klein's line on the right; however, it does not intersect on the left abnormal hip; (b) frog leg view in same patient, showing an apparent increase in the slip.

of prognosis, with a greater growth disturbance expected with a higher grade of injury.

6.7.2 Management

The growth rate and remodelling potential of the fracture differ even in a single long bone, which means that acceptable degrees of deformity will vary by bone, age of the child and distance from the physis. Accepted angulation in a 2-year-old

patient with a forearm fracture will be more than in a 14-year-old where the potential for remodelling is less (**Table 6.8**).

Growth plate injuries heal very quickly in whatever position they are in and should be reduced to anatomical alignment, ideally within 24 hours. Once reduced, most of these fractures are stable but they may require K wire fixation to maintain position during healing.

Table 6.8 *Factors that affect the potential for bone remodelling in children's fractures*

Factor	High remodelling rate	Low remodelling rate
Age group	<8 years	>8 years
Fracture site	Close to joint	Midshaft
Displacement and angulation of the fracture	In line with the joint movement	At right angles to the joint plane of movement
Proximity to joint	Knee, wrist and shoulder	Elbow, hip and ankle

6.8 Supracondylar humerus fracture

Supracondylar fractures are fractures through the thinnest part of the distal humerus and are most common in children. Anatomy of the growth plates around the elbow is shown in **Figure 1.6**.

6.8.1 Clinical features

Pain, swelling and deformity around the elbow are evident in displaced fractures and the child will be very reluctant to move the elbow. Significantly displaced bone fragments can cause puckering to the skin and vascular and nerve injuries. The following signs should be documented: radial pulse, motor function and sensation of the median, ulnar, radial and anterior interosseous nerves. Sensation is often difficult to assess, especially in young children, and litmus paper can be used to confirm the presence of sweating (absence of sweating indicates a possible nerve injury). Motor function can be assessed by observing finger and hand movements in very young children. Nerve injuries are uncommon and often resolve spontaneously (neuropraxia) (see section on peripheral nerve disorders later in this chapter, **Table 9.3 and Figure 9.8**). The most common injury is to the anterior interosseous nerve branch of the median nerve, which results in an inability to flex the IPJ of the thumb (flexor pollicis longus) and DIPJ (flexor digitorum profundus) of the index finger (**Figure 6.12**).

6.8.2 Management

Undisplaced fractures are managed with immobilisation in a plaster cast or sling. Displaced fractures require surgery to prevent malunion.

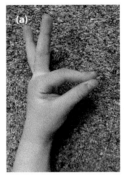

no flexion of the DIPJ

flexion of the DIPJ of the index and IPJ of the thumb

Figure 6.12 The OK sign: (a) injury; (b) normal.

Surgery

The fracture is manipulated into an anatomical position and wires are inserted to stabilise the fracture. During this procedure care must be taken to avoid piercing the ulnar nerve while inserting the wire on the medial side of the elbow. Stiffness of the elbow is common after injury, especially when the elbow needs to be immobilised. The elbow has a strong anterior joint capsule which stiffens rapidly after injury, resulting in loss of full extension of the elbow. Malunion of the fracture can lead to cubitus varus (gunstock) and cubitus valgus deformities (**Figure 6.13**). Cubitus valgus has a risk of tardy ulnar nerve palsy, where the nerve is stretched around the medial epicondyle due to the deformity (see *Section 9.9*).

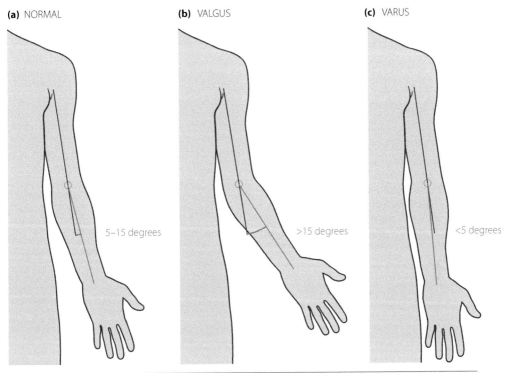

(a) NORMAL

5–15 degrees

(b) VALGUS

>15 degrees

(c) VARUS

<5 degrees

Figure 6.13 Supracondylar malunion: (a) normal carrying angle of 5–15°; (b) cubitus valgus, >15°; (c) cubitus varus, <5°.

6.9 Non-accidental injury

Non-accidental injury (NAI) is injury as a result of physical abuse leading to fractures and soft tissue injuries. No single form of injury is specific to NAI so a systematic approach must be adopted to identify this as a cause.

6.9.1 Aetiology

NAIs are caused by direct or indirect actions leading to physical harm. Causes include any form of violence – a punch, kick, blow, push or pull. The child may have been shaken or thrown or may have had a limb twisted or squeezed.

Common factors raising the risk of NAIs include:

- low socioeconomic status, but note that children from all socioeconomic backgrounds can be affected
- the child being the result of an unplanned pregnancy
- the child having special needs and/or a disability
- the child being young (less than 2 years old or before walking).

6.9.2 Clinical features

Clinical features suggestive of NAI are:

- bruises away from bony prominences, old bruises, bruises of different ages and bruises corresponding to finger marks
- bites
- burns, especially if they have a submersion line or a shape corresponding to a burning or hot object (e.g. electric ring or cigarette)
- fractures of various ages, i.e. in several stages of healing
- rib fractures
- bilateral fractures
- limb fracture in a non-walking infant.

Diagnosing an NAI is challenging because of the dependence on the parent or guardian for a history. It is important to check for consistency and feasibility of the histories given by different individuals.

> To get a clear history, questions should first be directed to the child if appropriate. The child should be asked to describe what happened in their own words before asking the caregiver. Watching the interaction between the child and caregiver can highlight concerns. If there is sufficient concern you should question the child on their own; it is considered a red flag if the caregiver does not permit this.

Suspicion of NAI should be raised in any of the following circumstances:
- there is a delay in presentation from the time the injury occurred
- the history is illogical (e.g. a femur fracture in an infant who is yet to stand or walk)
- the history is vague
- the parents or guardians are being overly defensive when questioned about the injury
- there are obvious features of abuse.

Any of these should prompt an assessment of medical history and past attendances to Emergency Departments. This may reveal frequent attendances and further raise suspicions.

> Disorders that are easily mistaken for an NAI include osteogenesis imperfecta, rickets and bleeding disorders. See *Section 5.3* for investigations to rule out metabolic bone disease.

6.9.3 Diagnostic approach

If there is any suspicion of NAI, the child safeguarding team should be involved at the earliest opportunity. They will then investigate and involve social services and the police if deemed necessary. Most hospitals have a protocol for escalation, usually termed 'Safeguarding Children Policy'.

> A child must not be left unattended with the suspected abuser; there must be a chaperone, to protect the child and as a safeguard for staff. The best approach is to be open and honest with the parents and let them know that you are referring them to the safeguarding children team. Be mindful that they may try to take the child away and things can escalate quickly. Refer to a senior colleague and involve the wider clinical team at the earliest opportunity.

6.9.4 Investigations

Radiographs are performed to confirm the type and pattern of bone injury. Whole-body skeletal surveys using radiographs can help to ascertain whether multiple fractures of differing ages are present.

6.10 Slipped capital femoral epiphysis

Slipped capital femoral epiphysis (SCFE) is a separation through the physis where the metaphyseal femoral neck is displaced from the femoral epiphysis that stays inside the acetabulum (**Figure 6.10**). Some children with SCFE will give a history of minor trauma, but the majority occur spontaneously.

6.10.1 Epidemiology

SCFE almost only affects children going through puberty, and they are at increased risk during a growth spurt. It is more common in boys but occurs earlier in girls due to their earlier onset of puberty. Overweight Afro-Caribbean boys between 12 and 15 years of age are at greatest risk.

6.10.2 Aetiology

The aetiology is unknown, but certain factors increase the risk of SCFE, such as obesity, hypogonadism, hypothyroidism and growth hormone treatment.

6.10.3 Clinical features

Patients often present as a 'limping child'. This term refers to children who have difficulty weight-bearing on a particular leg and are noticed to be limping without necessarily complaining of any pain. If they do present with pain, it can be in the knee, thigh or groin.

The differential diagnoses for limp in a child are described in **Table 6.9**.

> Knee pain is often a misleading symptom that disguises underlying hip pathology. The anterior branch of obturator nerve courses from the hip to the knee, supplying both, so pain in the hip can be perceived to be arising from the knee and vice versa.

6.10.4 Diagnostic approach

Clinical examination often shows no abnormal alignment of the leg, but it may be held externally rotated. Only in severely displaced slips would the leg be shortened. During hip flexion, there is a tendency for the hip to externally rotate.

6.10.5 Investigations

Radiographs of the pelvis (AP and frog lateral views, **Figure 6.11**) are obtained and may confirm the diagnosis. The frog lateral is most sensitive and will reveal the femoral metaphysis has displaced from the femoral epiphysis.

> If the radiograph appears normal and there is clinical suspicion, an MRI scan should be ordered as the slip may be subtle (often termed pre-slip).

6.10.6 Management

The child should be restricted from weight-bearing and an urgent specialist orthopaedic opinion sought.

Surgery

Surgery is offered to all patients. A single screw is placed across the growth plate, causing the growth plate to fuse and stabilising the slip.

Prognosis

Children with SCFE on one side have a 20–50% risk of developing it on the other side before they reach skeletal maturity. The child and family should be advised of this risk and operating on the other side to prevent a slip should be considered. The risk of AVN is higher in a more severely displaced SCFE.

Table 6.9 *Differential diagnosis for limp in a child*			
Features	**Septic arthritis**	**Perthes' disease**	**SCFE**
Usual age of presentation (years)	3–5	4–8	9–15
Clinical features	Signs of infection Severe hip pain Will not allow movement of hip due to pain Raised inflammatory markers and WCC	Child small for age Painful hip movement	Obese or tall and thin Hip in external rotation
Radiograph	Grossly normal May have increased joint space due to pus in the joint	Normal initially, later fragmentation and flattening of femoral head	Femoral neck metaphysis is displaced from the femoral epiphysis

6.11 Perthes' disease

6.11.1 Epidemiology

Perthes' disease is uncommon. It affects younger children between the ages of 4 and 8 years, and more commonly boys.

6.11.2 Aetiology

The cause of AVN (bone death due to a disruption of blood supply) of the femoral head from epiphyseal blood supply disruption in Perthes' disease is unknown. Perthes' disease progresses through four stages over several years:

- Initial – disruption of blood supply
- Fragmentation – dead bone is removed, making the bone weaker
- Re-ossification – new bone is formed
- Remodelling – the final shape of the femoral head is formed.

6.11.3 Clinical features

Pain in the hip or knee is common and can often present as a limp.

6.11.4 Investigations

Early in the disease no features may be seen on X-ray. An ultrasound may show a joint effusion.

Diagnosis is made on MRI. Late radiographic signs include reduced epiphyseal size and flattening of the femoral head.

6.11.5 Management

The long-term treatment aims to prevent permanent deformity of the femoral head, maintaining hip joint congruity and motion.

Non-surgical

Children should be kept non-weight-bearing until seen by a specialist paediatric orthopaedic surgeon. Avoiding high impact sports and reducing the force through the joint with bracing can help maintain the integrity of the femoral head shape.

Surgery

Osteotomies (cutting and realigning the bone) of either the femoral neck or pelvis can help maintain the shape of the femoral head within the hip joint.

Prognosis

Younger children have the best prognosis as they have the greatest potential to remodel. Those children who have severe deformity of the femoral head will progress to early OA and joint replacement in early adulthood.

6.12 Developmental dysplasia of the hip

Developmental dysplasia of the hip (DDH) occurs when the femoral head is not located in the acetabulum (cup of the hip joint); this leads to failure of the acetabulum to form correctly in the newborn.

6.12.1 Epidemiology

Girls and first-born children are more commonly affected and it often runs in families.

6.12.2 Clinical features

DDH is usually first noticed during the newborn 'baby check' examination when the hips are gently examined for instability. Late signs include

one leg being shorter than the other and uneven skin folds on the upper thigh.

6.12.3 Investigations

Ultrasound scans are the gold standard test, as very young children do not have ossified femoral heads. Ultrasound assesses how much the femoral head is covered by the acetabulum.

6.12.4 Management

Non-surgical

The Pavlik harness is used in babies under 6 months old. The harness relocates the femoral head inside the joint by flexing and abducting the hip and encouraging the acetabulum to develop normally.

Surgery

If the diagnosis is missed, surgery may be required to relocate the femoral head back in the joint. This can be done by manipulation or by an open reduction. Significant deformities may require osteotomies to realign the hip joint.

Prognosis

If treated early, a normal hip joint will form. Late presenting children can have a permanently dislocated hip and can develop arthritis in early adulthood.

OTHER INJURIES

6.13 Spinal injuries

Spinal fractures and spinal cord injury can be life-changing if they result in permanent disability.

6.13.1 Epidemiology

Spinal fractures and spinal cord injury occur mostly in the young from high energy road traffic accidents but are also common in the elderly, due to degeneration and osteoporosis of the spine.

6.13.2 Clinical features

Most trauma patients will be brought in by ambulance on a spinal board with a cervical spine collar supported by sandbags and tape (**Figure 6.14**). The spinal board keeps the rest of the spine straight when manoeuvring the patient, while a pelvic binder helps reduce the volume of the pelvis and can help tamponade bleeding. Neurological examination of limbs and the perianal area may reveal reduced motor function and sensation. See *Sections 2.3.6* and *9.3* for examination and clinical features of myelopathy and radiculopathy.

> Significant pain can distract the patient and the examiner from other injuries, therefore C-spine collars should not be removed until the patient has received a clear CT scan and they are able to comply with an examination.

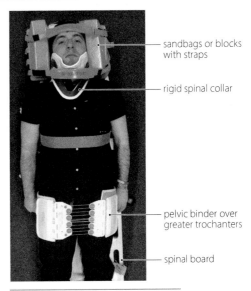

sandbags or blocks with straps

rigid spinal collar

pelvic binder over greater trochanters

spinal board

Figure 6.14 Trauma immobilisation.

6.13.3 Pathophysiology

Stability of the spine is described by F. Denis in three columns: the anterior column is the anterior two-thirds of the vertebral body; the middle column is the posterior one-third of the body; the posterior column is the pedicles, lamina and spinous process. If more than one column is damaged, the stability is compromised (**Figure 6.15**). The different spinal fracture patterns are due to different mechanisms of injury (**Table 6.10**).

Table 6.10 *Vertebral fractures*

Type	Mechanism	Description	Image
Wedge	Flexion or compression Low energy	Anterior column is crushed Stable	
Burst	Flexion or compression High energy	Involves anterior and middle column Likely unstable	
Chance	Flexion distraction High energy deceleration	All three columns Unstable	
Jefferson	Neck hyperextension or flexion High energy	Anterior and posterior arches of C1 vertebra Unstable	
Hangman's	Hyperextension and distraction High energy	Bilateral pedicle fracture of C2 vertebra Unstable	
Clay shoveller's	Sudden pull of the supraspinous ligaments Low energy	Spinous process avulsion fracture of cervical or thoracic vertebra Stable	

6.13.4 Investigations

Radiographs may be useful to assess alignment but CT scan is the imaging modality of choice to assess spinal fractures. MRI is useful to assess non-bony structures such as the cord and ligaments.

6.13.5 Management

The aim of treatment is to prevent injury to the spinal cord, so strict log-rolling (keeping the body in a straight line) is essential to prevent displacement of fractures.

Damage to the spinal ligaments can cause instability of the spinal column without a fracture. If there is a high index of suspicion due to mechanism of injury, cord injury or pain, then an MRI should be ordered.

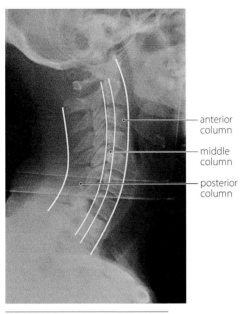

anterior column

middle column

posterior column

Figure 6.15 Three spinal columns.

Non-surgical

Stable fractures, such as wedge fractures that have not lost more than 30% of the vertebral body height, are treated with early mobilisation and a brace if needed for comfort.

Surgery

Unstable fractures and those with spinal cord injury need decompression of the spinal cord and stabilisation with screws and rods.

Prognosis

Fractures without spinal cord injury that are stable or that are surgically stabilised usually have a good outcome and function returns. Spinal cord injury is life-changing. Recovery of function is possible but variable; most patients reach full recovery potential by two years. Complete spinal cord injuries (complete disruption of the motor and sensory tracts) carry a worse prognosis than incomplete injury (some motor and sensory function).

6.14 Polytrauma

Polytrauma is injury to multiple limbs and or multiple systems, e.g. head and abdominal trauma. It is the result of high energy impact.

6.14.1 Epidemiology

The incidence of polytrauma in many countries is lower than a decade ago due to improvement in road and industry safety. However, road traffic accidents remain a significant cause of polytrauma. Although it tends to be younger males that are involved in such accidents, more elderly people are now sustaining high energy injuries due to the increase of the ageing population.

6.14.2 Aetiology

Most injuries are sustained due to the blunt impact of high energy trauma affecting vital organs such as the heart, brain, spleen and liver. Musculoskeletal injuries contribute to immediate and early fatality through secondary manifestations, e.g. an unstable cervical spine injury causing spinal cord injury and brainstem death, or pelvic and long bone fractures causing significant haemorrhage and circulatory collapse. Sepsis from open fractures leads to late complications and morbidity.

6.14.3 Clinical features and initial management

Pre-hospital care is vital to immediately resuscitate and transfer severely injured patients safely to hospital. The initial assessment and management are done concurrently, based on Advanced Trauma Life Support guidance (**Table 6.11**).

Table 6.11 *The Advanced Trauma Life Support (ATLS) algorithm follows the CABCDE assessment*

CABCDE assessment	Examination and action
Control of catastrophic haemorrhage	Apply pressure to the wound and elevate
	Tourniquet
	Artery forceps to clamp the vessel
Airway with protection of the cervical spine	Place your hands on either side of the head to stop C-spine movement
	Apply hard collar and secure with sandbags and tape
	Clear airway of debris
	Place oropharyngeal airway or intubate if not maintaining own airway
Breathing and ventilation	Give high flow oxygen
	Check equal chest wall movement and equal air entry
	Chest drains for pneumothorax
	Check respiratory rate and pulse oximetry
Circulation and haemorrhage control	Check pulse rate and blood pressure
	Apply pelvic binder
	Resuscitate with blood and platelets
	Check long bones and apply traction
Disability (neurologic) evaluation	Glasgow Coma Scale
Exposure of patient for examination	Full primary survey to include: ■ log-roll and spinal examination ■ per rectum and vaginal examination in pelvic fractures

Much of the current approach to management of polytrauma has been derived from military experience in conflicts, especially in the way that immediate care and transfer are carried out.

Once resuscitated and stable, a CT scan to include pelvis, abdomen, chest, head and neck should be done straight away, so that injuries can be quickly identified and treated.

Prognosis

Rehabilitation should start immediately during acute hospital admission to allow the patient to return to pre-injury levels of function. Family and employers need to be involved in this process to achieve the best patient outcomes.

6.15 Pelvis

6.15.1 Clinical features

High energy pelvic fractures can disrupt the pelvic veins, causing catastrophic haemorrhage. A pelvis binder placed over the hips reduces the volume of the pelvis to help tamponade (compress) the bleeding (**Figure 6.14**). The rectum and vagina should be examined because displaced fracture fragments can pierce the lumens, causing an open fracture. The urethra can also be damaged, and care should be taken when placing a catheter so as not to create a false passage; if in doubt use CT to guide placement. Fractures of the sacrum have a high incidence of causing damage to the sacral nerve roots leading to bladder and bowel dysfunction, so a full neurological examination should be completed; see *Section 2.3.6*.

6.15.2 Management

Urgent surgery is required if bleeding is uncontrolled. Unstable fractures can be stabilised with internal plate or screw fixation and/or external fixation. Weight-bearing is restricted until the fracture is healed, often taking up to 12 weeks.

6.16 Chest trauma

6.16.1 Clinical features

Displaced rib fractures can pierce the underlying lung and pleura, causing a pneumothorax (air within the pleural space) and haemothorax (blood within the pleural space). Pulmonary contusions (bruising) and lacerations can cause haemorrhage, resulting in haemorrhagic shock. The common symptoms of chest trauma are chest pain, shortness of breath and low oxygen saturation levels. Look at the chest wall movements for any asymmetry which may suggest a flail chest, which is a free-floating segment which moves paradoxically to the rest of the chest wall.

6.16.2 Management

The aim of treatment is to maintain ventilation by reducing pain to make it more comfortable for the patient to cough and clear secretions. This helps prevent complications such as pneumonia and acute respiratory distress syndrome. Chest drains are placed in the pleural space to drain both air and blood from the cavity. Surgical fixation of rib fractures is undertaken when the mechanical integrity of the chest wall is altered, such as a flail chest and if the patient is unable to maintain ventilation.

6.17 Open long bone fractures

Open fractures have a direct communication to the skin and are at risk of developing infection and non-union.

6.17.1 Clinical features

In addition to closed fracture features, the open fracture is associated with a wound. This may be a small puncture wound where the bone has pierced the skin or a large wound if a sharp or heavy object lacerates the skin. Wounds should be assessed for nerve and vessel injuries. Clinical photographs of the wound are helpful to document its size, skin loss and contamination.

6.17.2 Management

Antibiotics and tetanus boosters are given during the initial assessment and antibiotics are continued until the open wound is closed. Wounds contaminated with marine or agricultural sewage need urgent surgery to decontaminate them. Clean wounds can be dressed with saline-soaked gauze and fractures reduced and stabilised in a plaster back slab. In the next available theatre space, open fractures should be thoroughly debrided of any dead tissue and bone. Generally, internal fixation should not be completed unless the wound can be closed. In the presence of significant tissue damage, external fixation is used temporarily until swelling subsides or plastic surgery can cover the wound with a skin graft or flap.

6.18 Answers to starter questions

1. Bone density decreases with increasing age and therefore a lower amount of traumatic force is required to cause a fracture. These are termed fragility fractures. Deterioration in balance and mobility is also associated with ageing, making the elderly more prone to falls. Evidence suggests that fractures of the distal radius and proximal humerus are predictors of further fragility fractures in postmenopausal women.

2. Surgery for hip fractures provides excellent pain relief and allows patients to return to walking faster. Prolonged pain and bed rest makes nursing care difficult, increases the length of hospital stay and increases the risk of cardiovascular complications such as chest infection, DVT and pulmonary embolism. Non-operative management for hip fracture is rare in current healthcare practice but it is considered if the risks of surgery outweigh the benefits, or if the patient refuses surgery.

3. Smoking directly alters bone metabolism, affecting fracture union. In addition, it reduces blood supply to the peripheries, further compromising the ability to heal. This results in delayed or non-union which can be prevented by smoking cessation.

Chapter 7
Exercise-related injuries and soft tissue disorders

Starter questions

1. Why are women more at risk of anterior cruciate ligament injuries?
2. Why do children's 'growing pains' usually get better after puberty?
3. Why is tendinopathy difficult to treat?

Answers to questions are to be found in *Section 7.21*.

Tendons, ligaments, bursae and cartilage are all at risk of damage by both high energy trauma and chronic repetitive microtrauma. High energy injury can displace bones out of their joints, disrupt joint cartilage or tear tendons and ligaments. Repetitive injuries causing microtrauma to the tissues can turn into chronic injuries that are difficult to heal.

This chapter is divided into four separate parts covering disorders of the shoulder, soft tissue knee injuries, disorders of the hand and elbow, and disorders of the foot. Finally, fibromyalgia, a chronic musculoskeletal pain syndrome, is discussed.

Case 7.1 Painful deformed shoulder after trauma

Presentation

William March is a 20-year-old college rugby player who presents to the Emergency Department with an injury to his left shoulder which he sustained during a tackle. He had a sudden pain when his shoulder was wrenched above his head and is now unable to move his shoulder. He has noticed a hard swelling at the front of his shoulder.

Initial interpretation

Persistent inability to move a joint after trauma suggests a significant injury. The inability to move may be due to pain inhibition that occurs with soft tissue damage, fractures or due to mechanical reasons such as dislocation.

History

William remembers that his arm was out to the side with his hand above his head at the moment before his injury. It was forced into further external rotation during the tackle. He is right hand dominant and reports no previous injury to either of his shoulders or other joints.

Case 7.1 *continued*

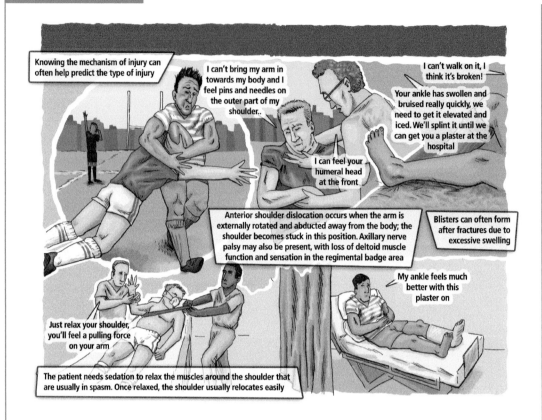

Examination

William is in severe pain and has a deformed shoulder. There is loss of the lateral shoulder contour which is formed by the humeral head. A hard and tender swelling is palpable in front of the shoulder. Sensation in the regimental patch, forearm and hand are normal. Capillary refill is less than 2 seconds and the radial pulse is present and symmetrical with the other side.

Interpretation of findings

William's deformed joint suggests a joint dislocation. In his case the humeral head has dislocated anterior and medially away from the glenoid. Anterior is the commonest direction of dislocation, accounting for the loss of lateral shoulder contour and the presence of anterior swelling. There is no evidence of nerve injury (the axillary nerve can be damaged in shoulder dislocation, resulting in loss of sensation in the lateral upper arm 'regiment patch' area, and weakness in the deltoid muscle).

Investigations

Radiographs of William's shoulder (AP, Y scapula and axillary views) have confirmed the anterior dislocation of the glenohumeral joint and have ruled out a fracture (see **Figure 7.1**).

Diagnosis

The diagnosis is a first-time anterior dislocation of the glenohumeral joint. William is given sedation and analgesia in the Emergency Department to allow manipulation and reduction of the injury. Radiographs are repeated to confirm reduction and that there are no fractures that were not seen on initial images. He is provided with a broad arm sling and advised to avoid extreme shoulder movements (in external rotation and abduction) because of the high risk of recurrent dislocation.

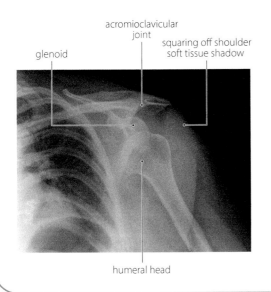

glenoid

acromioclavicular joint

squaring off shoulder soft tissue shadow

humeral head

He is referred for follow-up at the trauma clinic, at which time he will be counselled about the risk of further dislocation (which is very high). He may require early surgery and will certainly require physiotherapy before being allowed to return to contact sports.

Figure 7.1 AP radiograph left shoulder, showing an anterior dislocation of the glenohumeral joint. A loss of the rounded contour of the shoulder can also be seen.

Case 7.2 Four months of pain and weakness in dominant arm

Presentation

Alice is a busy right-handed 67-year-old retired cleaner. She enjoys taking an oil painting class but is finding it difficult to lift her dominant right arm to paint, as it is painful and weak. This has been going on for a few months but Alice has now come to her GP as she is unable to do up her bra and wash her hair properly.

Initial interpretation

A painful weak shoulder in the older generation without trauma could be OA or related to tears in the muscles and tendons around the shoulder girdle.

History

Alice has had no trauma to her shoulder but when she was a busy cleaner she used her shoulders to do a lot of overhead work. The pain and weakness in her shoulder have gradually come on over about 4 months and affect her dominant right side. The pain is worse when she is trying to do her housework, especially putting her clothes away in the wardrobe or when getting a plate out of the top cupboard. She has tried resting her arm and taking painkillers but the pain returns as soon as she uses her arm again.

Further history

Alice has symptoms suggesting subacromial impingement as well as the possibility of a small tear in the rotator cuff. It is often not possible to distinguish between these problems on clinical assessment but both are part of the same pathological process. After obtaining an X-ray to rule out OA, Alice's GP is able to give her an injection of corticosteroid into the subacromial space to relieve her pain and sends her for physiotherapy to improve her deltoid and rotator cuff strength. Alice finds this very useful and is symptom-free for a year before symptoms return. Alice's GP then sends her to a shoulder specialist for further assessment.

Case 7.2 *continued*

Examination

The right shoulder is tender and the supraspinatus and infraspinatus muscles, that lie on either side of the spine of the scapula, appear to have mild wasting compared to the contralateral left side. Alice is most tender around the right subacromial area and over the long head of biceps. She is able to forward flex and abduct her right arm to 90° actively, but this then becomes painful. She has normal external rotation of 30° and can internally rotate her hand to the level of her sacrum. Passively the range of movement of her shoulders is normal. Special tests actively testing the supraspinatus and infraspinatus tendons against resistance produce pain on the right side but are normal on the left. Testing of the subscapularis tendon shows no dysfunction. Right shoulder impingement tests (**Figure 7.5**) are positive but the acromioclavicular joint is pain-free on scarf test (**Figure 7.6**).

Interpretation of findings

Wasting of the muscles can be due either to loss of nerve supply to those muscles or disuse. The latter usually results from a chronic problem with the muscle or tendon. Unilateral involvement suggests a local problem. The supraspinatus, infraspinatus and teres minor muscles form a common tendon, known as the rotator cuff. It passes through the subacromial space and inserts on the greater tuberosity of the humerus. It becomes degenerate and can often have small degenerate tears, which causes inflammation and hypertrophy of the subacromial bursa. This in turn leads to a reduced subacromial space causing the rotator cuff to become trapped, known as impingement. Clinically there will be tenderness around the subacromial area and pain when the space is reduced by elevation and abduction of the arm, known as a painful arc. This is confirmed by eliciting positive impingement signs. A full range of passive movement but weakness and pain on active movement suggests tendon or muscle pathology, whereas OA will restrict active as well as passive range of movement.

Investigations

Radiographs of the shoulder do not reveal any OA.

Further investigations

At the hospital, the orthopaedic doctor suspects a full thickness rotator cuff tear as Alice is now only able to actively move her arm very little. An ultrasound scan is undertaken at the clinic which confirms a small full thickness tear of the supraspinatus tendon and a small partial thickness tear in the infraspinatus tendon.

Diagnosis

Full thickness tears are unlikely to heal and particularly if the patient has poor function, they may need surgery to repair or reconstruct the tendon. Surgery involves freeing up and widening the subacromial space to prevent further impingement, and repair of the tendons with sutures. Careful physiotherapy is required after rotator cuff surgery and the arm needs to be in a sling for 6 weeks.

Case 7.3 Painful swollen knee after a fall

Presentation

Kieran Kent, a 30-year-old electrician, is brought to the Emergency Department by his wife after falling from the second step of a ladder the previous day and injuring his left knee. He slipped off a step and as he fell, twisted his left knee and is now unable to go back to work. He is reluctant to weight-bear due to pain. He was unable to straighten his knee and noticed that his knee became swollen overnight.

Case 7.3 *continued*

Initial interpretation

Pain in the knee following a fall can be due to a direct impact (landing directly onto the knee) or indirect force (twisting). It is important to obtain a detailed history of the actual mechanism of injury, as this will help to predict the resulting injured structure(s). Mr Kent's inability to straighten his knee is termed a locked knee and indicates a mechanical block to extension. His delay in swelling indicates that there is unlikely to be a fracture or ligament injury that has bled acutely.

Timing of knee swelling:
- Immediate – acute intra-articular bleeding, e.g. fracture and cruciate ligament rupture
- 24 to 48 hours after injury – meniscal injury, surrounding soft tissue injury.

Examination

Mr Kent is experiencing quite a lot of discomfort. The resting position of his left knee is in approximately 30° of flexion. There is a large effusion and he has tenderness over the medial joint line. After provision of strong analgesia, he can demonstrate active and passive flexion of the knee to 110° but is not able to extend the last 30°. Examination of the ligaments did not reveal any instability.

Interpretation of findings

Mr Kent's locked knee is confirmed clinically. His history suggests a large, displaced meniscal tear and requires urgent specialist referral.

Investigations

Plain radiographs of Mr Kent's knee show evidence of joint effusion but no fracture.

Although an MRI would confirm the diagnosis of a meniscal tear, a locked knee requires early surgery and treatment must not be delayed.

Diagnosis

Mr Kent has a locked knee which is an indication for early arthroscopic (keyhole) surgery. The torn part of the meniscus causing the block to extension is repaired or removed. Mr Kent will have physiotherapy to restore his knee movement.

DISORDERS OF THE SHOULDER

The shoulder joint has a shallow glenoid socket and rounded humerus and is often described as a golf ball on a tee. The shoulder is very mobile due to its shape, making it prone to dislocation and overuse injuries.

7.1 Shoulder dislocation

7.1.1 Epidemiology

Shoulder dislocations are divided into two types:
- High-energy injury in adults (in the elderly this is often associated with a fracture of the proximal humerus)
- Atraumatic shoulder dislocation in patients who have hypermobile joints who can either self-dislocate (habitual) or dislocate after trivial trauma; these are often younger female patients.

7.1.2 Aetiology

Traumatic anterior dislocation is more prone when the arm is overhead or abducted and forced into external rotation. Posterior dislocation is rare and is caused by powerful contractions of the posterior shoulder muscles during seizure or electrocution.

Patients with hypermobility have a joint capsule that is lax but also have an imbalance of muscles around the shoulder. Incorrect muscle patterning around the shoulder can increase muscle force on either the anterior or posterior humeral head and cause dislocation.

7.1.3 Clinical features

Pain and loss of the outer contour of the shoulder are the most common symptoms. An anterior dislocation will present with the arm slightly abducted and externally rotated, whereas posterior dislocation will present with the arm held in internal rotation and adducted.

> The brachial plexus is vulnerable to injury in anterior shoulder dislocation (see **Figure 1.42**). The axillary nerve branch is the most commonly injured. Sensation in the regimental patch (over the lateral side of the shoulder) is reduced or absent in axillary nerve injury. Reducing the dislocation by traction can itself cause an axillary nerve injury. It is therefore important to document an axillary nerve function before and after any reduction manoeuvres.

7.1.4 Investigations

The most helpful radiographs are the scapular Y view and the axillary view (**Figure 7.2**), as they clearly show the glenoid and humeral head congruity. However, these radiographs are often difficult to obtain due to difficulty positioning the arm because of pain. The humeral head and glenoid should be inspected for fractures and depressions as they may affect stability of the joint once relocated.

7.1.5 Management

For anterior dislocations, a reduction should be performed under sedation in the Emergency Department. Multiple techniques are described; however, the simplest is the traction–countertraction method. An assistant provides countertraction with a towel around the patient

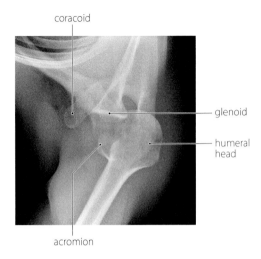

coracoid

glenoid

humeral head

acromion

Figure 7.2 Axillary view radiograph showing posterior displacement of the humeral head relative to the glenoid.

while gentle sustained longitudinal traction is applied to overcome the muscle spasm. Internal and external rotation can be applied at the same time to unhinge the dislocation. Once relocated, the arm is placed in a sling and is rested for a few weeks before beginning physiotherapy. For posterior dislocations, urgent reduction under general anaesthetic should be undertaken in theatre, as they are difficult to reduce and repeated attempts could lead to fractures. This will then allow open reduction if required.

Surgery

If a closed reduction cannot be achieved or the dislocation is associated with a fracture, an open reduction (where the shoulder joint is surgically opened) in the operating theatre should be performed as an emergency.

Prognosis

Young patients with traumatic dislocations are at high risk of further dislocations and should be followed up carefully. They are likely to have structural defects in the labrum, humeral head or glenoid. Surgery to restore these structures should be offered if diagnosed and there is recurrent instability. Atraumatic dislocators should be offered intense physiotherapy to retrain the muscles in the shoulder.

Patients with atraumatic shoulder dislocations should not be offered surgery, as they do not have a structural defect.

7.2 Rotator cuff disorders

The rotator cuff consists of four muscles around the shoulder (**Table 7.1**). They work together to keep the shoulder within its shallow joint and also to control movements of the shoulder (**Figure 7.3**).

7.2.1 Epidemiology

Degenerative rotator cuff tears are very common within the older population and are generally not symptomatic. Younger patients will often present

Table 7.1 *Rotator cuff examination tests*

Muscle	Action	Test	Description	Positive test
Supraspinatus	Abduction of the shoulder	Empty can	Patient holds arm extended at 90° in the scapular plane with thumb pointing downwards and tries to keep it there while examiner applies downward force on the upper arm	Pain and weakness elicited
Infraspinatus and teres minor	External rotation	External rotation lag	Patient flexes elbow to 90° and tucks arms into sides of body; examiner places arm in external rotation and asks patient to maintain this position	Position not maintained and arm returns to neutral
Subscapularis	Internal rotation	Gerber's lift-off	Patient places hand on lumbar spine, palm outwards, and tries to lift hand away from body as examiner places pressure on wrist	Pain and weakness elicited

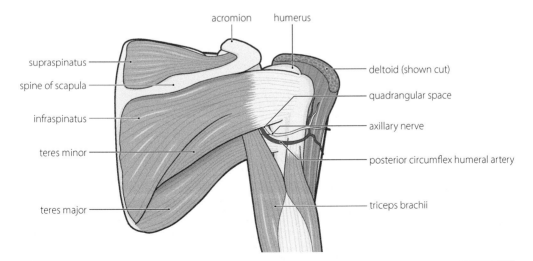

Figure 7.3 The four tendons of the rotator cuff insert onto the humeral head. A quadrangle-shaped space is created below teres minor; above teres major it is bounded medially by triceps and laterally by the humeral shaft. The posterior circumflex humeral vessels and the axillary nerve pass through this space.

after an acute traumatic tear with sudden pain and weakness in the arm.

7.2.2 Aetiology

Degeneration of the rotator cuff tendons is multifactorial but is mostly caused as a consequence of subacromial impingement (see *Section 7.3*). Blood flow to the tendons reduces as part of the ageing process. These factors result in these tendons becoming more prone to rupture.

7.2.3 Clinical features

Painful and weak active movements of the shoulder with normal passive movements are more likely to be rotator cuff disease rather than OA, which also affects passive movements. As the shoulder muscles work in tandem to move the shoulder it can be difficult to isolate specific shoulder muscles to test them individually (**Figure 7.4**).

7.2.4 Investigations

Initial workup should include an X-ray to rule out OA. However, if symptoms are severe and function is poor, assessment of the tendon with ultrasound or MRI can be useful to confirm the diagnosis and to plan surgical intervention.

7.2.5 Management

Most degenerative tears of the rotator cuff require no surgical treatment as there is usually more than one muscle in the shoulder which can compensate for the lost function. For example, supraspinatus, which is the most commonly affected muscle, can be compensated by using the deltoid muscle. Physiotherapy is key to recovering this function.

Often the impingement symptoms can be very painful, which can inhibit rehabilitation. A steroid injection into the subacromial bursa to reduce the inflammatory bursitis can

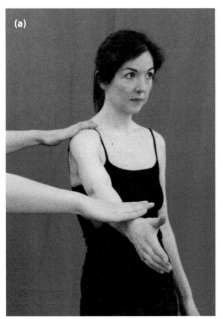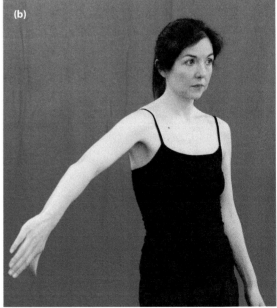

Figure 7.4 (a) The full can test elicits pain due to impingement or tears of the supraspinatus tendon, or may detect related muscle weakness. The arm is in an extended position with the thumb pointing upwards (holding a full can), then forward flexed at the shoulder to 90° in the 45° scapular plane. The examiner puts downward pressure on the arm and asks the patient to resist this movement. A positive test is pain in the supraspinatus tendon or subacromial region, or weakness; (b) this can be repeated in exactly the same way but with the thumb pointing downwards – the 'empty can test' (as if emptying out a can).

provide sufficient symptom relief until deltoid rehabilitation can begin.

Medication

NSAIDs are useful in the short term to help control pain and enable patients to start rehabilitation exercises.

Surgery

Surgery is offered if symptoms are severe or patients have failed to respond to conservative measures. It involves day-case arthroscopic surgery in which tendons can be repaired with sutures in conjunction with a decompression of the subacromial space. In difficult cases with large irreparable tears the cuff may require patch augmentation or grafting. Tendon transfers in the shoulder allow one muscle to take over the job of another; for example, the latissimus dorsi tendon can be substituted for the supraspinatus tendon.

Prognosis

Most patients improve with a simple steroid injection to the subacromial bursa and physiotherapy. Overall, those with successful rotator cuff repairs will experience the greatest return of their shoulder function.

7.3 Impingement

7.3.1 Aetiology

Impingement or entrapment of the supraspinatus and infraspinatus tendon is common in the subacromial space (**Figure 7.5**). As part of the ageing process, bony spurs can form in this area, inflaming the subacromial bursa (bursitis) and reducing the space for the tendons to glide.

7.3.2 Clinical features

The main clinical feature is pain around the acromion or deltoid region that is worse in the painful arc of movement between 60° and 120° of abduction. Patients with weakness should be investigated for a rotator cuff tear. Acromioclavicular joint pain is often confused with impingement pain. The scarf test (**Figure 7.6**) is positive in acromioclavicular joint disease. The scarf test is positive if pain is elicited over the acromioclavicular joint when the hand is placed on the opposite shoulder and the examiner pushes the arm into the body while stabilising the opposite shoulder.

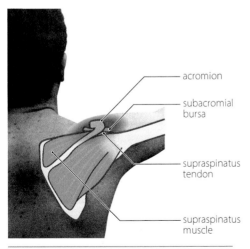

Figure 7.5 Shoulder impingement is caused by the space under the acromion becoming narrow, causing damage to the subacromial bursa and muscles of the rotator cuff.

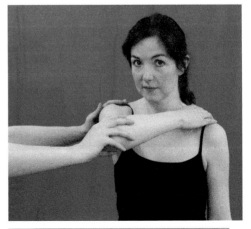

Figure 7.6 Scarf test for acromioclavicular joint pathology.

7.3.3 Investigations

Radiographs of the shoulder are used to rule out other conditions such as OA of the acromioclavicular or glenohumeral joints. A hooked shape to the acromion reduces the space for the tendons to glide and can be visualised on radiographs.

7.3.4 Management

Medication

Simple analgesia can help patients cope with their symptoms. A steroid injection directly into the subacromial bursa can improve the inflammation and pain.

Surgery

Ongoing symptoms that do not settle by injection could benefit from a subacromial decompression, where the undersurface of the acromion and bursa are surgically shaved away to leave room for the tendons to glide.

Prognosis

Good results are seen with steroid injection and physiotherapy. In resistant cases subacromial decompression usually gets patients back to normal function.

SOFT TISSUE KNEE INJURIES

The knee is vulnerable to injury as it relies heavily on the muscles and ligaments to prevent movement and dislocation. The tibial plateau is relatively flat and is made more congruent by the menisci that sit on top of it. The shearing and compressive forces on the menisci during sport make them susceptible to tears.

7.4 Anterior cruciate ligament injury

The ACL is a static stabiliser of the knee which prevents anterior translation of the tibia relative to the femur. Injury to this ligament destabilises the knee and makes it prone to further injury.

7.4.1 Epidemiology

There is a higher incidence of ACL injuries in men, but women participating in similar pivoting and jumping activities are more at risk due to the anatomical differences in their knees.

7.4.2 Aetiology

In adults, ACL tears cause significant bleeding and swelling in the knee (**Table 7.2**). In children the ACL can remain intact but the tibial spine where the ACL inserts on the tibia can be pulled away from the bone as an avulsion fracture.

The mechanism of ACL injuries are:
- non-contact pivoting injury to the knee
- traumatic valgus injury to the knee, e.g. a rugby tackle to the lateral side of the knee.

7.4.3 Clinical features

Patients report a painful popping sensation and immediate swelling at the moment of injury, followed by an inability to bear weight.

Examination reveals a painful joint with effusion. The anterior drawer test (*Section 2.3.4*) is positive. However, examination immediately after an acute injury can be difficult due to pain and swelling. Reassessment should be arranged when swelling has settled.

In delayed presentations, there is usually a history of a limp and of the knee giving way when performing activity involving pivoting or a sudden change of direction. There is also a subtle loss of complete extension of the affected knee, which is best checked from the end of the examining bed holding both the patient's heels.

An acute ACL rupture is often associated with simultaneous lateral meniscus and medial collateral ligament injuries.

Table 7.2 *Causes of painful swollen knee after trauma*

	ACL injury	PCL injury	Meniscal injury	Patellar dislocation	Quadriceps tendon rupture
Mechanism of injury	Sudden change in direction of knee and body using foot as pivot	Direct blow to knee when flexed	Twisting injury with knee in flexion (e.g. squatting)	Twisting and turning, similar to ACL and meniscal injury Direct trauma (less common)	Forceful eccentric contraction of quadriceps tendon (e.g. landing from a height)
Knee swelling	Immediate	Immediate	Within hours or next day	Correlates to severity	Swelling directly proximal to patella with palpable gap due to torn tendon
Examination	Positive anterior drawer test	Posterior sag Positive posterior drawer test	Effusion with joint line tenderness	If unreduced, patella located lateral to a flexed knee Following reduction, positive patella apprehension test	Inability to actively extend knee Extensor lag sign (knee fully extended passively, then with the withdrawal of support it sags into flexion)

7.4.4 Investigations

Plain radiographs show haemarthrosis, which can be seen as a white swelling in the suprapatellar pouch on a lateral view (**Figure 7.7**). Rarely, this is accompanied by an avulsion fracture of the lateral portion of the proximal tibia (Segond fracture, which is characteristic of an ACL rupture).

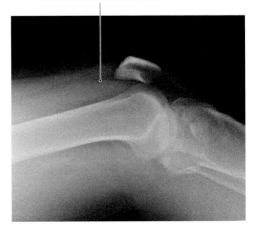

haemarthrosis fluid level line

Figure 7.7 Lipohaemoarthrosis of the knee in a patient with a tibial plateau fracture. A lateral radiograph of the knee with the patient lying horizontal. Blood and fat are denser than joint fluid and so sink to the lowest point, showing a distinct horizontal line between the two fluids.

MRI has 90% sensitivity and specificity in detecting an ACL rupture and will show discontinuity of the ACL on sequential images as well as any associated injuries.

7.4.5 Management

Physiotherapy and rehabilitation are the mainstay of ACL injury management. This should start early to maintain range of movement and quadriceps strength.

Surgery

Patients whose sports or work involve pivoting while weight-bearing, or who report recurrent instability despite rehabilitation, are more likely to need surgery to allow return to pre-injury activity levels. Surgery involves ACL reconstruction using grafts such as patella, hamstring, Achilles tendon or a synthetic ligament.

Prognosis

Patients usually regain full function after reconstruction of their ACL.

7.5 Posterior cruciate ligament injury

The PCL is a static stabiliser of the knee which prevents posterior translation of the tibia relative to the femur. The PCL is a stronger ligament than the ACL in resisting translation of the tibia.

7.5.1 Epidemiology and aetiology

PCL injuries are much less common than ACL injuries. The PCL tears after a significant posterior force is applied to the tibia when the knee is flexed (e.g. knee hitting car dashboard).

7.5.2 Clinical features

The initial symptoms are the same as the ACL injury. A posterior drawer test, where a posterior force is applied to the tibia (mimicking the mechanism of injury,) will show laxity compared to the opposite side (**Table 7.2**).

7.5.3 Investigations

MRI will show discontinuity of the ligament and any associated meniscal tears.

7.5.4 Management

Surgery

Most PCL injuries will regain stability of their knee with an intensive physiotherapy regime. Reconstruction is reserved for patients with high demand sporting activities or those with residual instability following rehabilitation.

Note the position of the tibia when the knees are flexed to 45°: a posterior sag can be seen in a PCL injury (**Figure 7.8**). This is important to note as it may produce a false positive anterior drawer test if you start with the tibia posteriorly subluxed and bring it forward to its normal anatomical alignment.

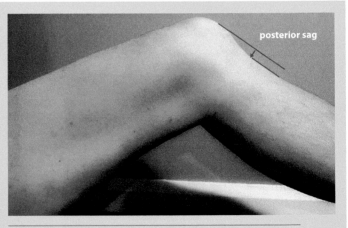

Figure 7.8 Lateral view of the knee showing the tibia sagging posterior on the femur.

7.6 Meniscal injuries

Meniscal injuries are very common and present at any age. In the majority of patients they do not heal but if they become troublesome with mechanical symptoms, they can be removed arthroscopically.

7.6.1 Epidemiology

Traumatic meniscal tears are common in young patients in high demand sports involving sudden twisting and pivoting. Degenerative tears are associated with OA and increasing age and do not normally involve an acute injury.

7.6.2 Aetiology

The menisci are resistant to compressive forces but are prone to tear when subjected to a shear force such as twisting. Joint space narrowing and loss of synovial cartilage in OA increase friction, and changes in the menisci as part of the ageing process also cause degenerative tears.

7.6.3 Clinical features

Pain, swelling and loss of extension are common features in both degenerative and traumatic tears. Pain is worse when weight-bearing. A locked knee is caused by a block to extension by a meniscal tear. The knee is held in flexion and cannot be straightened. Patients often have mechanical symptoms: they describe a clicking sensation and might need to shake their leg to get it straight again if it becomes intermittently locked.

7.6.4 Investigations

MRI is the investigation of choice for meniscal pathology. OA may be seen on a radiograph in older patients.

> MRI scans should not be ordered in the presence of OA or locked knee for suspected meniscal tear, as this will not influence treatment decisions. However, they may be helpful for surgical planning.

7.6.5 Management

Meniscal tear can be quite painful but symptoms often settle in a few weeks with rest, ice, elevation and rehabilitation with physiotherapy. Patients may benefit from surgery for ongoing pain or mechanical symptoms after a traumatic tear.

Surgery

Locked knees require early surgery and this should not be delayed by requesting MRI scans. Meniscal surgery is performed arthroscopically using cameras within the joint. Depending on the type, some tears can be repaired but most tears occur in the avascular zone and need to be removed as they will not heal.

Prognosis

Surgically repaired meniscal injuries need to be treated with care until healed, and weight-bearing should be reduced for at least 6 weeks. Patients who have had removal of a meniscal tear can mobilise straight away and often have instant relief of symptoms.

7.7 Cartilage disorders

Osteochondral defects are scuffs or divots in the synovial cartilage secondary to trauma such as a dislocated patella, where the patella is driven across the lateral femoral condyle. New hyaline cartilage cannot be formed once it is damaged, but new fibrocartilage can form at the site of the damage. Healing with fibrocartilage is dependent on whether the damage is above or below the level of the tidemark which is the division between the non-calcified cartilage (superficial injury) and the calcified cartilage (deep injury) (**Table 7.3**).

Depth	Tidemark	Vascularity	Healing
Table 7.3 *Cartilage injury and repair*			
Superficial injury	Non-calcified cartilage	Avascular	No healing
Deep injury	Calcified	Vascular	Healing, with formation of fibrocartilage

7.7.1 Clinical features

Defects in the cartilage can cause significant haemarthrosis because healthy bleeding bone is exposed. Pain, swelling and reduced range of motion are common in these injuries.

7.7.2 Investigations

Large defects entering the bone are visible on radiographs. However, the imaging modality of choice is MRI as it directly visualises cartilage and can pick up subtle injuries as areas of oedema within the bone.

7.7.3 Management

Surgery

Small lesions may be treated with a technique called microfracture; this attempts to stimulate the defect to fill in with fibrocartilage which is weaker than, and not as smooth as hyaline cartilage. Research is being undertaken on cartilage transplants in order that larger defects can be replaced with normal hyaline cartilage.

7.8 Baker's cyst

Baker's cysts are fluid-filled sacs at the back of the knee caused by an outpouching through the joint capsule due to fluid pressure in the knee.

7.8.1 Epidemiology

Baker's cysts are common and are almost always associated with either OA or RA.

7.8.2 Clinical features

A fluctuant swelling in the popliteal fossa may be noticed by the patient but is usually asymptomatic. Patients may feel a discomfort or clicking in their knee but this may be related to their underlying arthritis causing the cyst. In rare instances the cyst may burst; this can cause sharp pain and swelling in the calf which can be mistaken for a DVT.

A pulsatile swelling is likely to be a popliteal aneurysm. These should be investigated further, as there is a high risk of embolism.

7.8.3 Investigations

An asymptomatic Baker's cyst needs no further investigation. If the swelling rapidly increases in size, is pulsatile or painful, then MRI and ultrasound should be performed to exclude serious conditions such as tumour, aneurysm or DVT.

7.8.4 Management

Asymptomatic cysts do not need any treatment. Aches and swelling can be treated with simple ice, compression and analgesia. Treating the underlying arthritis is the mainstay of treatment. Cysts can be drained and injected with corticosteroid. Rarely, large cysts are surgically removed but there is a high level of recurrence.

7.9 Osgood–Schlatter disease

Osgood–Schlatter disease is an apophysitis, meaning inflammation of the bone tendon junction in a child. An apophysis is a secondary ossification site and therefore this is a syndrome of young adolescence (10–14 years).

7.9.1 Clinical features

Patients experience pain, swelling and tenderness over the tibial tubercle, where the patellar tendon inserts on the front of the tibia. Pain is worse during and after activities, when kneeling and resisting extension.

7.9.2 Investigations

Lateral radiographs of the knee show irregularity and fragmentation of the tibial tubercle.

7.9.3 Management

Activity modification to rest the patellar tendon should be considered, but this should be case-specific and balanced against symptoms. Once the apophysis fuses (usually around 14 years of age) pain should subside, so the condition is self-limiting.

The need for additional treatment is unusual but includes immobilisation in full knee extension in either a splint or cast, or surgery to remove any ossicles (small bone fragments) that are troublesome.

7.10 Bursitis

Inflammation of a bursa (bursitis) is caused by infection or overuse. The most common sites for bursitis are around the patella and the olecranon of the elbow.

7.10.1 Aetiology

Bursitis can occur at any age. Prolonged kneeling causes trauma to the bursa, resulting in inflammation; small skin breaks can also let in bacteria to the fluid-filled sac.

7.10.2 Clinical features

Pain, swelling, redness and heat around the knee are the most common symptoms. Knee range of movement is not normally affected. The most commonly affected bursae in the knee are the prepatellar bursa (in front of the kneecap; also known as 'housemaid's knee') and the infrapatellar bursa (just below the kneecap; also known as 'clergyman's knee') (**Figure 7.9** and **Table 7.4**).

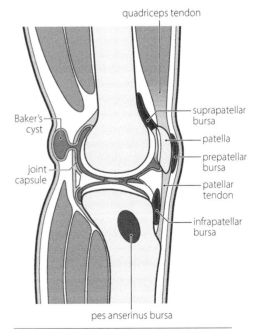

Figure 7.9 Fluid-filled bursae around the knee protect the tendons and patella from mechanical damage and are named after their location.

Table 7.4 *Types of swellings around the knee*

Pathology	Type of swelling	Redness and warmth	Tenderness	Range of movement
OA	Diffuse joint effusion	Mildly warm all over	Mild tenderness	Mild restriction
Septic arthritis	Diffuse joint effusion	Red and hot	Extreme tenderness	Unable to move
Haemarthrosis	Diffuse joint effusion	Mildly warm all over	Some tenderness	Some restriction
Prepatellar bursitis	Localised anterior to the patella	Mild warmth and redness anterior to patella	Localised mild tenderness	Not restricted
Infrapatellar bursitis	Localised inferior to the patella	Mild warmth and redness inferior to patella	Localised mild tenderness	Not restricted
Baker's cyst	Popliteal fossa at the back of the knee	None	Not usually tender	Not restricted

7.10.3 Investigations

The diagnosis is made on clinical examination. If white cell count and CRP are raised, this may indicate infection rather than inflammation. An aspirate of the fluid from the bursa for culture can be diagnostic as well as therapeutic.

7.10.4 Management

Bursitis generally improves after a period of rest. Analgesia, NSAIDs and ice can help with the pain and swelling. Infective bursitis needs treatment with antibiotics and can be surgically drained in refractory cases. Modification of activity or using knee-pads can help prevent further episodes. In rare cases of multiple recurrences, the bursa can be surgically removed.

DISORDERS OF THE HAND AND ELBOW

The hand is a complex array of tendons, ligaments and fascia, all of which can be affected by disease or injury. The hand and elbow are prone to overuse injuries especially in manual or repetitive jobs.

7.11 Dupuytren's contracture

Dupuytren's contracture (Dupuytren's disease) is a common disorder of the ulnar aspect of the hand and thumb and causes a progressive flexion deformity of the fingers due to thickening and contracture of the palmar fascia (**Figure 7.10**).

7.11.1 Epidemiology

This disease is ten times more common in males and is more likely in patients aged 50 and over. There is a strong genetic predisposition, especially in those of Viking ancestry.

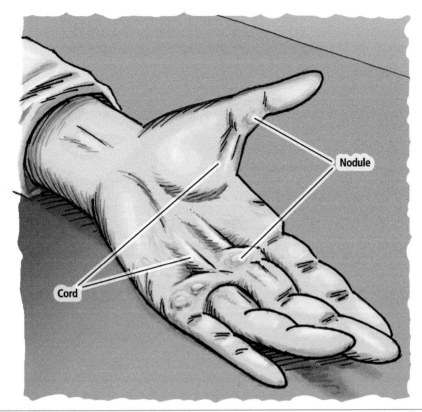

Figure 7.10 Dupuytren's contracture of the ring and middle fingers due to thickening of the palmar fascia with a visible node and cord.

7.11.2 Aetiology

Dupuytren's disease slowly lays down more type III collagen in the palmar fascia. Type III collagen is thicker than type I and, as more is laid down, the fascia becomes thick and shortened, contracting the fingers. Although commonly idiopathic there is an increased likelihood of developing these contractures in liver disease, diabetes and with medications such as phenytoin.

7.11.3 Clinical features

The little and ring fingers are the most commonly affected. Examination reveals tight bands of tissue within the palm and fingers, with the finger not able to be passively extended. Problems such as putting a hand in a pocket often cause painful knocks to the finger.

7.11.4 Diagnostic approach and investigation

Diagnosis is confirmed by clinical examination. Radiographs will rule out other causes of contracture such as OA, but are not used for diagnosis.

7.11.5 Management

Treatment depends on functional requirements and the extent of the disease.

Medication
For patients with single contractures, dissolving the collagen bands with injectable collagenase enzymes can improve their contractures.

Surgery
The mainstay of treatment is surgical excision of the tight collagen bands. Often due to the nature

of the contracture, skin loss following release may require further movement of skin on the hand in the form of advancement flap.

Dupuytren's disease almost always reoccurs but the rate of recurrence varies. Surgical management is delayed for when the fingers become a nuisance and normal daily tasks become difficult.

7.12 Ganglion (synovial cyst)

A ganglion or synovial cyst is a fluid-filled sac associated with a joint or a tendon. It is not lined with epithelium and thus is not a true cyst in the histological sense (**Figure 7.11**).

7.12.1 Clinical features

Ganglions are most commonly found around the wrist, hands and feet. They are believed to be outpouchings at points of weakness in the joint capsule or tendon sheath. Many ganglions form a small stalk with a one-way valve that lets fluid into the cyst but not back out again. Therefore, the ganglion becomes bigger and likely to recur unless the valve is disrupted. Ganglions are not in themselves painful but if they are knocked, they can be painful and burst, but often reoccur. On clinical examination they are mobile, compressible and are transluminescent.

7.12.2 Management

If not causing any symptoms and if radiographs do not show any underlying abnormality, a ganglion usually does not require treatment. Further imaging with ultrasound or MRI is advised if there are any red flag symptoms indicating the possibility of an alternative more serious diagnosis, such as pain, a sudden increase in size

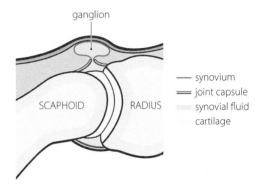

Figure 7.11 A dorsal wrist ganglion is an outpouching of synovium through the joint capsule filled with synovial fluid. The joint capsule will usually let fluid into the ganglion under pressure but will tightly close like a one-way valve, preventing fluids escaping the ganglion.

or a more unusual location away from a joint.

Surgery
Aspiration of the cyst can be effective but the fluid is likely to build up again. Recurrence after surgical excision is less likely but is still as high as 40%. In comparison, nearly 60% of ganglions resolve spontaneously without any treatment.

7.13 Tendinopathy

Tendinopathy is a chronic degenerative condition of a tendon, usually affecting a single site. The most common sites in the upper limb are the elbow epicondyles (epicondylitis), the wrist (de Quervain's) and the rotator cuff. Other common sites include the Achilles and patellar tendons, but any tendon can be affected. The cause of tendinopathy is multifactorial and therefore it can be very difficult to treat. The treatment principles of tendinopathy are to address any precipitating factors, provide pain relief and physiotherapy-based strengthening exercises. Surgical techniques are not reliably effective.

7.14 Epicondylitis

Epicondylitis is degeneration of the common tendon origins of the forearm muscles on the elbow's epicondyles (**Figure 7.12**). There are two types:

- lateral epicondylitis (insertion of the common extensor origin) – 'tennis elbow'
- medial epicondylitis (insertion of the common flexor origin) – 'golfer's elbow'

These are common among patients who are manual labourers or who do repetitive movements, for example musicians. As with all tendon pathologies, once it becomes a chronic pathology it is more difficult to treat.

7.14.1 Aetiology

Epicondylitis is a misnomer as it is very rarely an acute inflammatory injury. The most common presentation of epicondylitis is more chronic in aetiology. Repetitive twisting and bending of the forearm can commonly bring on epicondylitis. The extensor carpi radialis brevis (ECRB) muscle is the most lateral of the extensor muscles and as the elbow bends and straightens, the muscle and its common tendon rub against the bony contour. This can cause gradual wear and tear of the muscle and tendon over time.

7.14.2 Pathogenesis

Microtears are present within the tendons and muscles after repetitive use and if a sufficient amount of rest is allowed, these will normally heal. If the body is unable to keep up with the amount of healing required, as the tendon is repetitively traumatised over time this becomes chronic and a difficult injury to treat. As it progresses the body is less likely to continue this sustained attempt at healing and instead produces fibrous tissue that weakens and degenerates the tendons.

7.14.3 Prevention

Repetitive tasks, especially when the arm is in full extension, put extra strain on the extensor origin of muscles and should be avoided.

7.14.4 Clinical features

Pain and tenderness on the epicondyles are pathognomonic of epicondylitis (**Table 7.5**).

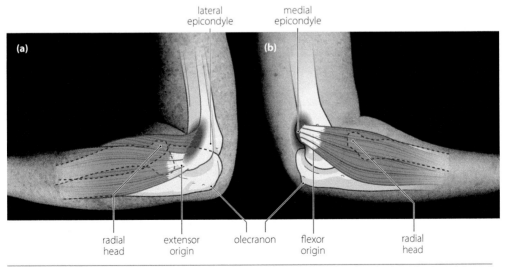

Figure 7.12 Extensor and flexor origins in the elbow: (a) lateral view showing the lateral epicondyle and origin of the forearm extensor muscles; (b) medial view showing the medial epicondyle and origin of the forearm flexor muscles.

Table 7.5 *Common features of epicondylitis*

	Lateral epicondylitis ('tennis elbow')	Medial epicondylitis ('golfer's elbow')
Location of pain and tenderness	Lateral epicondyle	Medial epicondyle
Muscle origin	Extensors	Flexors
Pain elicited	On resisted extension	On resisted flexion
Tasks avoided	Tasks in extension	Pronation and flexion

7.14.5 Management

Management is almost always conservative, with physiotherapy and symptom-reducing drugs. The main aim of physiotherapy is to retrain muscles in the elbow to work in normal harmony and avoid overusing other muscles. A splint is often useful because it enforces rest at the origin of the affected muscle.

Medication and physiotherapy

With medication, the aim is to dampen down any remaining inflammatory response to reduce pain, but it often doesn't solve the problem. Anti-inflammatory medications include a long-acting steroid injection to the epicondyle or oral NSAIDs.

Physical therapies aim to turn the chronic injury into an acute injury to restimulate the inflammatory process to reinvigorate the normal healing process. They include:

- deep tissue friction massage
- extracorporeal shockwave treatment
- ultrasound
- injections with plasma.

Surgery

Surgical treatment of tennis elbow involves releasing the ECRB muscle from its common extensor origin on the lateral epicondyle and restimulating the acute healing phase.

Prognosis

The success rate for all the treatments is highly variable. Surgery is a last resort because of its poor success rate.

7.15 De Quervain's tenosynovitis

De Quervain's tenosynovitis is a non-inflammatory process within the tendons of the first extensor dorsal compartment of the wrist (**Table 7.6**). Within this tendon sheath are the abductor pollicis longus and extensor pollicis brevis tendons which become thickened, degenerate and painful during movement.

7.15.1 Clinical features

Repetitive grasping and pinching activities usually precipitate this type of tendinopathy, producing pain and tenderness over the radial side of the wrist. Finkelstein's test, which passively stretches the tendons by ulnar deviating the hand with the thumb tucked in a grasp, usually precipitates the pain (**Figure 7.13**).

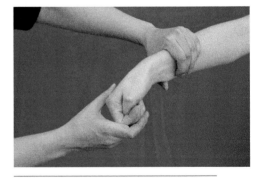

Figure 7.13 Finkelstein's test. The thumb is placed in the palm and the wrist is passively stretched towards the ulnar side, causing pain over the first dorsal compartment.

Table 7.6 *Extensor compartments at the wrist*

Compartment	Tendons	Action
I	Extensor pollicis brevis	Extension of thumb at MCPJ
	Abductor pollicis longus	Abduction of thumb at CMCJ
II	Extensor carpi radialis brevis	Extension and radial deviation at the wrist
	Extensor carpi radialis longus	
III	Extensor pollicis longus	Extension of the distal phalanx of thumb
IV	Extensor indicis	Extension of the index finger
	Extensor digitorum communis	Extension of the index to little fingers
V	Extensor digiti minimi	Extension of the little finger
VI	Extensor carpi ulnaris	Extension and ulnar deviation at the wrist

7.15.2 Management

Resting the tendons in a wrist splint is often enough to alleviate the symptoms.

Medication

Although this is a non-inflammatory condition, often friction of the tendons can cause inflammation of the tendon sheath and a local steroid injection may settle the pain symptoms. A resting splint and analgesics are also used.

Surgery

Surgery is only indicated very rarely when symptoms do not settle with conservative measures. This includes releasing the tendons from their sheaths, preventing the friction and inflammation.

7.16 Trigger finger

Trigger finger is a condition where the finger is locked or catches when the finger is flexed, making it difficult and painful to straighten. It is caused by inflammation and swelling of the flexor tendon synovium which can bunch and form a small bump in the tendon. This tendon bump can get caught in the pulleys of the finger, causing it to click or become trapped.

7.16.1 Clinical features

Patients describe a clicking or locked bent finger which suddenly pops out straight and is painful ('triggering'). Sometimes a nodule in the tendon can be felt when the finger moves.

7.16.2 Management

Resting the finger to reduce inflammation or taking NSAIDs is generally effective, and symptoms will improve over a couple of months. Steroid injection into the tendon sheath and using a splint can also reduce this inflammation. Surgically releasing the tendon sheath (A1 pulley) so the tendon can move freely is usually offered if conservative management fails.

DISORDERS OF THE FOOT

Akin to the hand, the foot is a complex structure of tendons, fascia and ligaments that are prone to sporting and overuse injuries. Generally, modification of activity, footwear and rest are the mainstay of treatment, with surgery only used in refractory disorders.

7.17 Bunions

Bunions, or hallux valgus, are a deformity of the great toe where the toe points away from the midline in towards the other toes (valgus) and causes the metatarsal head to move medially away from the other toes. Bunions are a common condition and present in all age groups.

7.17.1 Aetiology

Although associated with tightly fitting and high-heeled shoes, the aetiology of bunions is multifactorial. Hypermobility, flat fleet (pes planus), short first metatarsal and tight calf muscles are common causes of biomechanical instability and over pronation of the foot that precipitate the deformity.

7.17.2 Pathogenesis

Increased pronation of the foot increases pressure on the great toe, pushing it towards the other toes. The pull of flexor hallux longus tendon that inserts onto the great toe increases this deformity and over time the medial joint capsule around the MTP joint stretches.

7.17.3 Clinical features

The great toe is deviated towards the lesser toes and the metatarsal head deviates medially away from the lesser toes. A bump is also seen and may have skin changes where the bunion has rubbed on footwear. Some patients complain of pain, especially when walking.

7.17.4 Investigations

Radiographs of the feet when standing show the position of the foot when under the greatest stress and may reveal deformity not seen when not weight-bearing. OA is commonly associated with hallux valgus and if present would alter the surgical treatment plan.

7.17.5 Management

Modifying footwear and correcting flat feet with orthotics should be offered first before considering any surgical treatment. Most patients will get symptom resolution following these simple measures and surgical management is reserved for those who continue to have pain. Surgical options depend on the severity of the deformity and include tightening of the joint capsule (soft tissue rebalancing), realignment of the bone with an osteotomy, or joint fusion in those with OA.

7.18 Plantar fasciitis

Thickening and inflammation of the plantar fascia occur after chronic overuse or a sudden increase in activity. This causes pain and stiffness in the heel and sole of the foot and can be difficult to treat.

7.18.1 Epidemiology, aetiology and pathogenesis

Plantar fasciitis can occur at any age and is associated with repetitive stress. Increased stress on the plantar fascia can occur after wearing inadequately cushioned footwear, or from biomechanical deficiencies such as flat feet. Its pathogenesis is similar to tendinopathy, with an acute inflammatory stage. However, it generally turns into a chronic state and the body fails to continue its repetitive repair, making the plantar fascia thickened and weak.

7.18.2 Clinical features

Pain around the heel and sole of the midfoot when walking is the most common symptom. This pain may be worse in the morning when first getting out of bed or after prolonged walking.

7.18.3 Investigation and management

Diagnosis is made clinically but when there is diagnostic doubt, ultrasound or MRI can demonstrate the thickened plantar fascia.

Management

Using NSAIDs, ice and rest are the most important first-line treatments, supplemented with heel pad orthotics. Achilles and plantar fascia stretching exercises will improve most patients' symptoms.

Surgery

Corticosteroid injections are painful and carry a small increased risk of rupturing the plantar fascia, but do improve symptoms in some people. Releasing the plantar fascia surgically can help in very resistant cases.

Prognosis

Despite treatment, plantar fasciitis is often a chronic condition and can take up to 12 months to improve.

> **Plantar fasciitis and tendinopathy are common conditions but can be difficult to treat.** It is important to manage the patient's expectations. A patient may give up on their physiotherapy or orthotics if they do not see improvement in two weeks, but may persist with treatment if they understand that they might not see a benefit for a few months.

7.19 Achilles tendon rupture

In rupture of the Achilles tendon, there is a sudden force which tears the fibres of the tendon. This can be partial or a complete tear, where complete continuity of the tendon is lost.

7.19.1 Aetiology and clinical features

Achilles tendon rupture often occurs during a sporting activity, especially in people who don't often play sport. Patients report a sudden pain and snapping sound: *"it sounded and felt like I was shot in the calf"*. Swelling behind the ankle and an inability to perform active plantar flexion of the ankle (stand on tiptoes) are also common features. A gap or sulcus in the line of the tendon is palpable at the site of rupture. When the calf is squeezed, there is also a loss of plantar flexion of the ankle, indicating a positive Thompson or Simmonds' test (**Figure 7.14**).

The Achilles tendon is at higher risk of rupture when there is reduced blood flow and a reduction in the tendon's ability to regenerate after injury. These risk factors include:

■ chronic degeneration of tendon (tendinopathy)

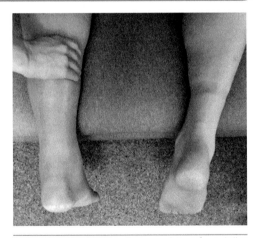

Figure 7.14 Thompson/Simmonds' test for Achilles tendon rupture: the foot is dangled over the edge of the bed and the calf is gently squeezed. If the foot plantar flexes this is a negative test and the tendon is intact (right); if there is no movement and the foot remains dorsiflexed the tendon is ruptured this is a positive test (left).

■ diabetes mellitus
■ steroid injection or supplement
■ fluoroquinolone antibiotics.

7.19.2 Management

Both partial and complete Achilles tendon tears can be treated non-operatively using a plaster cast or boot with the ankle plantar flexed and gradually brought up to neutral with serial casting over a 6–9-week period. Surgery to repair the tendon reduces the risk of re-rupture very slightly but has risks, such as poor wound healing. Surgery also does not necessarily allow an earlier return to activity. Physiotherapy after tendon injury or repair is essential to improve strength and range of movement of the ankle (**Table 7.7**).

Table 7.7 Achilles tendon healing			
	Inflammatory phase	**Fibroblastic phase**	**Remodelling phase**
Time	3–5 days	1–6 weeks	6 weeks to 9 months
Action	Fibrin clot	Collagen and matrix formed but is disorganised	Collagen and matrix formed into a cross-linked pattern

CHRONIC MUSCULOSKELETAL PAIN

7.20 Fibromyalgia

Fibromyalgia is a common condition characterised by chronic pain and tenderness affecting the soft tissue musculoskeletal structures, primarily the muscles. It is not associated with any inflammation or joint damage but is a pain disorder, thought to be caused by an amplification of the pain signals transmitted through the nervous system. It is associated with fatigue, non-refreshing sleep and poor concentration and is linked to other conditions such as irritable bowel syndrome and migraine. The condition can have a significant impact on a patient's quality of life and levels of function, although this can be improved with education and regular self-management.

7.20.1 Epidemiology

The prevalence of fibromyalgia is around 2–5% but it is underdiagnosed. Women are affected more than men. The condition is most commonly diagnosed between the ages of 20 and 50 years. Prevalence increases in patients who have relatives with fibromyalgia and those with other musculoskeletal disorders such as RA (sometimes termed 'secondary fibromyalgia'). There is also a link with lower socioeconomic status.

7.20.2 Aetiology

The aetiology is unknown. Fibromyalgia and other pain syndromes cluster in families. It is not clear how much of this is down to genetics or the shared physical and social environment. There are links to life events such as trauma or emotional stress and mental health problems.

7.20.3 Pathogenesis

The pathogenesis is unknown but the most commonly adopted explanation is that pain perception is altered due to either abnormal chemical signals in the nervous system or an exaggerated response in the brain resulting in an amplified pain response. There is no damaging pathological process such as inflammation within the affected joints or muscles and these structures remain normal.

Patients commonly report reduced quality and quantity of sleep which often precipitates an ongoing cycle of fatigue, pain and stress/anxiety/depression.

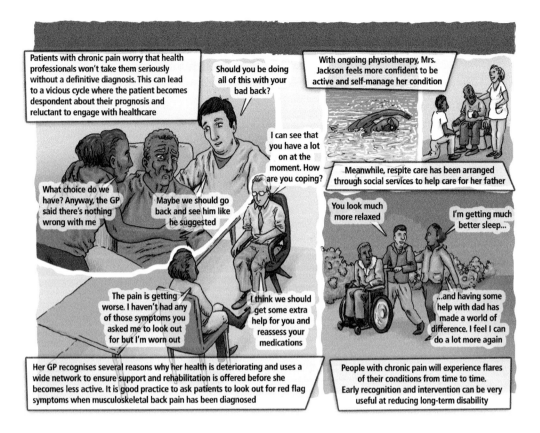

7.20.4 Clinical features

Symptoms can vary from person to person but include:

- pain (widespread)
- tenderness on examination (widespread, affecting large muscle groups on gentle palpation)
- fatigue
- sleep disturbance (difficulty getting to sleep/ frequent waking/early rising/non-refreshing)
- memory disturbance, cognitive problems, poor concentration (often described by patients as "brain fog")
- headaches
- dizziness
- aversion to bright lights/loud sounds
- concurrent diagnoses including anxiety, depression, irritable bowel syndrome and irritable bladder syndrome.

7.20.5 Diagnostic approach

The diagnosis of fibromyalgia is based on clinical features and the exclusion of other musculoskeletal conditions such as inflammatory arthritis or connective tissue disease. Patients will have a chronic history going back months or years of musculoskeletal pain and tenderness associated with fatigue, non-refreshing sleep and poor concentration with widespread soft tissue tenderness, often on only light palpation.

7.20.6 Investigations

Investigations are only carried out to rule out an alternative diagnosis, e.g. RA, Sjögren's syndrome or hypothyroidism.

7.20.7 Management

There is no cure or straightforward treatment for fibromyalgia. However, it is important to reassure patients that, with education, advice and support, they can self-manage their condition. Patients usually require a combination of bespoke treatments. Physical and psychological therapies are usually more effective at managing the condition than drug treatment. The principles of management are to:

- improve activity levels, stamina and muscle strength with graded exercise
- improve sleep using sleep hygiene techniques
- treat any concurrent or associated conditions, e.g. inflammatory arthritis, depression.

Physical therapies

A physiotherapist can help patients stay active and independent using exercises to strengthen muscles, improve posture and gradually increase levels of physical activity. This is usually the best way to help control symptoms. An occupational therapist can help manage daily activities and function. Pain management programmes and psychological therapies such as cognitive behavioural therapy may be helpful.

Drug treatments

Drugs may be used to help with pain (e.g. paracetamol, codeine), sleep or depression (e.g. amitriptyline, nortriptyline, duloxetine, gabapentin, pregabalin). Single or combination drug therapies may enable patients to start physical therapies but should not be used as the only treatment.

Prognosis

Prognosis is variable from person to person and may be influenced by other comorbidities. Education and sustained self-treatment can improve symptoms, function and quality of life and can manage the condition. However, relapses can occur, particularly during times of physical or emotional stress.

7.21 Answers to starter questions

1. The femoral notch is narrower in women, which impinges the ACL, causing it to become stuck in the notch and stretched. Ligaments in women are also more relaxed due to the effect of hormonal oestrogen, making the joints more mobile and likely to tear. The incidence of ACL injuries is also thought to vary according to the menstrual phase, although the reason for this is unknown.

2. In the absence of any red flag symptoms (see *Chapter 10*), apophysitis is a common cause of musculoskeletal pain in children and adolescents. The apophysis is a secondary ossification site and a site in which tendons insert onto bone. Excessive loading or repetitive movements can put strain on the apophysis, causing pain. As the apophysis remodels into adult bone and the growth plate closes, the pain subsides after puberty. This usually occurs earlier in girls than boys and is dependent on the site of the apophysis. In the calcaneus where the Achilles tendon inserts (Sever's disease) the apophysis fuses in girls between 12 and 14 years of age, and in boys between 15 and 17 years.

3. The causes of tendinopathy are multifactorial and therefore difficult to treat. The most common scenario is a history of repeated microtrauma such as repetitive movement causing tendon degeneration. If microtrauma is not stopped by resting, the tendon becomes degenerate as the ability to repair is overwhelmed by the repeated trauma causing fibrous granulation tissue to be substituted for healthy tissue. Tendons are relatively avascular and therefore healing inflammatory cells find it difficult to access the damaged area. The body's signalling system fails to recognise this as an injury and no further attempt of healing is started. Once in this state it becomes even more difficult to treat. Turning the degenerate tendon into an acute injury by deep friction massage, shockwave treatment or careful surgical microablations can restimulate the blood flow and inflammatory process and hopefully the tendon will heal normally.

Chapter 8
Infection

Starter questions

1. Why is septic arthritis a clinical emergency?
2. Why is it essential to recognise, diagnose and manage bone and joint infection promptly and efficiently?
3. Why is it important to identify the causative organism responsible for bone and joint infections, and how may this influence treatment?

Answers to questions are to be found in *Section 8.4*.

Bone and joint infections are potentially life- and limb-threatening, because untreated infection or treatment delay results in rapid destruction of bone and cartilage. This can lead to arthritis and/or deformity and permanent loss of function. A high index of clinical suspicion is required to ensure prompt diagnosis, early treatment and good outcome. For example, if a patient is elderly or immunocompromised or there is a history of recent infection, then bone or joint infection should always be considered as part of the differential diagnoses. Similarly, whilst infection is an uncommon cause of back pain, it is extremely important to recognise suspicious symptoms ('red flags') and be alert to the possibility of spinal infection, which is often a delayed diagnosis.

Identification of the causative organism through appropriate tissue sampling is key to successful management. Thus, aspiration of any potentially infected joint and microbiological testing of the aspirate should in general be performed prior to starting antibiotic treatment. Often patients require prolonged courses of combination antibiotic therapy and response may be slow. An infected prosthetic joint requires specialist orthopaedic assessment and management, as removal of the joint replacement may be necessary to eradicate the infection.

The musculoskeletal system can also be affected indirectly by infection in the form of reactive arthritis, where an infection elsewhere in the body triggers an inflammatory arthritis. This is discussed in *Section 3.5*.

Case 8.1 Acute, hot swollen joint

Presentation

Michael Green, a 35-year-old man, attends the Emergency Department with a painful, hot, swollen knee. It has developed quickly over the previous 24 hours and he is now unable to bend his knee or walk unaided.

Case 8.1 *continued*

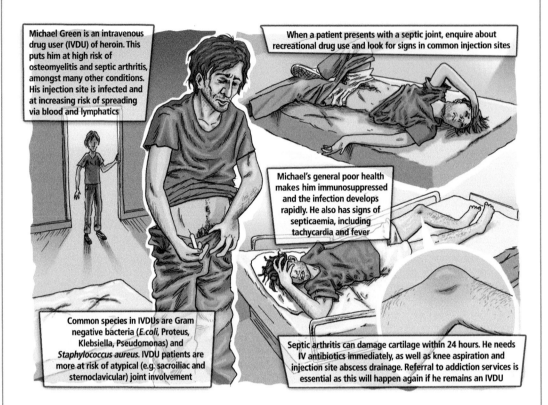

Michael Green is an intravenous drug user (IVDU) of heroin. This puts him at high risk of osteomyelitis and septic arthritis, amongst many other conditions. His injection site is infected and at increasing risk of spreading via blood and lymphatics

When a patient presents with a septic joint, enquire about recreational drug use and look for signs in common injection sites

Michael's general poor health makes him immunosuppressed and the infection develops rapidly. He also has signs of septicaemia, including tachycardia and fever

Common species in IVDUs are Gram negative bacteria (*E.coli*, Proteus, Klebsiella, Pseudomonas) and *Staphylococcus aureus*. IVDU patients are more at risk of atypical (e.g. sacroiliac and sternoclavicular) joint involvement

Septic arthritis can damage cartilage within 24 hours. He needs IV antibiotics immediately, as well as knee aspiration and injection site abscess drainage. Referral to addiction services is essential as this will happen again if he remains an IVDU

Initial interpretation

The speed of onset, and the degree of disability and functional impairment is concerning in such a young man. It is important to consider if there are any precipitating factors (e.g. trauma, recent surgery, infection or other illnesses) or if Michael has had anything like this before? He requires urgent further assessment.

History

Michael's left knee began hurting yesterday and quickly became more swollen during the day. The knee began to feel hot and he noticed redness over the joint. He had a disturbed night's sleep and neither paracetamol nor ibuprofen provided any significant pain relief. This morning he is in considerable pain and is having great difficulty bending the knee or bearing weight on his left leg.

Interpretation of history

Michael is describing inflammatory symptoms (pain, stiffness, swelling, heat, redness) which have occurred rapidly over a 24-hour period, resulting in loss of movement and functional disability. He has not responded to anti-inflammatory medications (paracetamol or ibuprofen) because of the severity of his symptoms.

Further history

Michael reports no previous problems with his joints. However, over the past week he has noticed a painful lump in his right groin and has been feeling feverish. He has never been in hospital before and denies taking any medications.

Examination

Michael looks unwell and appears to be in obvious pain. He is unable to get onto the examination couch without assistance because of extreme difficulty bending his left knee. His observations

Case 8.1 *continued*

are: temperature 38.4°C; pulse 112bpm; blood pressure 110/65mmHg. On inspection, the left knee is swollen and red; even on light palpation it is extremely tender and the joint feels hot; the knee is resting in a slightly flexed position and passive or active movement is not possible due to pain. There is a swelling in the groin which is about the size of a large egg; this is also tender and warm. There are multiple scars over both groins and also in both elbow creases. Other joints and general physical examination are normal.

Interpretation of findings

Michael is systemically unwell with a fever and tachycardia and has an acutely tender, hot, red, swollen left knee. Clinical findings also suggest the possibility of an abscess in his right groin and the scars over veins in his elbows and groins suggest IV drug use.

It is highly likely that he has septic arthritis affecting his left knee. This is a medical emergency and requires immediate aspiration and drainage of his left knee and IV antibiotics.

Investigations

Aspiration of the left knee reveals thick yellow/green fluid. Urgent microscopy and Gram stain demonstrate large numbers of polymorphs and Gram-positive cocci.

The blood results demonstrate:
- haemoglobin 11.2g/dl
- WCC 24.6 x 10⁹/L
- neutrophils 19.1 x 10⁹/L
- platelets 504 x 10⁹/L
- CRP 278mg/L.

This confirms high levels of inflammation and the neutrophilia suggests a bacterial infection.

Diagnosis

The diagnosis is septic arthritis of the left knee, probably due to *Staphylococcus aureus* infection. The cause is likely to be introduction of *Staphylococcus* from the skin during IV drug administration to the femoral vein in Michael's right groin and subsequent abscess formation, with bacteraemia and seeding of the infection in his left knee joint.

Immediately after aspiration of the left knee Michael should be started on high dose IV antibiotics including anti-staphylococcal and *Pseudomonas* coverage, whilst waiting for the culture and sensitivity results. The orthopaedic team should be contacted urgently, as he is also likely to need a washout procedure of his left knee, and he may need incision and drainage of the right groin abscess to help clear the infection. He should be closely monitored as he is at risk of developing septic shock and drug withdrawal.

He will require a prolonged course of IV followed by oral antibiotics in order to eradicate the infection and reduce the likelihood of joint damage, as septic arthritis can result in rapid joint destruction.

8.1 Septic arthritis

Septic arthritis is an infection of the joint space including the synovium. Usually only a single joint is involved but multiple joints can become infected, especially if the patient is immunocompromised. Prosthetic as well as native joints can be affected by septic arthritis, although this is usually referred to as prosthetic joint infection.

Acute septic arthritis is a clinical emergency, as demonstrated by *Cases 8.1* and *11.3*.

Joint symptoms causing an inability to bear weight or move the joint, in the presence of fever, raised WCC and ESR or CRP, are likely to be due to septic arthritis.

8.1.1 Epidemiology

Acute septic arthritis is more common in children, including neonates, than adults. Men are more frequently affected than women. There is a predilection towards the hip joint in children (the metaphyseal blood supply is within the joint capsule), although the knee is the most commonly infected joint in adults.

> Children with septic arthritis often don't directly localise their symptoms to the affected joint, e.g. hip pain may be referred to the knee, and they may also look well initially. Therefore, a limping child should have septic arthritis of the hip excluded as a priority.

8.1.2 Aetiology

There are several routes by which pathogens may gain access to a joint, including:
- haematogenous (via the bloodstream) from an infected site elsewhere in the body – this is the most common route
- extension of osteomyelitis from an adjacent metaphysis or epiphysis
- direct inoculation from iatrogenic intervention (e.g. surgical instrumentation) or penetrating injury.

Once in the joint, the pathogen triggers processes that cause rapid damage of articular cartilage (**Figure 8.1**). The typical causative organisms differ according to the patient's age and risk factors (**Table 8.1**). This information can be used to guide the choice of empirical antibiotic therapy until a definite organism has been identified and antibiotic sensitivities obtained.

There are a number of patient-related risk factors for septic arthritis associated with comorbid diseases, treatments and lifestyle factors (**Table 8.2**).

8.1.3 Clinical features

Patients with septic arthritis usually look unwell, are in pain and may manifest systemic signs of infection such as fever and tachycardia. Fever and tachycardia indicate a host versus pathogen response, whilst low blood pressure indicates the possibility of septic shock.

An infant might be restless and not feeding. Parents may report pseudoparalysis, i.e. reduced movement of the affected joint or limb, or not walking at all. Patients of any age usually have a short history of sudden onset of a painful, swollen and warm joint with inability to move the joint or bear weight due to extreme pain.

The surface overlying a septic joint is usually erythematous, warm and tender to palpation. However, this may not always be the case, particularly in a deep joint such as the hip, or if the patient is immunocompromised. The joint is swollen due to the large amount of inflammatory fluid within the joint and thickened synovium. Movement in all directions is painful due to distension of the joint and stretching of the capsule, and movement is restricted due to protective muscle spasm.

There is usually a large amount of fluid in an infected joint, therefore the patient often rests the joint in the position of most comfort and least tension:
- In a hinged joint, this is usually in a slightly flexed position.
- In the hip, the leg is usually slightly externally rotated, abducted and flexed.

> **Knee pain can be due to referred pain from the hip.** In suspected joint infection, physical examination should include all joints, but particularly the joints above and below the symptomatic site, as well as the whole patient, looking for a source of infection.

It is very important to enquire specifically about any risk factors for infection, for example:
- recent illness (particularly urinary, respiratory or GI infection)
- travel (exposure to more unusual infectious sources)
- sexual history (risk of STIs)
- IV drug use (needle and skin contamination)
- recent surgery
- previous orthopaedic procedures
- history of previous episodes
- history of potentially immunosuppressive illnesses or medications, e.g. corticosteroids, immunosuppressants or chemotherapy.

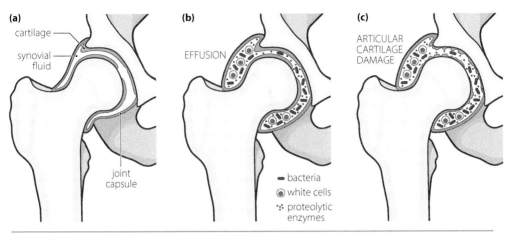

Figure 8.1 Pathogenesis of articular cartilage damage in septic arthritis: (a) normal joint; (b) early septic arthritis; (c) late septic arthritis.

Table 8.1 *Common organisms causing septic arthritis*	
Patient group	**Organism**
Infant	*Streptococcus*
	*Haemophilus**
Adolescent to adult	*Staphylococcus*
Sexually active	*Gonococcus*
Sickle cell anaemia	*Salmonella*
IV drug users	*Pseudomonas*
	Staphylococcus

* In unvaccinated infants and adults born prior to introduction of the vaccine in the early 1990s

Always ask about recent travel and take a sexual history, as this could help identify the cause of septic arthritis.

8.1.4 Diagnostic approach

An algorithm for diagnosis and treatment of a potentially septic joint is provided in **Figure 8.2**. A high index of clinical suspicion and thorough clinical assessment are required to inform an early diagnosis. This should always be confirmed by prompt aspiration of joint fluid (arthrocentesis) with urgent microscopy and Gram stain and subsequent culture for bacteria.

Table 8.2 *Risk factors for septic arthritis*	
Risk factor	**Examples**
Immunocompromised states	HIV, premature infant, organ transplantation, patients on steroids or other immunosuppressive treatments
Chronic systemic conditions	RA, diabetes mellitus, chronic renal failure
Obvious portals of infection	Skin ulceration, diabetic foot ulcers
Bone and joint surgery or intra-articular procedures	Steroid injections, arthroscopy, recent orthopaedic surgery
IV drug abuse	Injection through the skin into a blood vessel increases the risk of bacteraemia

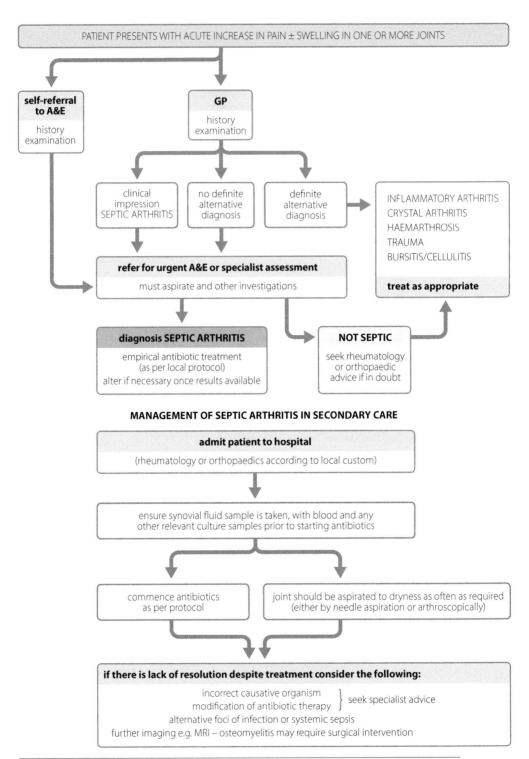

Figure 8.2 Algorithm for diagnosis of a potentially septic joint. Reproduced with permission of Oxford University Press from Coakley, G. *et al.* (2006) BSR & BHPR, BOA, RCGP and BSAC guidelines for management of the hot swollen joint in adults. *Rheumatology*, 45(8): 1039–1041.

8.1.5 Investigations

Arthrocentesis, as shown in **Figure 8.3**, is the essential investigation. It should be performed in all cases. Blood test results confirm systemic infection, and imaging is used to exclude other diagnoses or in cases of diagnostic uncertainty.

> In children, joint aspiration may be poorly tolerated without general anaesthetic, and therefore early referral to an orthopaedic surgeon is advised. An orthopaedic surgeon will consider further imaging such as ultrasound or MRI to confirm the presence of a joint effusion, and aspiration of the joint under anaesthesia.

Arthrocentesis

A sample of joint fluid is the most important diagnostic material and must be obtained in all patients, ideally before commencement of antibiotics to increase the likelihood of identifying the causative pathogen. Aspirated fluid must be sent urgently to the microbiology laboratory for microscopy, Gram staining and culture with testing for antibiotic sensitivity (**Figure 8.4**).

Microscopy should also look for crystals to exclude acute crystal arthritis, e.g. gout, which can have similar clinical features to septic arthritis.

A patient with a suspected infected prosthetic joint should be referred urgently to the orthopaedic team for further assessment *before* aspiration. If aspiration is required, it should be

GRAM STAIN POSITIVE (purple)	GRAM STAIN NEGATIVE (pink)
Staphylococcus aureus	*Neisseria gonorrhoeae*
Streptococcus	*Escherichia coli*
Clostridium	*Pseudomonas aeruginosa*

Figure 8.4 Gram stain of aspirated synovial fluid showing *Staphylococcus aureus*: Gram-positive (purple) cocci (round-shaped organisms) that clump together in groups like a bunch of grapes. Characteristic appearances of other organisms are also shown.

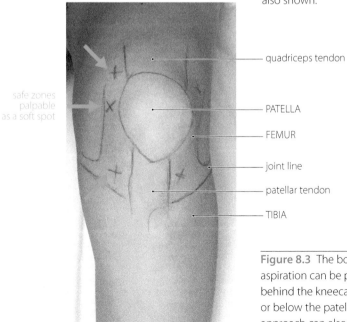

safe zones palpable as a soft spot

quadriceps tendon

PATELLA

FEMUR

joint line

patellar tendon

TIBIA

Figure 8.3 The bony landmarks for knee aspiration can be palpated. Safe zones enter behind the kneecap from either a soft spot above or below the patella. A direct lateral or medial approach can also be taken.

performed in a sterile environment, usually the operating theatre.

If arthrocentesis fails to draw fluid from the joint, ultrasonography is employed to localise any fluid and accurately guide aspiration. In deeper joints such as the hip, imaging-guided aspiration such as X-ray or CT is the preferred approach.

Blood tests

A septic screen (see *Section 2.5*) should always be done as part of the initial investigations to identify the causative pathogen. This requires sampling of multiple potential sources of infection, e.g. joint, blood, urine, skin, throat, sputum, and open wounds. It may confirm the site of infection and identify the pathogen and the most appropriate antibiotic(s) to be selected.

Typically, patients have raised white blood cells, neutrophils, ESR and CRP. These tests are also useful markers of treatment efficacy, as levels would be expected to fall in response to successful treatment.

U&Es should be checked regularly, as they may indicate deteriorating renal function which may occur with sepsis, and can guide fluid requirements.

Imaging

Plain radiography is rarely helpful in the diagnosis of septic arthritis but may show a joint effusion or demonstrate alternative diagnoses or incidental findings such as OA, chondrocalcinosis, fracture or, rarely, neoplasia. Signs that are more unusual include joint subluxation due to a large amount of intra-articular purulent fluid. Joint destruction may be visualised in cases of delayed diagnosis or prolonged symptoms, e.g. joint space loss, erosions and deformity.

Ultrasound is useful to confirm fluid in joints and can be used to guide arthrocentesis if 'blind' aspiration is unsuccessful.

MRI provides a more detailed assessment, visualising joint and soft tissue structures as well as bone (**Figure 8.5**), and is used when there is diagnostic uncertainty.

Paediatric patients may need sedation or anaesthesia to tolerate MRI as it takes time, they need to keep still and the scanner is a noisy and enclosed space. If a general anaesthetic is needed, it is often useful to transfer the child straight to the operating theatre for aspiration at the same time.

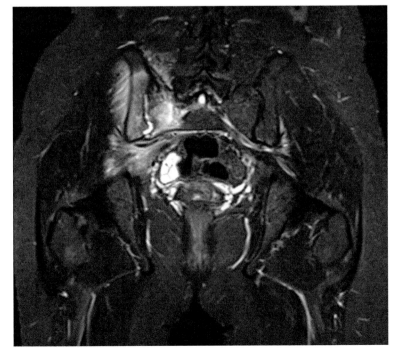

Figure 8.5 MRI demonstrating septic arthritis of the right sacroiliac joint. There is bright fluid in the right sacroiliac joint with extensive oedema in the bone on either side of the joint extending into the surrounding soft tissues.

8.1.6 Management

The aim is prompt treatment to eliminate the causative pathogen and chondrotoxic proteolytic enzymes from the joint space and synovium. Ideally, arthrocentesis is immediately followed by commencement of IV empirical antibiotic treatment and consideration of drainage of the joint to dryness by needle aspiration or arthroscopic washout.

> A negative Gram stain for joint fluid on microscopy does not exclude infection, particularly if there is strong clinical suspicion and/or the patient is elderly, immunocompromised or has received antibiotics prior to presentation.

Medication

If there is severe life-threatening sepsis, empirical IV antibiotic therapy is started immediately without waiting to aspirate the joint. In all other instances, empirical antibiotics are started straight after aspiration.

The choice of empirical antibiotic takes into account the specific clinical circumstances, local protocols and the advice of the local specialist microbiology service. Usually it comprises a combination of broad-spectrum antibiotics administered intravenously – for example benzylpenicillin with flucloxacillin, which will cover the most common causative organisms – whilst further microbiological information is awaited.

Once the causative pathogen(s) have been identified from the aspirate, the antibiotic selection is adjusted to match the confirmed sensitivity of the organism(s). A prolonged course is usually required, for weeks or even months.

Surgery

For the acutely septic joint, surgical washout should be performed as soon as possible to prevent the infection rapidly destroying the joint cartilage. An arthroscopic 'keyhole' technique is used or open arthrotomy is done to thoroughly wash out the joint with saline. Repeated washout procedures may be required, depending on the clinical course.

Management of infected prosthetic joints

In the infected prosthetic joint, management differs because there is no longer a threat to articular cartilage. Nevertheless, treatment is still urgent to prevent sepsis and, in acute infection, to save the primary prosthesis. More often, however, the joint has been infected for a long time before presentation because it has not been acutely painful. The decision then is whether the prosthesis needs to be removed and/or replaced. For these reasons, suspected infection in a prosthetic joint should be referred immediately to the orthopaedic team for assessment and aspiration.

Prognosis

Untreated septic arthritis quickly causes damage to articular cartilage and subsequent degenerative arthritis. Acutely, it may lead to systemic sepsis and septic shock. Outcomes can vary from return to normal function if treated promptly to severe cartilage damage leading to bony ankylosis. In prosthetic joints, recurrence of infection is more common, as bacteria avidly bind to the prosthetic joint material and are less susceptible to antibiotic treatment, so removal of the prosthesis and subsequent revision surgery may be required.

8.2 Osteomyelitis

Osteomyelitis is an infection of the bone. Left untreated, it results in local bone destruction, increasing the risk of fracture and deformity and can spread to cause systemic infection. There are several ways to classify osteomyelitis and one way is to describe its pathogenesis (**Table 8.3**).

8.2.1 Epidemiology

Osteomyelitis is an uncommon form of infection (approximately 20 cases per 100 000 patient years). The most common site is the spine in adults and long limb bones in children. It can

Table 8.3 *Classification of osteomyelitis on the basis of pathogenesis*

Cause	Mechanism	Example
Haematogenous	Infection travels from another source via the bloodstream	Endocarditis seeding bacterial emboli into the bloodstream
Contiguous	Inoculation from an adjacent tissue	Traumatic wounds, relating to orthopaedic implants, psoas abscess invading the lumbar vertebrae
Associated with vascular insufficiency	Diseases such as diabetes and peripheral vascular disease	Diabetic foot ulcers

present acutely as a new infection to the bone or as a chronic indolent infection following an initial insult that occurred at some time previously.

8.2.2 Aetiology

In osteomyelitis, there are several routes of infection:

- direct exposure to organism via an open wound resulting from trauma or an open fracture
- direct spread from a nearby structure such as soft tissue or joint infection
- secondary infection – the organism is seeded to bone from sepsis elsewhere.

Infection then spreads locally through the bone (**Figure 8.6**).

> Bacterial seeding usually occurs in the metaphysis due to tortuous capillaries in this region, causing the blood to slow and bacteria to diffuse into the bone.

Infection is usually bacterial; *Staphylococcus aureus* is the commonest organism (**Table 8.4**). About 5% of cases are caused by a mix of organisms. Chronic osteomyelitis can become persistent if inadequately treated; for example, if the antibiotic course is too short or the organism is not fully sensitive to the chosen antibiotic. This is more likely to occur in an immunocompromised patient, or in the presence of a prosthesis or metal from internal fixation of fractures. In rare cases of very persistent infection, organisms such as

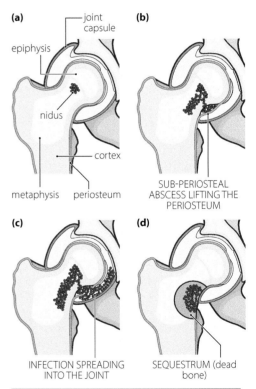

Figure 8.6 Pathogenesis and spread of infection in osteomyelitis: (a) a nidus is formed in the metaphyseal region: (b) a sub-periosteal collection forms, lifting the periosteum; (c) infection spreads to the joint; (d) sequestra (area of dead bone).

Mycobacterium and *Treponema* (syphilis) have been found to be responsible. In some cases, the infection comes and goes as a flare and is suppressed by antibiotics but is never fully cured.

Table 8.4 *Distinguishing features of osteomyelitis according to cause, including time of onset and haematogenous spread*

Origin	Organism	Feature	Onset
Skin*	*Staphylococcus aureus*	Most common organism	Acute or chronic
Colonisation of wounds	*Pseudomonas aeruginosa*	Wound is foul-smelling and green in colour; minimal systemic upset	Chronic
Urinary tract*	*Escherichia coli*	Haematogenous spread after urine infections	Acute or chronic
Oral cavity*	*Streptococcus* species	Common haematogenous spread after dental work	Acute
Airborne respiratory droplets	*Mycobacterium tuberculosis*	Consider in prolonged spinal infection	Chronic
Skin and mucous membranes*	Fungal infections, e.g. *Candida* and *Aspergillus*	Almost exclusively in the immunocompromised	Chronic
Soil, via intestinal tract	*Clostridium perfringens* (gas gangrene)	Severely unwell within hours	Acute

*Infection by the patient's native flora.

8.2.3 Clinical features

Patients usually have symptoms and signs of inflammation and infection. These may be subtle or incomplete in the immunocompromised patient or in chronic osteomyelitis. The classic clinical signs include:

- pyrexia and rigors
- redness, swelling and warmth over the infected area
- pain
- irritability in the young and delirium in the elderly
- worsening back pain in vertebral osteomyelitis
- night pain
- a non-healing ulcer or visible sinus tract in some patients.

However, not all patients exhibit these symptoms and signs of infection and a high index of clinical suspicion is important, e.g. in a patient with sepsis of unknown origin. Furthermore, there are differences between acute and chronic infections (**Table 8.5**).

Table 8.5 *Characteristics of acute and chronic osteomyelitis*

Condition	Feature
Acute	Swelling, pus formation, vascular congestion
Chronic	Large areas of necrosis and ischaemia and bone sequestra (areas of dead bone), or recurrence of acute case

8.2.4 Diagnostic approach

Particular points to consider in the clinical assessment are:

- Does the patient have any clues or risk factors for bone infection?
- Has there been recent surgery or are there other obvious portals of infection?
- Does the patient have other medical problems or medications that increase susceptibility to bone infection?

Such patients may deteriorate quickly, so prompt assessment and regular observation are important. If the patient is systemically unwell (e.g. pyrexia, tachycardia, hypotension), it is a medical emergency and you should assess as you would any septic patient. Additional investigations may help in cases of diagnostic uncertainty.

Tissue samples must be obtained for microbiological analysis to identify the causative organisms and inform antibiotic treatment choices. Preferably, this is done before initiating antibiotic therapy, because culture results can become negative once a broad-spectrum antibiotic is started, so the opportunity to identify the cause is missed. Early initiation of appropriate treatment increases the chance of achieving a good outcome.

8.2.5 Investigations

Diagnosing osteomyelitis often requires a combination of clinical assessment, blood tests, tissue sampling with microbiology analysis, and imaging.

Blood tests
Typically, patients have a raised WCC with a neutrophilia, raised inflammatory markers (e.g. CRP and ESR), and may have anaemia, as persistent inflammation can suppress red blood cell production.

Tissue samples
Samples and microbiology culture should be obtained from any potential sites of infection – e.g. wound swabs, urine, sputum or joint aspirate from a suspected septic joint – in order to attempt to identify the cause of infection.

Rarely, ultrasound or CT is required to accurately guide aspiration from a deep-seated abscess or intervertebral disc. A bone biopsy allows direct culture of organisms from the affected area. Biopsy is considered when the diagnosis is unclear or when the patient is not responding well to initial antimicrobial therapy.

> In suspected osteomyelitis, a full septic screen should always be included in the initial investigation, sampling multiple potential sources of infection – e.g. joint, blood, urine, skin, sputum, throat and open wounds – to identify the causative pathogen (see *Section 2.5*).

Imaging
Plain radiographs may show periosteal thickening, lytic lesions, loss of trabecular structure or new bone formation. However, they are often normal, particularly in the acute stages.

MRI is sensitive and often specific in identifying bone infection and can help determine the extent of involvement, particularly into adjacent bone and soft tissue structures (**Figure 8.7**). It can demonstrate bone destruction, bone marrow oedema and abscess formation (**Figure 8.8**). In the spine, it can help distinguish between infection and metastatic deposits.

CT is often less sensitive but may be useful in demonstrating soft tissue abscesses, sequestra and bone destruction, guiding a biopsy or aspiration and in patients who are unable to

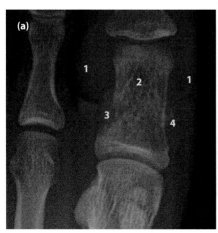
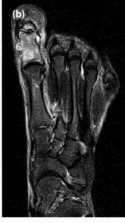

Figure 8.7 Osteomyelitis of the proximal phalanx of the great toe: (a) X-ray demonstrating soft tissue swelling ①, ill-defined lucency within the medullary bone ②, a breach of the bone cortex ③ and periosteal new bone formation ④; (b) MRI demonstrating oedema ⑤ with breaches of the cortical bone ⑥ and oedema extending through into the soft tissues ⑦.

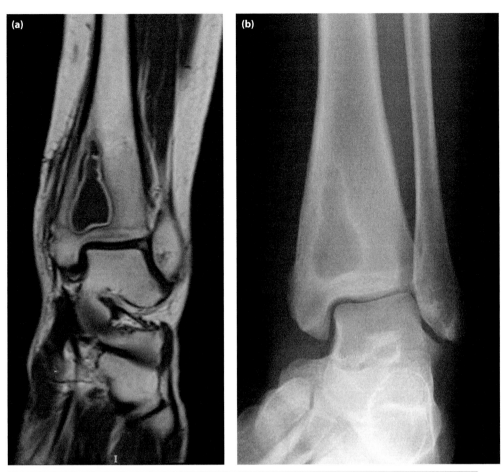

Figure 8.8 Osteomyelitis of the tibia with an intraosseous abscess (Brodie's abscess): (a) MRI showing a well circumscribed lesion in the medullary cavity of the distal metaphysis with an enhancing border but no direct communication outside the bone; (b) the lesion is visible but less obvious on X-ray; the surrounding bone looks normal and there is no obvious break in the cortex.

have an MRI scan, e.g. those with a pacemaker or metallic foreign bodies.

8.2.6 Management

Medical

In osteomyelitis, IV antibiotics are the mainstay of therapy. Often high doses of a combination of two antimicrobial agents are required for better bone penetration. Broad-spectrum antibiotics can initially be used to give coverage of the more common pathogens before results of sensitivities to the specific causative organisms are available.

The timing of the switch from IV to oral antibiotics will depend on the patient's clinical and biochemical response (e.g. CRP) but is not done until inflammatory markers have improved significantly and subsequent blood cultures have stopped growing bacteria.

Antibiotic therapy is usually required for at least 4–6 weeks, and in chronic cases much longer courses are needed.

> Assess for a good response to antibiotic treatment and ensure appropriate length of antibiotic therapy for good outcome.

Surgical

A poor response to antibiotic treatment may necessitate surgical debridement of the affected area. This is avoidable if the diagnosis is made early and treatment with the correct antibiotics is started promptly. Surgery is also indicated to remove any foreign body such as metal implants or sequestrum, as these act as a reservoir for bacteria to lie dormant, predisposing to recurrent infections.

Prognosis

Eradication of osteomyelitis is generally good with early diagnosis and accurate antibiotic management. Initiation of antibiotics before bony destruction occurs yields better outcomes. Eradication of osteomyelitis is poorer in the immunocompromised, elderly and patients with other comorbidities which may compromise healing, e.g. peripheral vascular disease or diabetes.

> Treating and eradicating deep infection, including osteomyelitis, in patients with diabetes is challenging due to the pathophysiological effects of diabetes. Complications include tissue necrosis and gangrene, which may require surgical amputation. Associated peripheral vascular disease may prevent surgical margins from healing, and patients can require further amputations of more proximal tissue.

8.3 Spinal infection

Infection of the spinal column is an emergency; it can be difficult to diagnose and needs to be considered with a high index of clinical suspicion. Delayed or suboptimal treatment may lead to bone destruction, spinal deformity and neurological compromise.

There are two types of infection of the spinal column:
- intervertebral discitis, i.e. infection of the disc
- vertebral osteomyelitis, which involves both the vertebra and the intervertebral disc.

8.3.1 Epidemiology

Intervertebral discitis is rare but is more common in children under 5 years of age.

Vertebral osteomyelitis is more common in adults aged 50–60 years, presenting more often in men than women.

8.3.2 Aetiology

Similar to other bone and joint infections, the potential sources of pathogens are:
- haematogenous spread (most common)
- iatrogenic (e.g. direct injection, surgery)
- direct spread (e.g. from adjacent retropharyngeal or retroperitoneal infection).

The reason discitis is more common in infants and younger children is that there is a blood supply into the nucleus pulposus of the intervertebral disc, allowing infection to enter directly from the bloodstream (haematogenous spread). The intervertebral disc becomes avascular in adulthood, making it an ideal harbour for infection, as the macrophages and phagocytic cells needed to fight infection are not delivered to the disc. The blood supply ends at the vertebral end-plate in adults; therefore infection first destroys one vertebral end-plate, subsequently extending to the disc space and then on to the adjacent vertebra (**Figure 8.9**).

Staphylococcus aureus is the most common organism in spinal infection. More recently, there has been an increased incidence of Gram-negative infections, particularly affecting the elderly. Certain patients may be more susceptible, for example:
- the elderly
- immunocompromised
- IV drug users
- diabetes mellitus
- malignancy
- recent urinary or chest infection.

8.3.3 Clinical features

Back pain is usually the predominant symptom. The onset of pain is usually gradual, of severe

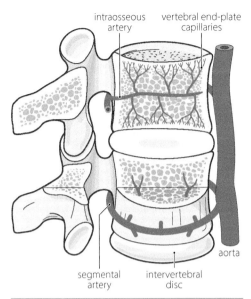

intraosseous artery   vertebral end-plate capillaries

aorta

segmental artery   intervertebral disc

Figure 8.9 The blood supply to the vertebral disc is supplied via the small capillaries of the end-plate; infection follows this vascular channel to the end-plate.

intensity and worsens with activity. Symptoms may vary in children and can be more non-specific in nature, including abdominal pain or loss of appetite.

Fever may be absent in the immuno-compromised, because such patients are less likely to exhibit the more classical symptoms and signs of infection.

Skin changes such as redness, warmth and swelling are usually much less obvious than in other bone infections, since the affected anatomical structures are situated much deeper below the skin. However, there may be point tenderness at the affected level and limited range of motion of the spine with spasm of the paraspinal muscles.

Careful assessment for neurological symptoms or signs is important, as these may indicate an associated epidural abscess or collection causing cord compression. Intercostal neuralgia may be a sign of thoracic-level infection. Paravertebral abscesses can track distally in the intermuscular planes and affect the sacroiliac or hip joints, so it is important to review any symptoms or signs at these sites. A Gibbus deformity can occur in

advanced TB, where bony destruction can result in wedge collapse of adjacent vertebrae and a kyphosis deformity. This may lead to pressure on the cord or nerve roots and even paralysis (Pott's paralysis).

8.3.4 Diagnostic approach

In a patient with new back pain, spinal infection should be suspected if:
- there are red flags for spinal cord compression; further assessment and investigation will be required (see *Section 2.2.10*)
- there are unexplained symptoms suggesting infection
- there is a recent history of infection elsewhere.

Often symptoms and signs are rather non-specific, particularly in children and the elderly. Any neurological symptoms and signs should prompt emergency referral for further clinical assessment and imaging assessment, usually with an MRI scan.

8.3.5 Investigations

Imaging is usually the most informative investigation in making a definite diagnosis, and MRI is the investigation of choice in most patients. Blood tests including raised CRP and WCC can provide clues towards an infective cause but are non-specific. As with other cases of musculoskeletal infection, identification of the causative pathogen is very important in selection of appropriate antibiotics and to increase the likelihood of a good outcome.

Imaging
Plain radiographs are often normal but may show loss of normal alignment. Loss of the normal lumbar lordosis (anterior curve) is often an indicator of paraspinal muscle spasm. Soft tissue changes such as loss of the psoas shadow may be subtle, suggesting a psoas abscess which can extend from an area of spinal infection. More obvious findings such as narrowing and irregular disc space, end-plate erosion or sclerosis and osteopenia can occur with ongoing chronic infection.

An isotope bone scan is highly sensitive in showing 'hotspots' of increased isotope uptake in areas of pathology, but lacks specificity for infection.

MRI, particularly with IV contrast, is the most sensitive and specific investigation for identifying spinal infection and is the most accurate imaging modality. Diagnostic findings include disc space narrowing, oedema in the adjacent vertebral bones, end-plate erosion and sometimes paraspinal, epidural and adjacent soft tissue inflammation (**Figure 8.10**).

Sometimes radiological-guided or even open surgical biopsy may be performed to provide a tissue sample for culture. If surgery is performed, tissue samples should be cultured to help identify causative organisms.

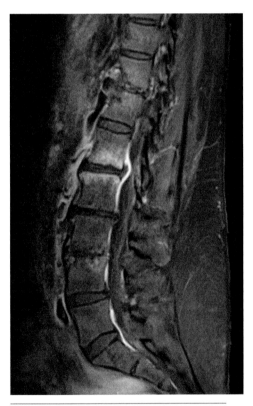

Figure 8.10 MRI demonstrating intervertebral discitis. There is oedema on either side of the L1/L2 intervertebral disc and some high fluid signal within the disc and enhancement of the surrounding soft tissues, indicating infection.

> The intervertebral disc space is classically preserved in metastatic spine disease, in comparison to infection, where it narrows.

Blood tests

Usually patients have a raised WCC, neutrophil count, ESR and CRP, consistent with active infection and inflammation.

Blood cultures are important to identify the organism responsible, as the most common cause is usually haematogenous seeding from an infection elsewhere. Careful tissue sampling and culture from any potential infected sites are crucial.

8.3.6 Management

The aim of treatment is to clear the infection and prevent spinal column destruction and neurological complications. Isolated infection can be managed non-operatively with appropriate antibiotics. Infection with the presence of neurological involvement, for example from an epidural abscess (infection around the spinal cord), almost always requires surgery.

Medical

Empirical IV antibiotics should be started based on the most likely organism. Blood, urine and sputum cultures should be obtained before commencing antibiotics, unless in severe sepsis, to increase the chance of isolating the causative pathogen. Nutritional support, analgesia and physiotherapy are important to aid recovery.

> In a non-responding spinal infection, TB should be considered. A long history of illness, HIV and back pain raises the likelihood. Culture for acid-fast bacilli is required to confirm the diagnosis.

Surgical

In the presence of a neurological deficit, surgery to remove or debride infected or necrotic tissue and decompression of the spinal cord or nerve root may be required. If bony destruction is advanced, the spine may become unstable; this may risk nerve or spinal cord compression and, in such cases, surgery is required to stabilise the spine. Options include removing the infected vertebral body (corpectomy) and stabilising the spine with instrumentation such as metal rods to provide supportive scaffolding. Antibiotics will still need to be administered after surgery.

Emergency surgery is required if there is any evidence of an associated epidural abscess or collection causing cord compression.

Prognosis

Response to treatment may be slow, and often prolonged courses of combination antibiotics are required. Potential complications of chronic severe infection include bone destruction, vertebral collapse, fusion and ankylosis of adjacent vertebral bones and spinal deformity.

Pott's disease is tuberculous infection of the spine and usually affects the thoracolumbar region. Collapse of two vertebral bodies and formation of an abscess in the area is known as a 'cold abscess' as it doesn't form an acute inflammatory response.

8.4 Answers to starter questions

1. Infection of a joint is usually due to bacteria rather than viruses. Within the joint, proteolytic enzymes produced by bacteria irreversibly damage the joint cartilage, resulting in premature degenerative changes, subsequent arthritis, deformity and loss of joint or limb function. Acutely, bacteraemia can lead to systemic septic shock.

2. Early recognition of bone or joint infection increases the chance of accurate diagnosis and isolation of the causative pathogen by appropriate investigations to guide antibiotic therapy. Poorly managed bone and joint infection leads to loss of joint function, with its negative effect on the quality of life of the patient. Treatment of chronic infection is costly, requiring lengthy antibiotics or multiple operations and a long hospital stay.

3. Identifying the causative organism allows the use of the most effective antimicrobial agent. There are 'usual suspects' or common causative organisms in certain at-risk patient groups. Empirical 'broad-spectrum' antibiotics are usually commenced in suspected bone or joint infection. Unless the patient is unwell (septic shock), it is best to start antibiotics after collecting specimens (blood culture, joint fluid aspirate, pus swab, etc.) to enable a higher chance of isolating the causative organism. In addition, isolation of the causative organism allows the use of more specific antibiotics, reducing the risks of antibiotic resistance and complications of broad-spectrum antibiotics.

Chapter 9
Spinal and peripheral nerve disorders

Starter questions

1. At what level of the spine is it safe to perform a lumbar puncture, and why?
2. Why is the thoracic spine more at risk of serious pathology than the lumbar spine?
3. Why are patients with diabetes more prone to developing peripheral nerve disorders?
4. Are nerve conduction tests always required for diagnosis of a peripheral nerve disorder?
5. Why does peripheral nerve compression cause pain as well as numbness?

Answers to questions are to be found in *Section 9.16*.

The spine is a flexible column of vertebral bones, separated by intervertebral discs, which supports the skull on the body, allows a range of upper body movements and protects the spinal cord (see *Section 1.10.2*). Like any other musculoskeletal structure, the spine is susceptible to pathological processes such as degeneration, infection, malignancy and fracture. However, because of its proximity to the spinal cord, any condition affecting the spine can also have serious neurological sequelae, including:

■ myelopathy – an upper motor neurone lesion affecting the cord

■ radiculopathy – a lower motor neurone lesion affecting the spinal nerves.

Peripheral nerves transmit the sensory, motor and autonomic communications from the brain and spinal cord to muscles and organs (see *Section 1.13*). They are susceptible to injury from sharp or blunt trauma, external compression and toxins because, unlike the spinal cord, they are relatively unprotected by the bony skeleton. Common examples include carpal tunnel syndrome and ulnar nerve compression.

Case 9.1 Acute thoracic back pain

Presentation

Janet Perry is 59 years old and is referred to the Acute Medical Unit with worsening back pain. She is unable to manage the pain with her current painkillers and is becoming distressed.

Initial interpretation

Although back pain is a very common presentation, it is crucial to find out more precise information about the nature and duration of Mrs Perry's symptoms and to enquire about red flags.

Case 9.1 *continued*

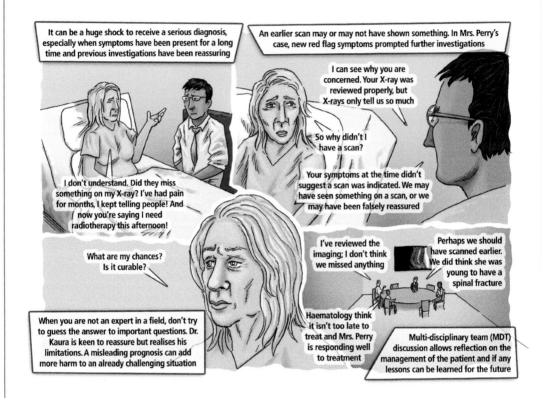

Any past medical history may also provide clues of an underlying pathological cause.

History

Mrs Perry has had back pain for six months. It is in the thoracic area of her spine and does not move anywhere else. She had an X-ray when she initially noticed the pain and was told she had a fracture due to thinning of the bones. This came as a surprise to her GP as she was not felt to be at risk for osteoporosis. In the past ten days her pain has become much worse and constant.

Interpretation of history

Thoracic back pain is a red flag, more likely to be caused by inflammatory, infective or malignant conditions than pain elsewhere in the spine. An acute-on-chronic pain raises concern that there is new pathology in the spine. She is young to have had an osteoporotic fracture without any specific risk factors for this.

Further history

Since her back pain began, Mrs Perry has been relatively immobile. She has lost half a stone in weight but thinks this is because she is eating less due to her pain. There has never been any trauma to her back. She doesn't report a fever, there are no bladder or bowel problems. She feels wobbly when she walks and has started to notice areas of numbness in her legs.

Examination

Mrs Perry is uncomfortable even lying at rest on the bed. Observations are normal. Examination reveals palpable tenderness of the thoracic and lumbar spine. Upper limb neurology is normal. Power is reduced in the lower limbs bilaterally to 4/5 on hip flexion and knee flexion and extension. There is reduced sensation within the dermatomes of L5/S1. Reflexes and tone are normal. Cardiovascular, respiratory and abdominal examinations are normal. However, palpation of the lymph nodes reveals a swollen cervical gland.

Interpretation of findings

Progressive thoracic back pain in a patient with weight loss and new neurology raises the suspicion of an infective or malignant process. Blood tests are important not only to establish whether there is an inflammatory response but also to look at bone markers including ALP and calcium which can be raised in malignancy affecting the bone. The neck lump could be unrelated but warrants investigation in a patient with red flag symptoms.

Investigations

FBC, LFTs, bone profile and U&Es were all normal. CRP was slightly elevated at 9mg/L. MRI of the spine demonstrated a tumour encompassing T7–T10 causing cord compression at levels T8–T9 (**Figure 9.1**). The biopsy of the neck lump was consistent with a non-Hodgkin's lymphoma. The spinal tumour was therefore also suspected to be lymphoma.

Diagnosis

The diagnosis here is non-Hodgkin's lymphoma affecting the glandular lymphatic tissue in the neck and the spine. The fracture first identified several months beforehand is likely to have been due to lymphoma that was, at that stage, undetectable radiologically. It is not unusual for there to be a delay in this diagnosis. Mrs

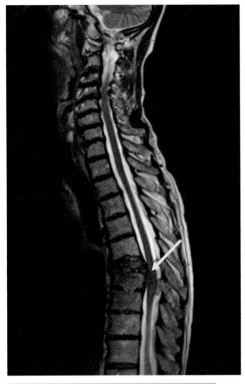

Figure 9.1 Sagittal MRI showing the tumour encroaching on the spinal cord (arrowed) and impacting on the vertebrae and discs.

Perry underwent emergency radiotherapy to the affected area of the spine, was commenced on high dose oral steroids to reduce swelling around the nerves and subsequently started chemotherapy for non-Hodgkin's lymphoma with curative intent.

Case 9.2 Numbness and pain in the hands

Presentation

Bill Taylor is a 55-year-old man who presents to his GP with symptoms of intermittent pain, numbness and weakness in both his hands over the last few months. He is finding it difficult to get dressed and to continue his work as a joiner.

Initial interpretation

When considering possible causes of limb numbness and weakness, it is important to consider pathological processes affecting the central nervous system (e.g. stroke, multiple sclerosis, Guillain–Barré syndrome) and peripheral nerves. In this instance a

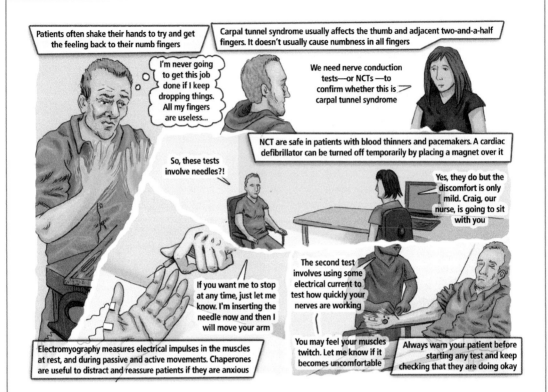

peripheral nerve compression is more likely as the weakness is intermittent and only the fine finger movements are affected, but myelopathy should also be considered.

History

Mr Taylor has a BMI of 32 (a healthy BMI is 18.5–24.9). His past medical history includes diabetes mellitus type II and hypertension, for which he takes metformin, simvastatin and lisinopril. He is experiencing pain during the night which wakes him from sleep and feels he needs to shake his hands to get them to 'wake up'. His little finger is not affected. After reading his morning paper he finds it difficult to fasten the buttons on his shirt and often drops his morning cup of tea. At work he feels his hand becomes painful and useless after long bouts of sawing.

Interpretation of history

Obesity and diabetes are risk factors for carpal tunnel syndrome. Repetitive tasks such as sawing

can exacerbate symptoms. Waking due to pain and numbness in the hands is common in carpal tunnel syndrome and patients can develop little tricks like shaking their hands to help relieve their symptoms.

Examination

Mr Taylor is examined using the look, feel, move approach. He has:

- wasting of the thenar muscles (**Figure 9.2**)
- loss of fine touch and two-point discrimination on index finger and thumb; normal sensation on the dorsum of first web space and the ulnar border of little finger
- weakness of thumb abduction against resistance; normal finger abduction and extension power
- negative Hoffman's test (see *Section 9.3.1*). Phalen's test (**Figure 2.22**) is positive after 20 seconds. Tinel's sign (**Figure 2.23**) is also positive.

Case 9.2 *continued*

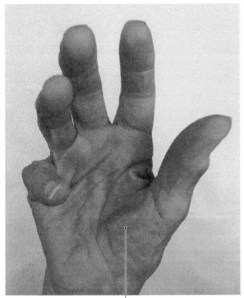

thenar eminence
muscle wasting

Figure 9.2 Thenar muscle wasting is seen in carpal tunnel syndrome.

Interpretation of findings

Weakness and wasting of thenar muscles that are supplied by the median nerve points to significant nerve compression, present for many months. Only the median nerve supplies sensation to the tip of the index finger and therefore loss of two-point discrimination in the index finger can only be due to median nerve dysfunction. A negative Hoffman's test suggests there is no myelopathy.

Investigations

No additional investigations are usually necessary. However, nerve conduction studies can be used when the diagnosis is uncertain, if suspecting more than one nerve compression or to determine the anatomical level of compression. EMG studies are rarely used in this case but can help measure the severity of nerve damage, which can be helpful for prognosis.

Diagnosis

Median nerve compression in the carpal tunnel is known as carpal tunnel syndrome (CTS) and is usually a clinical diagnosis. Due to his significant symptoms (persistence, functional impact, muscle weakness and wasting), Mr Taylor is referred to an orthopaedic hand surgeon for consideration of surgical decompression. In the meantime, resting night splints to keep the wrist extended are provided for symptomatic relief. Established numbness and wasting are indicative of possible permanent nerve damage, which will not improve after surgery. Patients should therefore ideally be referred before this happens.

9.1 Mechanical back pain

The term mechanical back pain is used for symptoms originating from the joints, bones or soft tissues around the spine, which does not necessarily have a specific or serious cause. It is the most common diagnosis for back pain, affecting 8 out of 10 people in their lifetime. It is a frequent reason for time off work and causes more disability worldwide than any other condition. It can occur anywhere along the spine, but the lumbar spine is most commonly affected.

Most back pain is self-limiting but you must always ask specific questions to ensure no red flag symptoms are present, as these may indicate a serious underlying cause. You should also ensure that all patients with mechanical back pain know it is important to seek medical attention if they develop any of these red flag symptoms.

9.1.1 Epidemiology

80% of the population will have at least one episode of lower back pain in their lifetime and

15–20% have at least one episode of back pain per year. Onset is most frequent between 35 and 55 years of age. Back pain is rare in children but increases in adolescence. There are no sex differences in prevalence.

9.1.2 Aetiology

The most common cause of back pain is mechanical, making up 80–90% of cases. Other causes include osteoporosis, infection, fracture, degeneration and malignancy. The risk factors for mechanical back pain are:
- obesity
- smoking
- depression
- work-related stress
- posture (e.g. prolonged standing or awkward lifting)
- tall stature
- increasing age.

9.1.3 Prevention

Prevention of mechanical back pain is by addressing risk factors. Strengthening and flexibility exercises are useful but not many people incorporate these into their daily lives. Good work practices are essential, e.g. training in manual handling and lifting, provision of equipment and advice from occupational health on appropriate workstations.

9.1.4 Pathogenesis

Mechanical back pain can be caused by degeneration of the intervertebral discs and facet joints or injury to muscle or ligament structures. Local inflammation, triggered for example by an awkward movement or excessive weight load, causes pain and leads to inactivity and subsequently to loss of muscle strength. The patient is then susceptible to further injury.

9.1.5 Clinical features

Pain may start suddenly, after a sudden movement, or may build up gradually. It tends to be isolated to one area of the back, typically the lumbar spine, but it can move, for example to the buttocks and sometimes down the leg in the case of sciatica. Movement of the back, including when coughing, exacerbates pain. Numbness and weakness in the legs is uncommon but can happen intermittently.

Examination is difficult if the patient is in pain. Spinal tenderness is not usually present and the neurological examination is normal. Note that power and range of movement can be altered due to pain even in the absence of a specific neurological cause, but the reflexes should be normal.

Checking for saddle anaesthesia and anal tone is vital if there is any suspicion of serious pathology, e.g. myelopathy or cauda equina syndrome.

'Red flag' symptoms, which suggest a serious underlying cause, are:
- age of onset <20 years or >55 years
- recent violent trauma, or minor trauma in someone with osteoporosis
- constant progressive pain, severe at night
- thoracic pain
- past medical history of malignancy, prolonged use of corticosteroids, drug abuse, HIV or immunosuppression
- systemically unwell (e.g. weight loss, fever)
- widespread neurological symptoms (e.g. loss of bladder or bowel control, saddle anaesthesia).

9.1.6 Diagnostic approach

A detailed history must include ruling out any red flag symptoms. Examination should include a thorough neurological assessment. If no red flag symptoms or signs are present, and there is a reasonable suspicion of mechanical back pain, then no further investigations are required. All patients should be advised to seek further medical attention if they develop any red flag neurological symptoms. This is called a 'safety net'.

Urgent neurosurgical referral is required in the presence of saddle anaesthesia, disturbances in bowel or bladder control, weakness or sensory disturbance affecting the legs, as these findings may indicate cauda equina syndrome.

9.1.7 Investigations

Investigations are not often necessary unless the diagnosis is in doubt or there are red flag symptoms or signs.

MRI is the gold standard for imaging the back because it gives great detail on all of the structures. A plain X-ray is only useful if a vertebral fracture is suspected. These X-rays give more than 100 times the dose of radiation that a chest X-ray does and are often not diagnostic.

Blood tests are useful if an infectious or inflammatory cause is suspected. A raised ALP is not specific but can be a sign of increased bone turnover in malignancy.

9.1.8 Management

Patients should be encouraged to stay as active as possible. Short-term use of analgesia can be useful to enable patients to participate in exercise. Ideally, all patients would see a physiotherapist for guidance on back strengthening and flexibility exercises. All patients should receive written information on exercises and self-management.

Medication

Paracetamol and NSAID tablets may help relieve pain.

Prognosis

90% of cases are self-resolving within 6 weeks. These patients may go on to experience recurrences of pain and the remaining 10% of patients go on to experience chronic back pain. Yellow flags can identify those patients more at risk for developing chronicity. These include emotional factors (low mood, social withdrawal, anxiety), high expectation of medical treatment rather than active physiotherapy, and a belief that back pain is disabling.

SPINAL DISORDERS

In the spine, two elements of the nervous system are compressible:
- In myelopathy, the spinal cord itself is compressed.
- In radiculopathy, the spinal nerve roots (the radicals) are compressed.

Compression of the spinal cord most commonly occurs in the cervical region; it causes myelopathy symptoms at or below the compression level. In contrast, compression to a nerve root most commonly occurs in the lumbar spine at L4 or L5 levels; it causes radiculopathy symptoms specific to the distribution of that nerve root. Myelopathy and radiculopathy are terms used to describe the symptoms experienced by the patient rather than the disease process itself.

9.2 Radiculopathy

Compression of a spinal nerve root causing radicular symptoms is most commonly caused by:
- a prolapsed spinal intervertebral disc
- a tumour – either in the nerve sheath itself, an osteosarcoma, or from metastatic spread of a primary tumour elsewhere
- infection causing inflammation of the nerve.

A prolapsed disc is the usual cause, compressing the nerve as it exits from the spinal cord through the lateral foramen.

Radiculopathy has pure lower motor neurone symptoms and signs arising from the nerve root with weakness, hypotonia, hyporeflexia, muscle atrophy and sensory symptoms with numbness or tingling.

9.2.1 Clinical features

Compression of a specific nerve root causes radiculopathy, with sensory symptoms in the skin (dermatome) supplied by the nerve root and weakness in the muscles (myotome) innervated by that nerve root. Pain can be sharp, burning or shooting, worsened by movement and coughing and sneezing, and often spreads into the area supplied by the nerve root.

For example, if there is a C7 radiculopathy, there is pain and sensory symptoms from the neck down to the middle finger of the hand, weakness of elbow and wrist extension and loss of the triceps reflex.

In L5 radiculopathy, there are symptoms of sciatica, with pain radiating down the back of the leg below the knee, restricted straight leg raising, weak great toe dorsiflexion, and reduced sensation in the anterolateral leg and on the dorsum of the foot.

Table 9.1 summarises the typical clinical findings when an intervertebral disc prolapse results in nerve root compression and radiculopathy.

9.2.2 Diagnostic approach

Careful clinical assessment and correlation of findings with MRI are essential to confirm the diagnosis, identify the cause and to inform any surgical management.

9.2.3 Management

Most radiculopathies are caused by a prolapsed disc and will settle spontaneously with conservative management using analgesia, physiotherapy and positive reassurance. Surgical decompression is required in cases of severe motor loss, e.g. foot drop, or persistent or progressive symptoms.

Table 9.1 *Clinical findings of the most common sites of intervertebral disc prolapse*

Site of disc prolapse	Spinal root affected	Clinical signs
C6/C7	C7	Pain radiates from the neck down the arm to the middle finger
		Numbness occurs in the middle finger
		Weakness occurs in elbow extensors and wrist flexors
		Triceps reflex is lost
L4/5 Lateral disc	L4	Pain from back to mid-calf
		Numbness in lateral thigh, anterior knee and medial leg
		Weakness in ankle dorsiflexion
L4/L5 Paracentral disc	L5	Pain from back into leg/foot
L5/S1 Lateral disc		Numbness occurs in lateral calf and great toe
		Weakness occurs in extension of the great toe
L5/S1 Paracentral disc	S1	Pain from back into leg/foot
		Numbness occurs in the posterior calf and little toe
		Weakness occurs in plantarflexion of the ankle
		Ankle reflex is lost

9.3 Myelopathy

The most common cause of myelopathy is cervical spondylosis, where degenerative changes in the intervertebral disc (often with subsequent prolapse), arthritis with osteophyte formation and bony and ligamentous thickening, combine over time to cause narrowing of the spinal canal and compression of the spinal cord. Acute compression can also occur due to trauma, infection or ischaemia. Myelopathy is the functional deficit that results from the spinal cord being compressed (an upper motor neurone lesion) and hence unable to transmit signals appropriately.

9.3.1 Clinical features

The site, severity of compression and speed of onset will determine the clinical features. Characteristically in cervical radiculopathy there will be lower motor neurone signs (e.g. weakness, flaccid tone, reflex loss) at the level of the lesion (e.g. a C6/7 disc protrusion will affect the C7 nerve root). Upper motor neurone signs in myelopathy (spastic tone, increased reflexes) are below the level of the lesion. Pain may or may not be present. Symptoms tend to evolve slowly, initially with mild numbness and weakness but over time progressing to more severe weakness and functional loss, e.g. poor gait or loss of dexterity, depending on the level of the lesion.

For example, cervical myelopathy due to spondylosis usually causes gradual onset of limb weakness, progressing to spasticity and hyperreflexia, especially in the legs, classically with clonus and positive Hoffman's and Babinski signs.

> **Hoffman's sign** – in a positive test, flicking the middle fingertip results in flexion of the thumb and index finger.

> **Babinski sign** – in a positive test, stroking the sole of the foot from the lateral border to medial across the metatarsal heads with a sharp object results in extension of the big toe.

9.3.2 Diagnostic approach

MRI is essential to confirm the diagnosis, identify the cause and to inform surgical management.

9.3.3 Management

All patients with myelopathy symptoms should be referred urgently to hospital for specialist assessment and MRI scanning. This is because spinal cord compression is serious and can lead to permanent ischaemic cord damage and irreversible functional loss, so urgent surgical decompression is usually required.

9.4 Intervertebral disc prolapse

A prolapsed, herniated or slipped disc occurs when the inner disc extrudes through the fibrous capsule and bulges out, causing inflammation and compression of the accompanying nerve root (**Figure 9.3**). Disc prolapse causes pain in the nerve root that is compressed. Patients commonly suspect that they have 'slipped a disc' when they suffer a bout of acute back pain; however, this is actually only the case in 5% of acute back pain presentations.

9.4.1 Epidemiology

Symptomatic disc protrusion has a prevalence of 2%. The male to female ratio is 2:1 and the area most commonly affected are the discs between L4–L5 and L5–S1. Interestingly, there is radiological evidence of disc protrusion in up to 25% of asymptomatic patients. The most common age range for symptomatic disc prolapse is between 30 and 50 years of age.

9.4.2 Aetiology

The aetiology is not clear. Some people may have a predisposition to a prolapsed disc if their annulus fibrosus is inherently weak. Risk factors that increase the chance of a prolapsed disc include repeated heavy lifting, obesity, smoking, increasing age and participation in weight-bearing sports.

9.4.3 Prevention

There is no definitive way to prevent a prolapsed disc, other than to reduce individual risk factors and to address occupational causes.

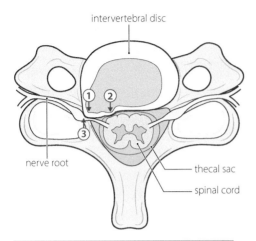

intervertebral disc

nerve root

thecal sac

spinal cord

Figure 9.3 Disc prolapse impinging on a spinal nerve in the right intervertebral foramina. ① = the intervertebral disc has prolapsed and herniated to the right side; ② = disc prolapse will also compress the spinal cord and compress the cerebrospinal fluid in the thecal sac; ③ = the herniated disc compresses the spinal nerve root exiting from the spinal cord.

9.4.4 Clinical features

The patient will report an acute onset of back pain which is exacerbated by walking or sitting for prolonged periods. Lying down flat will lessen the pain. In many cases the patient reports sciatica. Sciatica is a term to describe pain originating from the back, going into the buttock, thigh, lower leg or foot. The prolapsed disc is thought to cause direct pressure and nerve irritation. However, discectomy to relieve the pressure on the nerve is not always effective at relieving pain. On examination, pain will limit movement and power. However, neurological examination is generally normal apart from numbness within a dermatome pattern. If more significant neurology is present, the prolapse could be more severe. Straight leg raise can reproduce the pain in the leg or the back.

9.4.5 Diagnostic approach

Often the clinical diagnosis of sciatica is sufficient to diagnose a prolapsed disc. Most patients benefit from conservative management and are only investigated if symptoms do not settle.

9.4.6 Investigations

If pain is ongoing or there are any red flags, then an MRI scan is performed (**Figure 9.4**) to assess whether the diagnosis is correct, the extent of the prolapse and if the site of the prolapse corresponds to the patient's reported symptoms.

9.4.7 Management

Initial management is conservative, utilising self-management, exercise-based treatments, physiotherapy and analgesia.

Medication
Paracetamol and NSAID tablets may help relieve pain. Analgesia that targets neuropathic pain, e.g. amitriptyline and pregabalin, may be helpful. Epidural steroid injections may help with pain control in refractory cases.

Surgery
In cases where there is a clear correlation between symptoms, clinical signs and imaging, removal of the herniated disc (discectomy) can be performed.

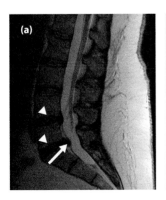

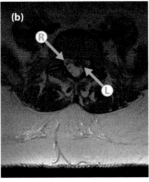

Figure 9.4 MRI showing L5–S1 intervertebral disc herniation: (a) sagittal view with herniation arrowed; (b) axial view showing displacement of the transiting left S1 nerve root Ⓛ, while the right S1 nerve root Ⓡ remains normal.

This tends to help peripheral radicular symptoms but is less effective at relieving back pain.

Prognosis

Most patients recover in weeks to months with conservative management. Up to a third of patients can go on to have pain for more than one year and a proportion of these can have chronic back and leg pain.

9.5 Cauda equina syndrome

Cauda equina syndrome is a spinal emergency as it can cause rapid and permanent loss of bladder and bowel function. It is caused by irritation or compression of the lowest lumbar and sacral nerve roots in the spinal canal after the spinal cord ends below the L1 vertebra. The most common cause is intervertebral disc prolapse, but other causes include tumour, abscess, haemorrhage or, more rarely, demyelination.

9.5.1 Clinical features

There is a lower motor neurone pattern of weakness affecting the most distal muscles of the leg in the ankle and foot (e.g. weakness, flaccid tone, reflex loss) and altered sensation in the perineal, perianal and genital regions, which are supplied by the spinal nerve roots. In addition, autonomic signals are disrupted to the bladder and bowel, leading to sphincter disturbance with loss of tone and function, e.g. urinary or faecal incontinence or retention.

9.5.2 Diagnostic approach

Urgent spinal MRI is essential to confirm the diagnosis, identify the cause and inform surgical management (**Figure 9.5**).

9.5.3 Management

Urgent referral to a spinal surgeon or neurosurgeon for decompression surgery is required in order to reduce the risk of permanent neurological deficit and bladder and bowel incontinence.

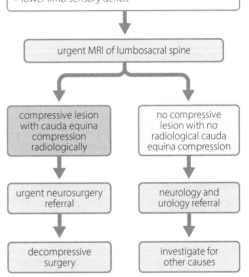

Figure 9.5 Cauda equina syndrome diagnostic approach.

9.6 Cervical and lumbar spondylosis

Degenerative OA affecting the cervical or lumbar spine is also known as spondylosis. As part of this disease process there is loss of facet joint cartilage and the intervertebral discs degenerate and may rupture and prolapse. The loss of their cushioning can disrupt the biomechanics of the vertebral column. As a result, new bone grows as a repair and mechanical response, forming bony spurs (osteophytes), and there is hypertrophy of bone and the spinal ligaments.

It is a common condition, affecting over 50% of the population over 50 years of age, but as with other sites affected by OA, the clinical presentation is variable, ranging from asymptomatic to severe disabling symptoms.

9.6.1 Clinical features

Spondylosis causes gradual onset of pain and stiffness at the affected site with features of mechanical back pain. Symptoms are often chronic although acute exacerbations may occur. Occipital headache can be a symptom of cervical spondylosis.

Complications include compression of the spinal nerve roots in the intervertebral foramina (radiculopathy) and narrowing of the spinal canal (spinal stenosis) with compression of the spinal cord (myelopathy) or the lowest lumbar and sacral nerve roots (cauda equina syndrome).

9.6.2 Diagnostic approach

Clinical evaluation with particular attention to neurological assessment is key to making the diagnosis and identifying complications. If there is evidence of OA in other joints then this increases the likelihood of spondylosis. Determine if there are any particular precipitating factors that may increase the risk of spondylosis, e.g. occupation, obesity, previous injury or surgery.

An MRI scan will be required for further assessment if there are symptoms or signs suggesting neurological complications (**Figure 9.6**).

9.6.3 Management

Management is similar to mechanical back pain with the focus on active self-management with exercise, analgesia and positive reinforcement. Physiotherapy is helpful. Other options for persistent or progressive symptoms include epidural corticosteroid injection, targeted nerve root corticosteroid injection and surgery, e.g. discectomy, laminectomy (removal of additional bone) or laminoplasty (bone spread apart to reduce pressure).

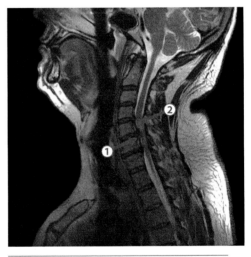

Figure 9.6 Sagittal MRI scan showing multiple disc prolapse ①, degenerative changes and cord compression in the cervical spine. The high signal within the cord is myelomalacia ②.

9.7 Spinal stenosis

Spinal stenosis is narrowing of the spinal canal, which can result in compression of the spinal cord (myelopathy) or the lowest lumbar and sacral nerve roots (cauda equina syndrome).

The most common cause is lumbar spondylosis, although there can be other acquired and congenital aetiologies, e.g. scoliosis, ankylosing spondylitis or disc pathology.

9.7.1 Clinical features

Onset is usually gradual, but patients typically have chronic progressive lower back pain, pain in both buttocks and the back of both legs. Depending on the site of compression, patients may also develop symptoms of myelopathy, radiculopathy or cauda equina syndrome.

Neurogenic claudication is characteristic of lumbar spinal stenosis. This is due to compression of the lumbar and sacral nerve roots which supply the lower limb muscles and results in symptoms often described as tiredness and heaviness affecting the buttock and hamstring muscles (and sometimes calves). Patients will often lean forward as if pushing a shopping trolley, as this widens the spinal canal, relieving some of the pressure on the nerves and helping these symptoms.

> It is important to distinguish between neurogenic and vascular claudication. If the patient experiences relief when they lean forward this points to a neurogenic claudication. If rest rather than changes in posture help, then vascular claudication is more likely.

9.7.2 Diagnostic approach

Clinical evaluation may be non-specific but it is important to pay particular attention to neurological assessment to identify any complications and to exclude peripheral vascular disease if there are symptoms of claudication. The diagnosis is confirmed with an MRI scan (**Figure 9.7**).

9.7.3 Management

Patients must be reminded to stay active and reassured that activity will not cause damage. Physiotherapy and analgesia are the mainstay of conservative treatment with use of NSAIDs and neuropathic pain-modifying agents, e.g. amitriptyline and pregabalin. Corticosteroid injections into the epidural space or targeted nerve root corticosteroid injection in cases of localised radiculopathy may be helpful.

Surgery

Decompression surgery is reserved for those who are not improving with conservative management or who have significant or progressive neurological impairment. Surgery involves removal of the tissues that are contributing to the compression (lumbar laminectomy, discectomy ± spinal fusion). Close correlation of symptoms with MRI scanning is important to plan the most effective surgical treatment. Often diagnostic injections are performed to identify the level or area of compression before surgical decompression is undertaken. The response to treatment and prognosis is variable.

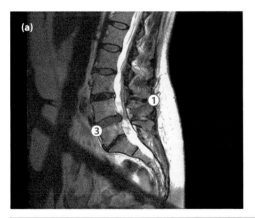
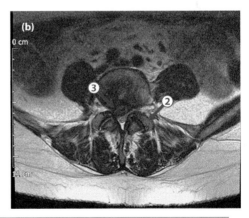

Figure 9.7 T2-weighted MRI sequences of the lumbar spine: (a) sagittal; (b) axial. Lumbar canal stenosis secondary to combined disc prolapse and facet joint hypertrophy has led to compression of the cauda equina and nerve roots and a decrease in the anteroposterior diameter of the spinal canal. ①, compressed thecal sac with effacement of CSF and near-complete effacement of cauda equina; ②, hypertrophic facet joint; ③, prolapse of disc.

PERIPHERAL NERVE DISORDERS

Peripheral nerve disorders are divided into mononeuropathies, which are a dysfunction of a single nerve, and polyneuropathies, which are a dysfunction of several peripheral nerves, usually indicating a systemic metabolic, toxicity or inflammatory problem. This section will consider the most common mononeuropathies.

Mononeuropathies have several features in common:

■ They are caused by changes in local anatomy such as swelling of adjacent tissues, displacement, entrapment, external compression or trauma.
■ The location of the pathology is at anatomically vulnerable sites.
■ There can be precipitating mechanical factors such as certain movements, unusual posture and repetitive actions which can be related to activity or occupation.

■ Most cases respond well to treatment and prognosis is good.

Figure 9.8 illustrates the mechanism of nerve fibre injury.

Clinical features

Clinical features relate to the specific nerve that is affected with reduced power and tone in the muscles supplied by the nerve, and sensory disturbance in the distribution of the nerve.

Table 9.2 reviews the causes, sensory and motor signs for the most common peripheral nerve disorders. Sensation is tested in specific areas, as it is common for the skin to be supplied by more than one nerve.

The most common symptoms are:

■ pain
■ numbness

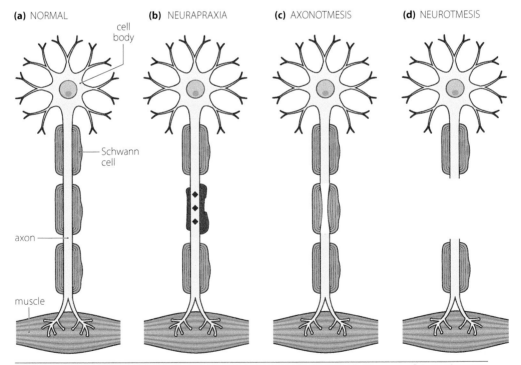

(a) NORMAL   **(b)** NEURAPRAXIA   **(c)** AXONOTMESIS   **(d)** NEUROTMESIS

cell body

Schwann cell

axon

muscle

Figure 9.8 Nerve fibre injury: (a) normal nerve; (b) compression injury creates areas of demyelination, producing a conduction block; (c) traction injuries damage the axon but the Schwann cells are intact; (d) nerve is in discontinuity, with damage to both Schwann cell and axon in penetrating injuries.

■ paraesthesia.

If it occurs, weakness presents late.

Management

Most mononeuropathies respond well to analgesia, mechanical support with splinting or orthoses, and avoidance of precipitating behaviours or activities. If symptoms are persistent or progressive, nerve decompression surgery can be performed. Direct trauma which results in a discontinuity of the nerve has a poorer prognosis, but direct surgical repair is possible. Traumatic nerve injuries are described by the Seddon classification (**Table 9.3**).

The term neurapraxia is used when a nerve suffers temporary loss of communication following traumatic injury.

Table 9.2 *Common peripheral nerve disorders*

	Median nerve	**Ulnar nerve**	**Radial nerve**	**Common peroneal nerve**	**Tibial nerve**
Common injury	Carpal tunnel compression	Cubital tunnel and ulnar tunnel compression	Spiral groove of the humerus and between supinator muscle	Fibular neck	Tarsal tunnel
Sensory supply compromised	Tip of index finger	Tip of little finger (cubital tunnel only)	Dorsum 1st web space (hand)	Dorsum 1st web space (foot)	Plantar aspect of foot
Motor function compromised	Thumb abduction	Finger abduction or thumb adduction	Wrist and finger extension	Ankle dorsiflexion	Toe flexion

Table 9.3 *Seddon classification of traumatic nerve injuries*

Type	Pathology	Aetiology	Severity	Recovery
Neurapraxia	Intact nerve with conduction block	Compression or ischaemia	Least severe	Complete (weeks to months)
Axonotmesis	Nerve intact with axon discontinuity	Traction injury	Moderate	Partial/full (months to year)
Neurotmesis	Axon and nerve discontinuity	Severed nerve	Severe	None without surgery

9.8 Carpal tunnel syndrome

The carpal tunnel is a space on the volar aspect of the wrist bound by carpal bones and enclosed by its roof, the transverse carpal ligament. The median nerve originates at the medial and lateral cords of the brachial plexus, travels down the anterior aspect of the forearm and enters the hand through the carpal tunnel. Several tendons also pass through it. Compression of the median nerve in the carpal tunnel is called carpal tunnel syndrome (CTS) and causes pain, weakness and numbness affecting structures in the hand supplied by the median nerve.

9.8.1 Epidemiology

CTS is common, affecting up to 5% of the adult population. It is three times more prevalent in women and 50% of pregnant women develop symptoms. Risk factors also include inflammatory arthritis, hypothyroidism and obesity. Diabetic patients are fifteen times more likely to develop CTS.

9.8.2 Aetiology

In CTS, the median nerve and several tendons passing through this space become compressed, leading to ischaemia and loss of the sensory and motor communications (**Figure 9.9**). Most cases (90%) are idiopathic, but compression secondary to oedema in pregnancy is common, as are mechanical factors such as repetitive tasks.

Causes of CTS can be remembered by the mnemonic '**PRAGMATIC**':
- **P**regnancy
- **R**heumatoid arthritis
- **A**cromegaly
- **G**lucose (diabetes)
- **M**echanical (fractures)
- **A**myloid
- **T**hyroid (underactive)
- **I**nfection
- **C**rystals

9.8.3 Clinical features

The sensory fibres are first involved, but often sensation is completely normal between episodes. Two-point discrimination can be reduced, specifically on the palmar aspect of the index finger but can also be reduced in the thumb and middle finger. The little finger is supplied by the ulnar nerve; hence it is spared in CTS.

The median nerve supplies motor function to the 'LOAF' muscles of the hand (**Table 9.4**). Weakness and wasting in these muscles are

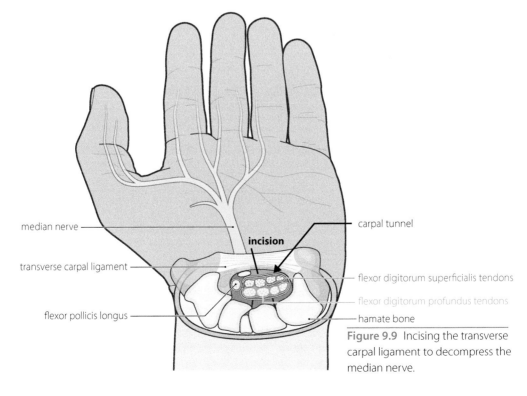

median nerve

carpal tunnel

incision

transverse carpal ligament

flexor digitorum superficialis tendons

flexor digitorum profundus tendons

flexor pollicis longus

hamate bone

Figure 9.9 Incising the transverse carpal ligament to decompress the median nerve.

Table 9.4 *'LOAF' muscles of the hand: motor function is supplied by the median nerve*

Muscle	Action
Lateral two lumbricals	Flexion of the MCPJ with extension of the PIPJ and DIPJ of the index and ring finger
Opponens pollicis	Opposition of the thumb
Abductor pollicis brevis	Abducts the thumb
Flexor pollicis brevis	Flexes the thumb at the MCP joint

hallmarks of CTS and indicate long-standing compression. Flexion of the wrist narrows the carpal tunnel and if held in this position for up to 30 seconds can bring on symptoms (Phalen's test; see **Figure 2.22**). Tinel's sign is positive (see **Figure 2.23**) if the area over the carpal tunnel is gently percussed and symptoms are reproduced.

9.8.4 Diagnostic approach

CTS is a clinical diagnosis, made from the patient's history and physical examination. Scoring systems may be used to help make a diagnosis and to distinguish whether further tests are required (**Table 9.5**).

9.8.5 Investigations

CTS is most commonly idiopathic, but underlying causes should be considered. Interestingly CTS may develop before a formal diagnosis of diabetes. In cases of diagnostic uncertainty, a diagnosis of CTS can be confirmed with NCS and EMG. Other imaging techniques such as ultrasound can be used to look for median nerve flattening and hypertrophy, as well as any structural cause within the carpal tunnel.

9.8.6 Management

Initial treatments include night splints to prevent flexion of the wrist while sleeping (**Figure 9.10**)

Table 9.5 *A clinical questionnaire for the diagnosis of CTS: a score ≥ 5 is strongly suggestive of CTS; a score > 3 suggests diagnostic uncertainty, and nerve conduction studies can be useful in this instance*

Symptom	Score for 'yes'
Pain:	
Wrist pain woken you at night?	1
Any neck pain present?	−1
Tingling and numbness in hand:	
Woken you at night?	1
Worse on waking?	1
Occurs when reading a newspaper, steering a car, knitting, etc.?	1
Alleviated by wrist splint?	2
Do you use any specific movements to make the tingling, numbness go away?	1
Is tingling and numbness in your little finger always absent?	3
In a current pregnancy, has tingling and numbness in hand:	
been severe?	1
NOT been severe?	−1

Adapted from Kamath, V. and Stothard, J. (2004) Erratum to: a clinical questionnaire for the diagnosis of carpal tunnel syndrome 2003; 28: 455–459. *J Hand Surg*, 29: 95.

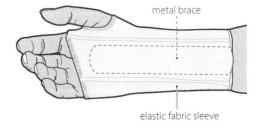

metal brace

elastic fabric sleeve

Figure 9.10 Carpal tunnel splints are effective, especially if worn at night, as they prevent flexion of the wrist and increased pressure within the tunnel.

and local corticosteroid injections or NSAIDs to reduce inflammation in the carpal tunnel. Should conservative methods fail, or if there are progressive symptoms or established sensory or motor loss, carpal tunnel decompression surgery should be performed. This involves incision of the transverse carpal ligament to relieve pressure on the nerve (**Figure 9.9**).

Prognosis

Most patients will have resolution of their symptoms with supportive conservative management. Surgical decompression is usually effective. However, if the nerve has been compressed for a long time or there is established motor weakness, function may not return, and symptoms may persist.

9.9 Cubital tunnel syndrome

The ulnar nerve is prone to compression at two points along its long course from the medial cord of the brachial plexus to the hand. Compression occurs at the medial side of the elbow through the cubital tunnel and at the medial side of the wrist through the ulnar tunnel (Guyon's canal).

Cubital tunnel syndrome is caused by compression of the ulnar nerve in the cubital tunnel, an area posterior to the medial epicondyle of the elbow. The nerve is superficial here as it winds round the medial epicondyle. It is not protected by the bony skeleton, which makes it particularly prone to injury at this site.

9.9.1 Epidemiology

Cubital tunnel syndrome is more common in people who spend long periods with their elbows flexed or resting on a desk, e.g. prolonged holding of a telephone or reading a book. It is also common in those using tools at work that vibrate and make repetitive movements. Tardy ulnar nerve palsy can develop after a supracondylar elbow fracture, as

the resultant valgus deformity at the elbow can stretch the nerve (see *Section 6.8* and **Figure 6.13**).

9.9.2 Aetiology

The medial epicondyle and the olecranon process are covered by the tendinous origins of the two heads of the flexor carpi ulnaris muscle to form the cubital tunnel. The ulnar nerve in this area is relatively unprotected and can be compressed from external sources or, more commonly, from the overlying tendons (**Figure 9.11**).

9.9.3 Clinical features

Pain and numbness in the little and ring finger are the most common symptoms and are especially present at night, as the elbows are usually flexed.

> The ulnar nerve supplies all the small muscles of the hand, except the 'LOAF' muscles (**Table 9.4**). Thus chronic ulnar nerve palsy will cause wasting in the hypothenar muscles but the 'LOAF' thenar muscles are spared.

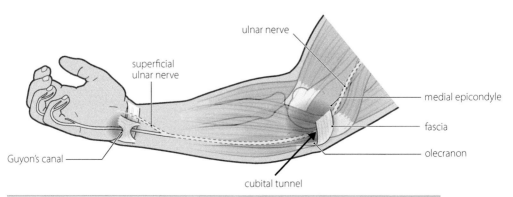

Figure 9.11 Ulnar nerve compression at the elbow (cubital tunnel) and wrist (Guyon's canal).

Froment's test will demonstrate weakness of thumb adduction, as this is controlled by the interosseous muscles innervated by the ulnar nerve (**Figure 9.12**). In a positive Froment's test, there is weakness of thumb adduction and compensatory flexion of flexor pollicis longus (FPL) to stop a piece of paper being pulled from between the thumb and finger.

Tinel's test over the cubital tunnel can reproduce pain and numbness in the little finger, similar to hitting the funny bone.

9.9.4 Diagnostic approach

The diagnosis of cubital tunnel syndrome is made clinically. NCS and EMG are helpful for determining the site of compression.

9.9.5 Investigations

Further investigation is not usually required, although X-ray or MRI may be used to rule out compression from a bony cause or soft tissue mass.

9.9.6 Management

Modification of activities and using resting elbow splints are effective at alleviating symptoms. If symptoms do not improve or are severe, surgical decompression of the cubital tunnel is performed by incising the aponeurosis which covers the two heads of flexor carpi ulnaris.

> **Compliance with splints can be difficult**, as some patients find them uncomfortable at night or difficult to wear at work.

Prognosis

In most patients, cubital tunnel syndrome resolves without surgery. When surgery is needed it is effective in around 80% of patients.

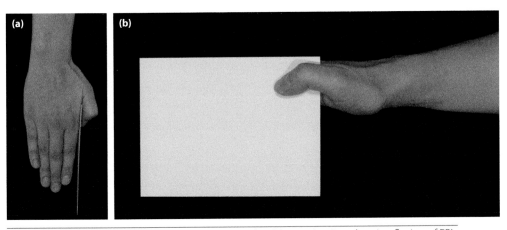

(a) **(b)**

Figure 9.12 Positive Froment's test in ulnar nerve palsy: (a) superior view showing flexing of FPL; (b) lateral view showing the same compensatory FPL function.

9.10 Ulnar tunnel syndrome

The ulnar nerve and artery pass through the ulnar tunnel (Guyon's canal) at the wrist. The ulnar tunnel is bound on each side by the hamate and pisiform bones and covered by the palmar carpal ligament, which is an extension of the flexor retinaculum. Small ganglions, fractures and leaning on bicycle handlebars can all cause compression in this area.

9.10.1 Clinical features

Symptoms are similar to cubital tunnel syndrome. However, the sensation on the dorsum of the little finger may be spared, as the dorsal branch of the ulnar nerve divides 5cm proximal to the wrist and does not enter the ulnar tunnel, so there is no loss of sensation in the area it innervates (**Figure 9.11**).

9.10.2 Management

Initial treatment includes modification of activities and splinting. Surgical decompression of the ulnar tunnel is recommended if symptoms do not improve, or persist or progress.

9.11 Radial nerve compression and injury

The radial nerve supplies the posterior compartments of the arm and forearm and controls the extensor function of the hand, wrist and elbow. Compression and injury of this nerve is common in the axilla, around the humeral shaft and as it passes through the supinator muscle in the forearm.

> **The radial nerve is prone to injury following midshaft humeral fractures:** it can become compressed or lacerated by fracture fragments around the spiral groove. Documentation of radial nerve function is essential on presentation with this type of injury as it can affect up to one in five cases.

9.11.1 'Saturday night palsy' or 'Crutch palsy'

Compression to the radial nerve in the axilla as it passes around the spiral groove can result in a radial nerve palsy.

9.11.2 Aetiology

As a continuation of the posterior cord of the brachial plexus, the radial nerve winds round the spiral groove of the humerus. This close proximity to the humeral shaft makes it vulnerable to compression from external pressure, e.g. falling asleep with an arm hanging over a chair or axillary walking crutches (**Figure 9.13**).

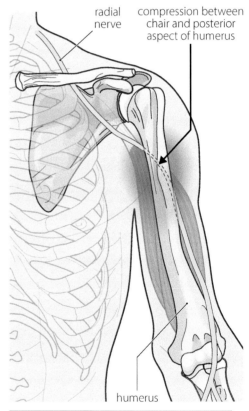

radial nerve — compression between chair and posterior aspect of humerus

humerus

Figure 9.13 'Saturday night palsy' occurs when the radial nerve is compressed in the axilla.

9.11.3 Clinical features

Proximal radial nerve palsies cause finger and wrist drop (**Figure 9.14**) due to weakness of finger and wrist extension, and loss of sensation over the dorsum of the first web space.

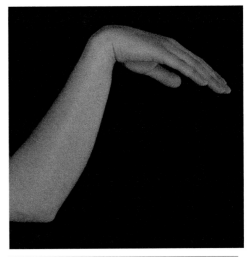

Figure 9.14 Wrist and finger drop in radial nerve palsy.

9.12 Posterior interosseous nerve syndrome

The posterior interosseous nerve is a continuation of the deep branch of the radial nerve supplying all the extensor muscles of the forearm except brachioradialis, anconaeus and extensor carpi radialis longus.

9.12.1 Aetiology

The posterior interosseous nerve can become compressed as it pierces the supinator muscle at the elbow. Microtrauma from repetitive supination movements and space-occupying lesions such as ganglions and lipomas are the most common causes of posterior interosseous nerve syndrome.

9.12.2 Clinical features

Finger extension is weak. However, wrist extension is preserved when the wrist is radially deviated, as extensor carpi radialis longus is supplied more proximally by the radial nerve. The posterior interosseous nerve does not supply any sensation to the skin and therefore numbness is not a feature.

9.12.3 Diagnostic approach

Radial nerve palsies almost always require NCS and EMG to differentiate between simple neurapraxia and nerve discontinuity by trauma. MRI can diagnose soft tissue compressive lesions.

9.12.4 Management

In neurapraxia, symptoms will resolve within a few weeks to months, but can take up to 18 months to resolve. Resting splints and physiotherapy are used to prevent contractures whilst the nerve recovers. Discontinuity of the nerve requires surgical repair and prognosis is less favourable. If no improvement is seen, then repeat nerve conduction studies can be useful to show the extent of nerve regeneration, and can aid prognosis.

9.13 Tarsal tunnel syndrome

The tibial nerve supplies most of the small muscles of the foot and the sensation on the plantar aspect of the foot. It is commonly compressed by space-occupying lesions such as ganglions, bone spurs and varicose veins as it travels through the tarsal tunnel behind the medial malleolus. The tarsal tunnel is formed by deep bone surfaces of the calcaneus, talus and distal tibia as the floor, and an inflexible band of tissue called the flexor retinaculum as the roof. This means that any increased pressure in the tunnel from any cause will eventually cause nerve compression (**Figure 9.15**).

> Contents of the tarsal tunnel can be remembered with this mnemonic: '**T**om, **D**ick **A**nd **V**ery **N**aughty **H**arry'
> - **T**ibialis posterior tendon
> - Flexor **D**igitorum longus
> - Posterior tibial **A**rtery
> - Posterior tibial **V**ein
> - Tibial **N**erve
> - Flexor **H**allucis longus

9.13.1 Clinical features

Ankle pain with burning and numbness in the sole of the foot are typical symptoms, especially after exercise or prolonged standing, but symptoms can be varied and diagnosis difficult. Performing Tinel's test by lightly tapping over the nerve in the tarsal tunnel reproduces symptoms.

9.13.2 Diagnostic approach

It is usually a clinical diagnosis, but in cases of diagnostic uncertainty NCS and EMG can be helpful. An MRI scan can be used to identify any precipitating cause.

9.13.3 Management

Correcting any foot deformities with orthoses to relieve pressure on the tibial nerve can be helpful, as patients with a flat overpronated foot are more susceptible. Surgery to remove compressive lesions and to release the retinaculum can be considered if physiotherapy and corticosteroid injections do not improve symptoms.

> Unlike wrist splints, foot orthoses are tolerated better by patients and compliance is higher.

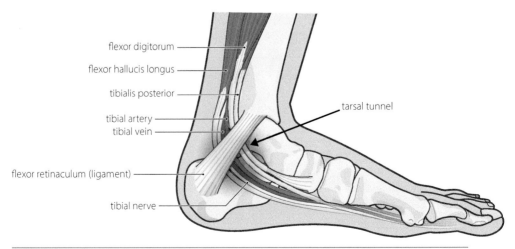

flexor digitorum
flexor hallucis longus
tibialis posterior
tibial artery
tibial vein
tarsal tunnel
flexor retinaculum (ligament)
tibial nerve

Figure 9.15 Medial view of the ankle showing compression of the tibial nerve in the tarsal tunnel.

9.14 Foot drop

Foot drop is the inability to dorsiflex the foot against gravity. It is commonly caused by pathology affecting the common peroneal nerve or its superficial or deep branches.

The common peroneal nerve is a continuation of the sciatic nerve. It winds around the head of the fibula, branching into:

- superficial peroneal nerve, to supply all the muscles of the lateral compartment of the lower leg and sensation to the dorsum of the foot
- deep peroneal nerve, to supply the anterior compartment of the lower leg and sensation to the first dorsal web space of the foot.

The peroneal nerve is susceptible to injury all along its course, as it runs relatively superficially. This is particularly the case at the fibular neck where compression can occur from an above-knee cast or tight boot or crossing the legs, and injury or fracture at the proximal fibula.

Other causes of foot drop include:

- L5 spinal nerve root compression
- mononeuropathy, e.g. vitamin B12 deficiency, diabetes, mononeuritis multiplex

- injury to the ankle dorsiflexor muscles, e.g. tibialis anterior.
- compartment syndrome.

9.14.1 Clinical features

Ankle dorsiflexion is weak. Patients present with a high stepping gait and exaggerated flexion of the hip and knee to prevent their toes catching on the ground. They are not able to walk on their heels. Sensation to the first web space is reduced if the deep nerve is affected and to the dorsum of the foot if the superficial peroneal nerve is affected.

9.14.2 Management

Definitive treatment depends on the cause. Peroneal nerve compression can be released by surgical decompression. Physiotherapy is helpful to improve muscle strength and restore gait. An ankle–foot orthosis to keep the foot in a neutral position and at right angles to the ankle (a 'cock-up splint') is helpful to use when walking during the rehabilitation and recovery phase.

9.15 Morton's neuroma

Morton's neuroma is thickening of the interdigital nerve between the toes. It most commonly occurs between the third and fourth then second and third toes. Middle-aged women are most often affected and it is more common in people who wear tight-fitting footwear or pursue running-based sports. Symptoms include forefoot pain and sensory symptoms such as burning and

shooting pain in the toes. Clinical examination by squeezing the forefoot over the metatarsal heads reproduces symptoms and produces a palpable click known as 'Mulder's click' as the nerve tissue is pushed between the metatarsal heads (**Figure 2.11**). Treatment options include foot orthoses, local corticosteroid injection or surgical excision.

9.16 Answers to starter questions

1. Lumbar punctures in adults are performed at, or lower than, L3/L4 as the spinal cord terminates at L1/L2. Putting a needle into the vacant cauda equina space is relatively safe because the loose nerve fibres can move if pushed by the needle. In infants, the spinal cord may still lie at L3,

so the procedure must be performed lower down.

2. Lumbar back pain is more common than thoracic back pain, so the total numbers of serious pathology as a percentage are lower. The thoracic spine is less mechanically affected than the lumbar spine and therefore, statistically, it is more common

to have non-mechanical reasons for pain here. However, musculoskeletal pain remains the most common cause for lumbar and thoracic back pain.

3. Diabetes increases the risk of developing peripheral nerve syndromes as well as trigger finger, Dupuytren's contracture and frozen shoulder. The definitive cause of this association is unknown but insults to nerves and their vascular supply occur when they are exposed to high levels of glucose in the blood. Demyelination as well as axonal damage occurs, making the nerve more sensitive to even minor degrees of compression.

4. NCS and EMG are useful when the clinical diagnosis is uncertain or to distinguish the level of compression; for example, distinguishing between cubital and ulnar tunnel syndrome when a patient presents with ulnar nerve symptoms. Generally, CTS can be diagnosed from history and clinical examination.

5. There are several different types of sensory receptors within the PNS, which include nociceptors and mechanoreceptors. Nociceptors are stimulated by pain and are only covered in a small amount of myelin. They transmit more slowly than the mechanoreceptors (which detect sensation), that are fully covered in myelin. The nociceptors can become unusually sensitive when compressed, leading to increased pain.

Chapter 10
Tumours and malignancy

Starter questions

1. Why do primary bone tumours develop most commonly in children?
2. Why is multiple myeloma most commonly diagnosed in the over-70s?

Answers to questions are to be found in *Section 10.4*.

The most common tumours to affect bones are metastases from other primary tumours. Tumours originating from bone-derived cells, i.e. primary bone tumours, are rare. They can present in all ages but are most common in children or the elderly. There are no specific risk factors and primary bone tumours are often missed as they are mistaken for simple muscle strains in otherwise fit young individuals.

There are multiple types of bone tumours and multiple ways to classify their characteristics. Even distinguishing between benign and malignant tumours does not always equate to how destructive the tumour can be or its prognosis.

In metastatic bone disease, secondary bone tumours originate from primary tumours in other organs and spread to bone. Haematological cancers such as multiple myeloma originate in the bone marrow.

Case 10.1 Non-traumatic limb pain in a child

Presentation

Kamal is a fit and active 12-year-old boy who plays for his local football club. He is always getting bumps and scrapes on the football field but has now had pain and swelling round his knee for 3 weeks and has no specific trauma that he can remember. He is also getting pain at night and it wakes him from sleep even though he is taking painkillers.

Initial interpretation

It is normal for children to get bumps and scrapes on the football field, but red flag symptoms in this history include: no obvious trauma, night pain and swelling. Simple sports injuries do not usually cause significant sleep disturbance.

Examination

Kamal limps into the GP's examination room; he has an evident swelling around his knee with an effusion present. His knee is tender to touch, especially his distal femur, but it is not red or warm. No lumps or bumps are felt and an examination of ligaments shows the knee is stable. He does not have a temperature.

Interpretation of findings

Bony tenderness in a child warrants investigation. Differentials include fracture, osteomyelitis

Case 10.1 *continued*

(infection of the bone) or bone tumour. Absence of redness and heat does not exclude infection or tumour as a cause, as this can be present or absent in both pathologies.

Investigations

In the first instance, Kamal is sent for a plain radiograph of the knee and blood tests, including inflammatory markers. CRP and WCC are normal (a raised CRP and WCC would make osteomyelitis a more likely diagnosis). The radiograph shows a mixture of lytic and sclerotic areas of bone around the distal femur metaphysis. There is significant periosteal reaction and soft tissue calcification. The radiologist at the hospital sends an urgent report to Kamal's GP that there are significant abnormalities on the radiograph and that an urgent orthopaedic referral is required (**Figure 10.1**).

Diagnosis

Within a week Kamal is seen at the regional hospital that has a specialist orthopaedic tumour service. Further imaging in the form of MRI, CT (of the knee, chest, abdomen and pelvis) and isotope bone scans are undertaken to further characterise and stage the cancer. MRI shows a large soft tissue mass adjacent to the bone but it appears not to spread outside the fascial compartment of the anterior thigh. CT shows no distal spread to other organs.

Primary bone tumours can present innocuously in children and are often missed, at a high cost. This is a diagnosis that should not

be missed, as early detection and treatment can improve survival. This is a typical history for an osteosarcoma, as it presents in a male teenager around the knee. When planning curative surgery, it is critical that all cancer cells are removed and for that reason surgical excision of the tumour is extensive and often requires joint replacement surgery or amputation. Osteosarcomas have one of the lowest survival rates of bone tumours: 65–70% at 5 years. There can be significant morbidity following aggressive surgery. Patients and their families will need support for many years even following successful treatment.

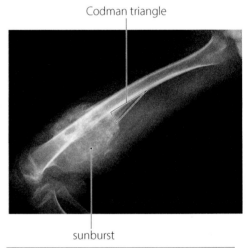

Codman triangle

sunburst

Figure 10.1 Radiograph showing osteosarcoma of the distal femoral metaphysis characterised by a sunburst appearance. A Codman triangle is formed as the periosteum lifts up due to growth of the underlying tumour.

Case 10.2 A suspicious fracture

Presentation

Carol Gledhill is 70 years old and has been getting pain in her hip over the last two weeks. She had not fallen or done anything physically exerting to trigger the pain. She enjoys gardening but she

would have expected it to have improved by now if she had overdone her pruning. She has now decided to contact her GP about her symptoms as it is becoming more painful every day. Pain is felt in her groin and is worse when walking. Painkillers ease the pain a little but the pain is keeping her

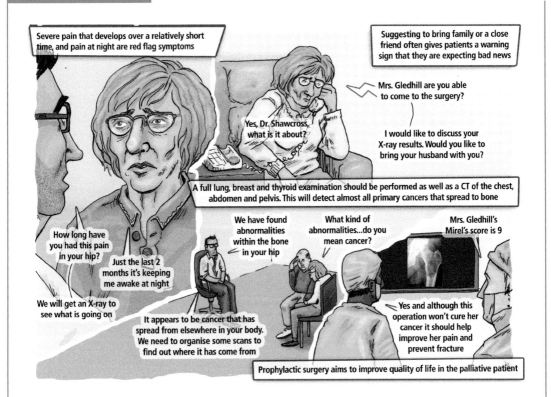

Severe pain that develops over a relatively short time, and pain at night are red flag symptoms

Suggesting to bring family or a close friend often gives patients a warning sign that they are expecting bad news

Mrs. Gledhill are you able to come to the surgery?

Yes, Dr. Shawcross, what is it about?

I would like to discuss your X-ray results. Would you like to bring your husband with you?

A full lung, breast and thyroid examination should be performed as well as a CT of the chest, abdomen and pelvis. This will detect almost all primary cancers that spread to bone

How long have you had this pain in your hip?

Just the last 2 months it's keeping me awake at night

We will get an X-ray to see what is going on

We have found abnormalities within the bone in your hip

What kind of abnormalities...do you mean cancer?

Mrs. Gledhill's Mirel's score is 9

It appears to be cancer that has spread from elsewhere in your body. We need to organise some scans to find out where it has come from

Yes and although this operation won't cure her cancer it should help improve her pain and prevent fracture

Prophylactic surgery aims to improve quality of life in the palliative patient

up at night. She has had no sign of fever but has had no sign of fever but has been getting a little more tired lately. She is putting that down to the painkillers, not sleeping well and the extra effort it is taking her to walk. She has not noticed any other symptoms.

Initial interpretation

Hip pain is common secondary to OA in this age group, often starting with a niggle and gradually over months becoming worse. However, acute pain without trauma is a red flag symptom, especially if suffering significant pain at rest. Be mindful that knee and spinal pathology can refer pain to the hip.

Examination

Carol is using her husband's walking stick as she walks to the examination couch. There are no obvious skin changes or swelling to the hip area or back. Examination reveals a near-normal range of movement but it is painful to move in all directions. Carol finds it difficult to raise her heel

from the bed with her leg straight. She is very tender to touch over the groin.

Interpretation of findings

OA generally has a restricted range of movement and pain mostly occurs at the extremes of movement and not through the whole range of movement. Tenderness in the groin is specific to the hip joint, which impacts on her ability to flex the hip and raise her leg. Pain around the greater trochanter is less indicative of hip joint pain. There is no pain radiating to the hamstring or calf, which could indicate radicular symptoms from irritation to the sciatic nerve, e.g. from a prolapsed lumbar disc.

Investigations

Radiographs are ordered by Dr Shawcross, Carol's GP, as he has concerns that this may be something more than a flare of OA. Dr Shawcross is contacted by the radiologist at the hospital who informs him that a large lytic lesion is seen in the

Case 10.2 *continued*

intertrochanteric region of the hip bone and has severely weakened the bone structure.

Diagnosis

Solitary lytic lesions in this age group are almost always secondary bone tumours. Examination and investigation must now turn to identifying the primary tumour. If multiple lytic lesions were identified, then further tests would be required to diagnose multiple myeloma or a primary bone disease process such as fibrous dysplasia or infection.

10.1 Primary bone tumours

The two largest groups of primary bone tumours are named according to the cells from which they arise:

- Chondromas – tumours arising from chondrocytes, the cartilage-forming cells
- Osteomas – tumours arising from osteocytes, the bone-forming cells.

10.1.1 Types

The classification of primary bone tumours is based on cell type, architecture, and matrix production (**Table 10.1**). Benign cartilage (chondrocyte) tumours are termed chondromas and benign bone (osteocyte) tumours are termed osteomas. Malignant tumours are suffixed with -sarcoma. For example, a malignant chondrocyte tumour would be a chondrosarcoma. Overlap in these conditions is common and, therefore, classification can be complex. There are multiple types of bone tumours but only the most common are discussed here: the general features and principles of diagnostic workup are the same.

Table 10.1 *Common primary bone tumours*

Tumour type		Age (years)	Common sites	Percentage of cases	Prognosis/5-year survival (%)
Benign	Osteochondroma	10–30	Knee, proximal femur and humerus	64	Latent
	Chondroblastoma	10–30	Knee, proximal humerus and calcaneus	11	Active
	Giant cell tumour (GCT)	20–50	Knee, distal radius, pelvis	21	Aggressive
Malignant	Osteosarcoma	10–30	Knee and proximal humerus	35	70%
	Chondrosarcoma	50–80	Pelvis, knee and proximal humerus	25	10–90%, depending on grade
	Ewing's sarcoma	5–30	Pelvis and long bones	16	25–80%, depending on grade
	Chordoma	30–80	Spine	8	68%

10.1.2 Epidemiology

Most bone benign and malignant tumours occur in the young (typically the second decade), because this is a time of significant growth and cell turnover. The faster the cells multiply, the greater the chance for mutations to occur. The cell type also determines which age group is affected; for example, osteosarcoma usually occurs in adolescence, chondrosarcoma over the age of 40 years and myeloma in the elderly.

10.1.3 Clinical features

Pain is the most common symptom, but the patient may also present with a mass. Most tumours occur around areas of high bone growth around the knee and also the proximal humerus. Night pain is a red flag symptom which should prompt urgent investigation.

10.1.4 Diagnostic approach

If a patient presents with symptoms that raise the suspicion of a tumour, for example nocturnal pain or pain without a history of trauma, radiographs should be obtained at the outset.

10.1.5 Investigations

Once a tumour is identified on plain radiographs, urgent referral to the regional bone tumour service for MDT discussion is essential. Isotope bone scans, MRI and staging CT will be able to assess local and distal spread of disease to aid surgical planning and medical treatment.

Blood tests are required to rule out anaemia and hypercalcaemia. ALP adds prognostic value. Biopsy will confirm the diagnosis by cell type and grade.

> Bone biopsy is usually done by specialist surgeons in the bone tumour service, to prevent seeding of cancer cells during biopsy.

10.1.6 Management

Surgery

Surgical excision – or curettage – and bone grafting is the mainstay of treatment in symptomatic benign lesions. Destructive aggressive benign lesions such as GCT may require amputation if too large to remove. Recurrence of benign lesions is common.

A malignant tumour requires surgery if its location permits it, because this can reduce local spread as well as metastases. However, wide excision is not always possible and the stage of the tumour may be too advanced for surgery to change the prognosis.

> **Benign tumours sound innocuous;** however, they can be even more destructive and debilitating than malignant tumours. GCTs, for example, can erode and destroy joints rapidly. Multiple enchondromas can cause skeletal deformity and disability.

Medication

Chemotherapy has a role in certain primary bone tumours. In some, such as Ewing's sarcoma, it is an effective treatment. In others, it can be used as an adjunct: either pre-surgery, to reduce the size of the tumour to be excised, therefore potentially sparing the limb, or post-surgery, to reduce recurrence or where complete excision was not possible. Chemotherapy is also combined with radiotherapy in certain tumours, e.g. in incompletely excised Ewing's sarcoma.

Chemotherapy is also used for palliative treatment in inoperable tumours, to reduce symptoms.

Radiotherapy

Radiotherapy uses high energy X-rays directed to a concentrated area. It is used to control spread and recurrence of certain bone tumours and is effective as primary treatment in Ewing's sarcoma when combined with chemotherapy. It is also used to treat the distant spread of such tumours, e.g. lung metastases from Ewing's sarcoma.

Prognosis

Prognosis varies with different tumours. Overall 5-year survival for all malignant bone tumours is around 65%. High grade tumours with metastatic spread have a poor prognosis. Those patients who have a successful surgical excision in low grade tumours can expect up to a 92% 5-year survival.

ALP is released from bone following destruction by osteosarcoma. It is used as a marker of prognosis, as survival is better in those with near-normal values.

10.2 Multiple myeloma

Multiple myeloma is a cancer of the bone marrow specifically affecting the plasma cells that produce antibodies. Multiple myeloma is a disease of old age, with most patients presenting over the age of 70.

10.2.1 Pathology

Multiple myeloma occurs after a rapid proliferation in plasma cells that produce paraprotein, an abnormal antibody. The abnormal cells and antibodies interfere with the normal function of the marrow, reducing its capacity to make normal cells. The paraproteins can become lodged within the renal tubules, causing renal failure, and the destruction of the bone releases calcium into the circulation.

10.2.2 Clinical features

Two-thirds of patients with multiple myeloma present with bone pain, the most common site being the spine. Multiple myeloma may also present with a fracture following trivial trauma. Anaemia, hypercalcaemia, renal failure and an increased susceptibility to infections occur as a consequence of the disease.

Diagnostic criteria mnemonic **'CRAB'**
- **C**alcium >2.75mmol/L
- **R**enal failure
- **A**naemia Hb <10g/dl
- **B**one pain (lytic lesions or compressive spine wedge fractures)

10.2.3 Diagnostic approach

Patients over the age of 70 presenting with lethargy, bone pain or a pathological fracture should be investigated for myeloma. Wedge compression spine fractures can occur due to osteoporosis, but myeloma should always be suspected in these cases. Myeloma is also suspected in elderly patients with raised calcium, creatinine and ESR and low haemoglobin.

A diagnosis of multiple myeloma requires either of the following conditions to be fulfilled:

1. A plasma cell tumour (proven by biopsy) or at least 10% of the cells in the bone marrow are plasma cells, and at least one of the following:
    - high blood calcium level
    - poor kidney function
    - low red blood cell counts (anaemia)
    - lytic lesions found on imaging studies
    - an abnormal area in the bones or bone marrow on an MRI scan
    - increase in one type of light chains in the blood so that one type is 100 times more common than the other.
2. 60% or more plasma cells in the bone marrow.

10.2.4 Investigations

Myeloma is confirmed with both blood and urine tests for paraprotein and a bone marrow biopsy. Blood tests show a raised level of paraprotein, usually of IgG origin, or other constituents of immunoglobulins such as free light chains. Urinary paraprotein, known as Bence Jones protein, is also raised. Marrow biopsy, usually from the sternum or pelvis, will show abnormal plasma cells; more than 10% is diagnostic. Radiographs can show lytic lesions in the bones.

10.2.5 Management

Management is usually multidisciplinary, often led by Haematologists. Patients may require joint specialist care, such as when a patient admitted for a pathological fracture for orthopaedic assessment is subsequently diagnosed with myeloma.

Medication

Chemotherapy and steroids comprise the standard medical therapy, and for those fit enough, an autologous stem cell transplant can prolong life. Bisphosphonates are used to prevent fractures, and to treat hypercalcaemia and bone pain. Supportive therapies include dialysis for renal failure and transfusions for anaemia.

Surgery

If a spinal fracture becomes unstable or painful, vertebroplasty (injecting bone cement into the affected vertebrae) can improve pain. Surgery may also be required to stabilise impending or established pathological fractures of long bones.

Prognosis

Five-year survival of all age groups is around 35%.

10.3 Metastatic bone disease

Distant spread of cancer cells to bone can occur by lymphatic or haematogenous routes, or by local invasion (**Figure 10.2**).

10.3.1 Aetiology

There are five cancers that commonly metastasise to bone: prostate, breast, lung, thyroid and kidney. They can form blastic (dense bone) or lytic (resorbed bone) lesions, visible on plain radiography (**Table 10.2** and **Figure 10.3**).

10.3.2 Clinical features

The typical presentation is bone pain, including thoracic pain, often persisting at night, pathological fracture or metastatic spinal cord compression. It is considered a medical emergency if patients have neurological symptoms in their legs with bladder and bowel dysfunction, and they require urgent assessment. These symptoms suggest spinal cord compression and these patients often also have concurrent hypercalcaemia.

10.3.3 Diagnostic approach and investigations

In a patient presenting with bone pain, especially nocturnal, the initial investigation is plain radiography, as metastatic lesions are almost always visible. Isotope bone scan or MRI may be required, to better characterise the lesion or to identify whether the metastasis is solitary or multiple. Metastatic bone disease can also be discovered during staging investigations for patients already diagnosed with cancer. In addition, incidental findings can occur during routine imaging for an unrelated condition.

Once a metastasis is diagnosed on radiograph, there needs to be a thorough workup. In patients without a previous diagnosis of cancer, the primary tumour needs to be identified. This will include a full clinical assessment including breast, chest, abdomen and rectal/prostate examination, as well as blood tests to check for anaemia, raised inflammatory markers, raised calcium levels and specific

Table 10.2 *Types and radiographic appearances of bone metastases*

Primary tumour	Prostate	Lung, thyroid or kidney	Breast
Type of bone lesion	Osteoblastic	Osteolytic	Mixed
Radiograph appearance of bone lesion	Dense/sclerotic	Resorbed	Dense and resorbed

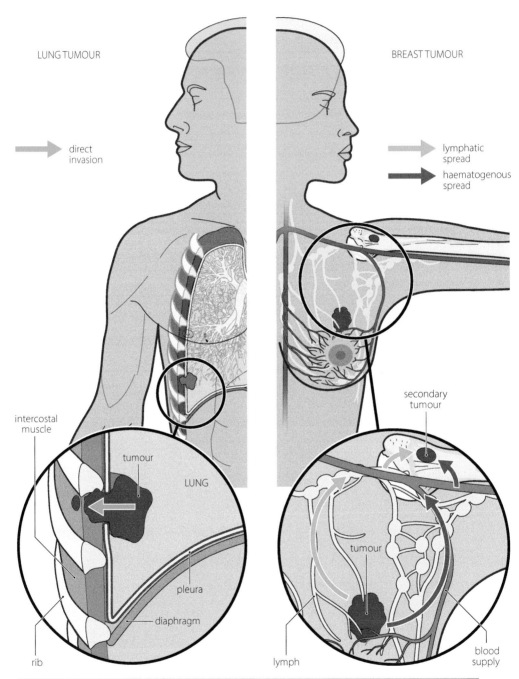

Figure 10.2 Mechanism of metastatic spread of cancer cells: (a) lymphatic; (b) direct local invasion; (c) haematogenous.

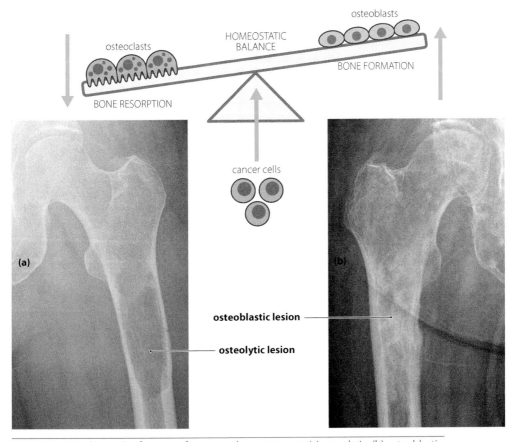

Figure 10.3 Radiographic features of common bone tumours: (a) osteolytic; (b) osteoblastic.

tumour markers (e.g. CA 19-9 for pancreas, CA 125 for uterine, ovarian and breast, CEA for bowel and PSA for prostate). CT of chest, abdomen and pelvis should be performed to help diagnose the primary cancer and for staging.

10.3.4 Management

Medication

Metastatic bone disease is painful, so initial management often requires the use of opioid analgesic medication. The best treatment for bone metastases is the treatment of the primary cancer. Therapies may include chemotherapy, hormone therapy and immunotherapy, including monoclonal antibodies.

Chemotherapy may be required to reduce local spread of some primary tumours. Chemotherapy can also help to reduce the size of tumours. Hypercalcaemia often needs treating with bisphosphonates, a medication that binds to osteoclasts to reduce calcium levels in the plasma. Bisphosphonates also help to reduce pain. The use of high dose steroids can have an important role in reducing oedema associated with spinal metastasis causing spinal cord compression.

Radiotherapy

Solitary or a small number of bone metastases can be treated locally by radiotherapy. This reduces pain and can prevent pathological fractures.

Surgery

A single metastasis to bone could potentially have curative surgery. An example of this is renal cell carcinoma, where excision of the primary tumour (with a nephrectomy) combined with wide local excision of the single bony metastasis is curative. More often surgical treatment is for pain control and to treat or reduce the risk of pathological fracture. Mirels' score, which assesses the risk of fracture (**Table 10.3**), is used as a guide to whether surgery should be undertaken. However, the medical condition of some patients may prevent them from being suitable for an anaesthetic and therefore surgery. Surgical treatment for spinal metastases in the form of vertebroplasty can help to reduce pain.

Prognosis

By the time patients develop bone metastases, their cancer may have advanced and spread to other organs. This is often a sign of poor prognosis and curative treatment at this point is rare. The prognosis, however, depends on many factors such as the type of primary tumour, whether there is any local or distal spread, and how well it responds to treatment.

Table 10.3 *Mirels' scoring system for assessing fracture risk in long bones with metastases*				
Points	**Site of lesion**	**Size of lesion**	**Nature of lesion**	**Pain**
1	Upper limb	<⅓ of cortex	Blastic	Mild
2	Lower limb	⅓–⅔ of cortex	Mixed	Moderate
3	Trochanteric region	>⅔ of cortex	Lytic	Functional

The minimum score is 3, maximum 12. A score of >9 indicates high risk of fracture, warranting prophylactic fixation. With a score of <7 fracture is unlikely, therefore non-surgical treatment is indicated. Those with a score of 8 are treated according to the judgement of the clinical team.

10.4 Answers to starter questions

1. Childhood is a time of growth and development. This rapid cell turnover increases the chance of cells acquiring mutations that lead to malignant transformation. Most primary bone tumours in children occur around joints with the highest growth, e.g. the knee and proximal humerus.

2. The very late onset of multiple myeloma is likely due to the cumulative effects of genetic mutations, which initially lead to a premalignant plasma cell proliferative disorder known as monoclonal gammopathy of undetermined significance (MGUS). Further mutations give a 'second hit' that leads to multiple myeloma and end organ damage.

Chapter 11
Musculoskeletal emergencies

In the musculoskeletal system, there are several emergency diagnoses that must not be missed and must be referred for urgent treatment by a hospital specialist. These usually present with a rapid deterioration in symptoms and, if not treated promptly, can leave patients with significant morbidity.

> A common cause of litigation is failure to recognise disorders that cause permanent damage if not treated promptly. Documentation in the emergency setting must be clear and concise and should include timings of referrals.

This chapter covers the common emergencies and those that should be escalated to seniors early to allow for timely diagnosis and treatment.

Case 11.1 Unilateral headache and blurred vision

Presentation

Lillian James had to abandon her hair appointment when she developed a severe right-sided headache made worse by the hairdresser brushing her hair. On return home her vision became blurred in her right eye. She tried to rest, thinking she had a migraine and that her symptoms would improve. Her daughter came to check on her after she finished work and tried to persuade Lillian to eat her evening meal, but her jaw was aching as she started to chew. Lillian's vision suddenly deteriorated and her daughter took her straight away to the Emergency Department.

Initial interpretation

Headache is a very common symptom; however, sudden loss of vision is an emergency and needs to be seen in hospital immediately. Loss of vision can be caused by structural eye problems such as retinal detachment, or a problem with the optic nerve or its blood supply. Facial pain may indicate trigeminal neuralgia but scalp tenderness is less common in this condition. The combination with claudication jaw pain points more towards a problem with the blood supply to these areas.

History

Lillian is 70 years old and a retired secretary. Her past medical history includes hypertension which is well controlled. She likes to keep active but has been feeling very tired recently and her muscles have felt quite stiff, weak and aching. This is especially when she is doing overhead activities such as hanging clothes in the wardrobe.

Interpretation of history

Symmetrical pain and stiffness in the girdle muscles of the shoulders and hips are symptoms of PMR, an inflammatory disorder affecting the muscles and soft tissues (see *Section 4.10*).

Case 11.1 *continued*

15% of patients with PMR will develop temporal arteritis; however, 50% of patients with temporal arteritis will also suffer from PMR.

Examination

Inspection of Lillian's scalp reveals a prominent temporal artery which is very tender to touch. Lillian cannot see out of her right eye. Fundoscopy reveals a swollen pale optic disc and narrowing of the retinal arteries with some small retinal haemorrhages (**Figure 11.1**). Cranial nerve examination is otherwise normal.

Interpretation of findings

Fundoscopy findings are consistent with decreased blood flow to the eye from the ophthalmic artery. Inflammation of the temporal artery causes prominence; tenderness and reduced pulsation are signs of temporal arteritis.

Investigations

High CRP and ESR shows that there is an inflammatory process in the body, but this does not specifically diagnose PMR and temporal arteritis. A high platelet count also suggests an inflammatory process.

Diagnosis

The diagnosis is confirmed following biopsy and histopathological analysis of a sample of the temporal artery, which demonstrates inflammation in the vessel wall which may include giant cells (hence the alternative name 'giant cell arteritis'). Tertiary centres are now offering temporal artery ultrasound scans. Treatment must not be delayed for confirmation on biopsy, due to the risk of permanent vision loss. High dose steroid treatment dampens down the inflammatory processes in the arteries, gradually allowing the blood to flow again, and should be started immediately. This form of vasculitis only affects large vessels such as the temporal artery, ophthalmic artery and branches of the

PROMINENT TEMPORAL ARTERY

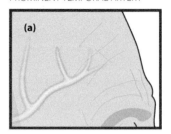

superficial temporal artery

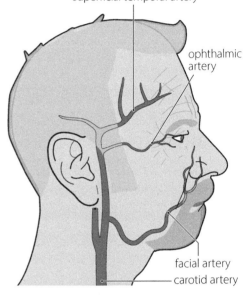

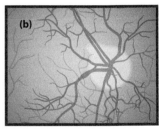

PALE, OEDEMATOUS OPTIC DISC

Figure 11.1 Temporal arteritis signs and symptoms: (a) raised and inflamed superficial temporal artery; (b) pale optic disc.

aorta but does not affect the medium and small vessels of the kidneys and skin and other organs (**Table 11.1**).

Table 11.1 *An example of the emergency management of temporal arteritis; the dosage is increased if symptoms or inflammatory markers worsen*

	Medication	**Timing**
Immediate (in high risk sight-threatening situations)	IV high dose (500–1000mg) methylprednisolone	3 days
Maintenance	High dose 40–60mg oral prednisolone	4 weeks
	Reduce by 10mg every 1–2 weeks	Until 20mg
	Reduce by 2.5mg every 2–4 weeks	Until 10mg
	Reduce by 1mg every 1–2 months	

Case 11.2 Back pain and difficulty walking

Presentation

Jane Haikney is 72 years old and likes to keep active; she very rarely visits her GP. Thus her GP is surprised when Jane requests a home visit as she has significant pain in her thoracic region and has had difficulty mobilising. She has had multiple falls and recently has felt very clumsy when she walks. She has had ongoing lower back pain for many years and has been told she has 'wear and tear' in her spine.

Initial interpretation

Isolated lower limb clumsiness and losing the feel of proprioception are red flags and suggest significant spinal cord compression in either the lumbar or thoracic spine.

History

Jane had successful treatment of breast cancer in her 50s with a mastectomy and anti-oestrogen treatment. She has been taking painkillers for OA in her lower back for many years, but now her pain has moved to the middle of her back. She has not been passing much urine but has noticed a couple of times that her bed sheets are wet despite not feeling she has passed any urine.

Although very embarrassed, she also tells her GP that during the night she had an episode of faecal incontinence.

Examination

Power in both of Jane's legs is reduced as well as sensation to both light touch and pin prick. Her knee and ankle jerks are brisk on both sides and her plantar reflexes are upgoing. Rectal examination reveals loss of sensation on both sides of the saddle area; anal tone and wink are absent. Her arms are unaffected.

Interpretation of findings

Loss of anal sensation and tone as well as urinary incontinence are the clinical manifestations of compression on the cauda equina, a lower motor neurone syndrome, or spinal cord compression. Urine incontinence in patients is often due to overflow from a distended bladder that is unable to contract to empty. Brisk reflexes are a sign of an upper motor neurone syndrome and are seen in cord compression above the level of the cauda equina nerve roots. Patients with cervical spine cord compression would have weakness affecting all four limbs. Jane is likely to have spinal cord compression at the level of her thoracic spine, as

Case 11.2 *continued*

her pain radiates from this area and she has upper motor neurone signs below this level (**Figure 11.2** and **Table 11.2**).

Investigations

Jane is referred as an emergency to spinal surgeons who perform an urgent MRI scan. The history suggests that Jane is at risk of osteoporosis but she also has a previous history of cancer. Collapse due to osteoporosis of the vertebral body, spondylosis, invasion by tumour and central disc protrusion are common causes of atraumatic cord compression. The MRI confirms that there is tumour invasion of the vertebrae with spinal cord compression and myelopathic (ischaemic)

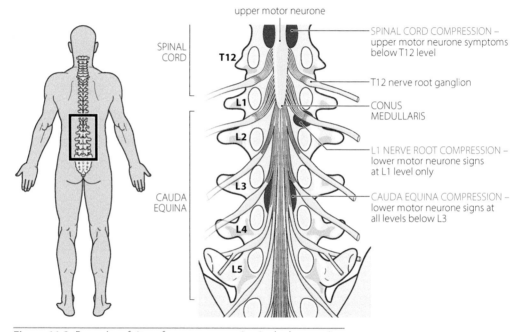

Figure 11.2 Examples of sites of nerve compression in the lower spine.

Table 11.2 *Signs and symptoms of compression at different spinal levels*

Level involved	Spinal cord	Single nerve roots	Cauda equina
Pattern	Upper motor neurone with signs below level of compression	Lower motor neurone with signs only at the specific nerve root	Lower motor neurone with signs below level of compression
Reflexes	Brisk	Absent	Absent
Sensation	Reduced	Reduced in single dermatome	Reduced
Motor	Reduced	Reduced in single myotome	Reduced
Bowel and urinary incontinence	Common	Only if sacral nerve roots affected	Almost always

changes within the cord at T10. She has other multiple lesions including her lumbar spine vertebra.

Diagnosis

It is likely that Jane's breast cancer has returned and metastasised to bone. Staging CTs are performed to confirm the diagnosis and to assess

extent of disease. Urgent IV steroid treatment and radiotherapy are used to reduce oedema around the cord to improve her symptoms.

In certain cases, with long life expectancy or intractable pain, surgery to debulk the tumour and/or stabilisation may be of benefit. Single lesion metastatic deposits can be excised and are curative in certain tumours, e.g. renal cell.

Case 11.3 Sudden pain in knee

Presentation

Paul Plumley attends his out-of-hours GP after suddenly developing pain in his right knee. Paul had been a keen runner in the past but now in his 60s has had to work on his golfing handicap due to OA in his knees. Earlier that day Paul's knee started to become painful at the twelfth hole and by the sixteenth it was very swollen; he had

to get a golf buggy to return to the clubhouse. Paul thought his OA was flaring so he took some ibuprofen, elevated his knee and applied some ice.

Initial interpretation

Initially this sounds like a potential flare of OA or degenerate meniscus. Paul has done his initial

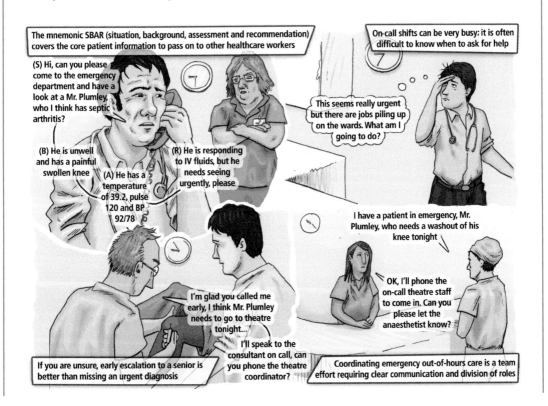

at-home treatment correctly. This problem should settle in a few days.

History

Paul has kept fit most of his life and is taking aspirin and atorvastatin for primary cardiac prevention. He enjoys a few pints of beer after a round of golf and working in his allotment. Last week he caught his leg on a rose thorn but it healed up and he thought nothing of it.

Interpretation of history

Three differentials are possible here. First, as Paul takes aspirin there is a small chance this has caused bleeding into his knee joint (haemarthrosis) following a long round of golf. Alcohol and a high purine diet can precipitate an episode of gout. Even a small cut gives an entry point through the skin for bacteria which can spread through the bloodstream to the knee joint.

Further history

Later that evening Paul's knee becomes very hot and he is unable to weight-bear despite taking ibuprofen, paracetamol and codeine. He feels feverish and unwell, prompting him to attend the out-of-hours GP.

Examination

Paul's temperature is 38.8°C and pulse rate 110bpm. The GP notices that the scratch on Paul's leg, which had almost healed, is red and hot. Paul's knee has an obvious effusion but he won't let the GP touch or move his knee as it is too painful.

Interpretation of findings

Paul has signs of a systemic inflammatory response secondary to infection, with a raised temperature and pulse rate.

Haemarthrosis and gout are unlikely to produce a systemic response if only one joint is affected; septic arthritis or osteomyelitis are much more likely.

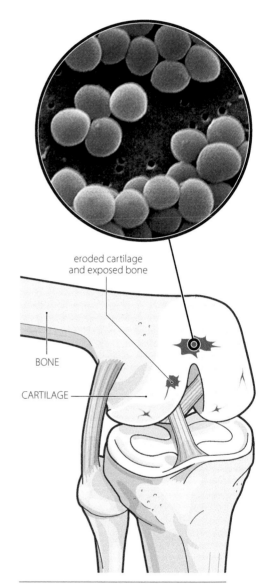

eroded cartilage and exposed bone

BONE

CARTILAGE

Figure 11.3 Bacterial *Staphylococcus aureus* septic arthritis causing destruction of the articular cartilage.

Investigations

Paul is sent urgently to the hospital to see the Orthopaedic team. They aspirate 50ml of purulent fluid from the knee and it is sent for urgent microscopy. Within half an hour the report shows that there are many polymorphs +++, no crystals and multiple small cocci bacteria in clumps.

Fluid sent for culture will take a few days to grow any bacteria and show antibiotic sensitivities, but treatment should not wait for these results to be available, if septic arthritis is suspected.

Diagnosis

The cause of Paul's knee pain is a bacterial septic arthritis, with the most likely pathogen being *Staphylococcus aureus* introduced through the break in the skin (**Figure 11.3**). Appropriate broad-spectrum antibiotics under the advice of the microbiology team are only given once there is a sample of the joint fluid sent to the lab.

Antibiotics can then be narrowed to a specific target once the culture results are known in a couple of days' time. If antibiotics are given prior to aspirate, the sample is often sterile and therefore it is not possible to narrow down the antibiotics to a more effective choice. The bacterial load within the knee is reduced with an arthroscopic washout in the operating theatre.

If a patient is septic you should not delay giving antibiotics while you wait for an aspirate sample.

Case 11.4 Pain following high energy fracture

Presentation

Daniel Petrescu is a 38-year-old man who has fallen from his bicycle at 20mph, sustaining a midshaft tibial fracture. He is currently on the orthopaedic ward in a long leg plaster and surgery is planned for tomorrow. Following application of his plaster he felt a lot more comfortable but the pain in his lower leg is now throbbing.

Initial interpretation

Initial treatment of a fracture is to give analgesia, reduce the fracture and hold it in a reduced position. This provides comfort for the patient. Daniel has had a high energy injury and should be given adequate analgesia.

History

Daniel is fit and well and does not take any medications.

Further history

The F1 doctor prescribes 1000mg paracetamol, 60mg codeine, 800mg ibuprofen and 10mg of oral morphine. Daniel's pain eases a little but he is asking for more morphine an hour later.

The F1 doctor is concerned that his pain is out of proportion to what is normal for this fracture. She decides to split the plaster in case it is too tight. Daniel's pain is eased again and the foot of the bed is raised to reduce any further swelling. Later that evening the pain increases again and the orthopaedic registrar is called to see Daniel.

Examination

Daniel is very uncomfortable; he has a raised pulse rate at 115bpm and he is sweating. His calf is very tender and swollen and he is unable to move his toes due to pain. Passive extension of the toes causes Daniel significant pain but passive flexion is not as bad. Sensation and both pulses in the feet are normal.

Interpretation of findings

Pain despite adequate analgesia and out of proportion to the injury is the first symptom in compartment syndrome. If this is treated early no other symptoms should manifest. There are four compartments within the lower leg and one or all of them can be affected at one time (**Figure 1.44**). Increasing the pressure by passively stretching the compartment causing

Case 11.4 *continued*

pain, is diagnostic of compartment syndrome (**Table 11.3**). In this case the flexor (deep posterior and superficial posterior) compartment is affected.

Investigations

Compartment syndrome is a clinical diagnosis and if suspected, the patient should be taken urgently to theatre for decompression. In cases where it is difficult to obtain a history, e.g. in an intubated patient, a pressure monitor can be inserted to measure the intracompartmental pressure. Normal compartment pressures range from 0–8mmHg; pressure >30mmHg or within 30mmHg of the diastolic blood pressure is diagnostic of compartment syndrome. CK is a marker of muscle cell death and can give an indication of severity, but is not used for diagnosis.

Diagnosis

Daniel has compartment syndrome of his lower leg and is taken to theatre within the hour to have his decompression surgery. Long incisions are made on either side of his tibia, allowing access to all four compartments within the lower leg.

Table 11.3 *Signs and symptoms of compartment syndrome: 'All the Ps' is a simple way to remember the late signs*

Symptoms	Timing
Pain out of proportion to injury	Early
Paraesthesia	Intermediate
Pain on **p**assive stretch	Early
Tense swelling	Early
Paralysis	Late
Pallor	Very late
Pulseless	Very late
Perishingly cold	Very late

The fascia is incised in all four compartments and the wounds are left open to allow the swelling to subside (**Figure 11.4**). Daniel is rehydrated during surgery to dilute myoglobulin (a muscle breakdown product) to prevent renal failure. He will return to theatre in a few days to have the wounds closed or skin grafted.

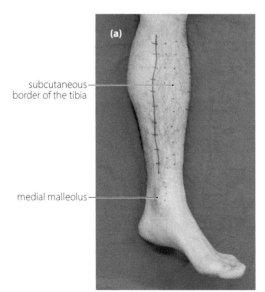
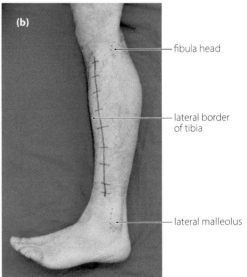

(a) subcutaneous border of the tibia — medial malleolus

(b) fibula head — lateral border of tibia — lateral malleolus

Figure 11.4 Fasciotomies are performed to release the pressure in all four compartments of the leg through two incisions on either side of the tibia.

Case 11.5 Open fracture

Presentation

Gary Morrison is 25 years old and is out training with the army when he slips down a steep slope. His foot is caught underneath a rock and his leg twists. He noticed blood on his trousers, his leg is deformed and bone is seen visible in the wound just proximal to his ankle. The paramedics realign his leg and place him in a splint and transfer him by helicopter to the nearest hospital.

Initial interpretation

Gary has sustained an open fracture to his lower leg. The initial resuscitative treatment is to give analgesia and realign the bone for comfort and to prevent further injury.

History

The 'SAMPLE' history technique is used to quickly hand over important information in patients with trauma (**Table 11.4**).

Examination

In the Emergency Department Gary is assessed by the trauma team. Both dorsalis pedis and posterior tibial pulses are present. Sensation in the foot is normal and he is able to move his ankle a little but it is painful. There is an open wound 4cm in length over the lateral part of his lower tibia and although there is no skin loss, the wound appears dusky round the edges. The wound is clean and photographs are taken so others are able to see the wound without having to take down the dressings multiple times. It is then wrapped in saline-soaked gauze and placed in an above-knee cast to prevent any movement of the fracture. Neurovascular function post cast immobilisation is normal.

Interpretation of findings

Although there does not appear to be any skin loss, the soft tissue injury beneath is likely to be severe due to the mechanism of injury, and the edges of the wound are dusky. Involvement of plastic surgeons is appropriate at this point for planning of wound coverage following a full debridement of the wound. As no plastic surgeons are available at the current hospital, it is advised by BOAST (British Orthopaedic Association's Standards for Trauma) to transfer the patient early to a hospital that has this expertise.

> Even though the wound appears clean, IV antibiotics and tetanus cover are given early to reduce infection. Poor wound healing and ongoing bone infection are two of the most important complications of open fractures.

Investigations

The initial radiographs show displaced multifragmentary distal tibial and fibular fractures which extend into the ankle joint.

Table 11.4 *SAMPLE history*	
	Handover
Signs and symptoms	Open fracture to left lower leg, sensation and pulses are normal
Allergies	No allergies
Medicines	No medicines
Past medical history	Fit and well
Last ate	4 hours ago
Events surrounding trauma	Fall down slope, deformed open lower leg fracture reduced on scene

Diagnosis

On transfer to the regional trauma centre, Gary is prepped for theatre for that afternoon. A debridement is performed of all the devitalised tissue and a large skin defect of 7 × 5cm is left. As skin closure is not feasible, a temporary external fixator is used to stabilise the fracture while further planning for skin coverage with muscle flaps is planned by the plastic surgeons. A CT scan is performed following surgery to assess the fracture configuration, in order to help plan for definitive surgery.

Case 11.6 Progressing painful swollen hand

Presentation

Pamela Wallace is a 55-year-old who presents to the Walk-in Centre with a painful, red, hot and swollen index finger which has quickly progressed to involve her hand.

Initial interpretation

A red, hot and swollen digit indicates inflammation. Spreading quickly to other parts of the hand suggests infection is the most likely cause.

History

The previous day Pamela had been out with her friends for a picnic in the park when she leant on a rusty nail which pierced the palm of her index finger. There was a small puncture which seemed innocuous. Pamela gave it a good wash when she got home and dressed it with a plaster.

Interpretation of history

An entry point for bacteria to get to the deep structures of the hand makes the diagnosis of infection most likely.

Examination

Pamela's finger is very swollen and fusiform in shape. She is holding her index finger and wrist in flexion for comfort. The wound from the nail is very small and almost healed and there is no discharge. Palpation on the palm and finger is exquisitely tender and pain increases on passive extension of the fingers and wrist. Further palpation down the forearm is also starting to feel uncomfortable. Pamela's observations are as follows: temperature 37.8°C, pulse 105bpm regular, respiratory rate 22/min and blood pressure 100/72mmHg.

Interpretation of findings

This patient has four cardinal signs of flexor tendon sheath infection:
1. Fusiform swelling of finger
2. Tenderness over flexor tendon sheath
3. Finger held in flexion
4. Pain on passive extension.

Pyrexia and tachycardia are signs of systemic infection.

Investigations

A radiograph is performed which does not demonstrate any residual foreign body or osteomyelitis. Blood tests reveal a neutrophilia with a WCC of 15×10^9/L and a CRP of 210mg/L.

Diagnosis

Pamela has a clear case of flexor tendon sheath infection and the definitive treatment is to surgically drain the infection to prevent destruction of the tendon. Whist waiting to go to theatre the arm is elevated above the level of the heart and IV antibiotics are administered. Infection within the sheath is a surgical emergency, as early treatment is required to prevent permanent tendon damage.

The flexor tendons are surrounded by sheaths which protect the tendons and help them glide (**Figure 11.5**). These sheaths are often interconnected and therefore an infection in one part of the sheath can spread very quickly to the rest, including into the palm and forearm. The infective process can damage the tendon, making the tendon become scarred and fibrosed in the sheath and thus preventing the smooth gliding movement.

Surgical drainage is performed urgently. The sheaths are opened and if severely infected, may be left open to further aid drainage. It is not uncommon for multiple washouts to be performed to get the infection under control and sometimes catheters are left *in situ* to allow continuous drainage. Early physiotherapy is key to preventing stiffness and to regain function in the hand and this can start even when the wounds are still open.

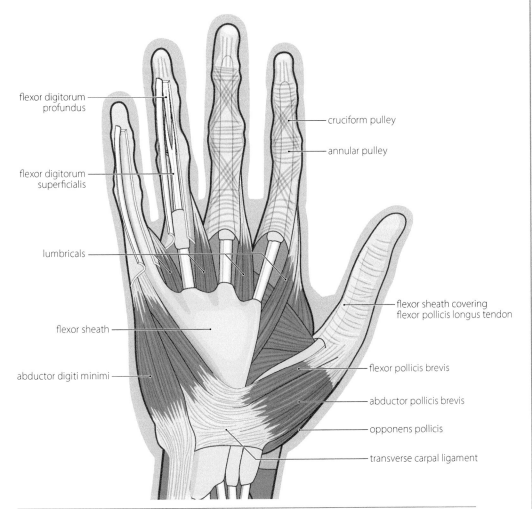

Figure 11.5 The flexor sheath surrounds the FDS and FDP tendons in each finger. The tendons are surrounded by cruciate and annular pulleys that allow the tendons to glide.

Chapter 12
Self-assessment

12.1 SBA questions

Chapter 3: Arthritis

1. A 47-year-old woman attends the rheumatology clinic with a 4-month history of pain, stiffness and swelling in the small joints of her hands and feet.
   What is the most likely diagnosis?
   A. Calcium pyrophosphate arthropathy
   B. Gout
   C. Osteoarthritis
   D. Psoriatic arthritis
   E. Rheumatoid arthritis

2. A 22-year-old man is referred to the rheumatology clinic with lower back and buttock pain associated with prolonged morning stiffness. A diagnosis of axial spondyloarthritis (ankylosing spondylitis) is suspected.
   Which of the following HLA antigens is most commonly associated with this condition?
   A. HLA-B27
   B. HLA-B51
   C. HLA-DR3
   D. HLA-DR4
   E. HLA-DRB1

3. A 23-year-old man attends the GP surgery with a 6-month history of lower back pain.
   Which one of the following features, taken from the history, would suggest an inflammatory cause?
   A. Evening stiffness
   B. Improvement with exercise
   C. Reduced range of movement
   D. Response to analgesia
   E. Sudden onset

4. A 46-year-old woman presents to her GP with painful swollen fingers. On examination there is symmetrical swelling of the distal interphalangeal joints of both hands, pitting in her nails and a scaly rash over both elbows.
   What is the most likely diagnosis?
   A. Calcium pyrophosphate arthritis
   B. Osteoarthritis
   C. Psoriatic arthritis
   D. Reactive arthritis
   E. Rheumatoid arthritis

5. You suspect a diagnosis of rheumatoid arthritis in a patient in clinic.
   Which single autoantibody test is the most specific for this condition?
   A. ANA
   B. Anti-CCP
   C. Anti-La
   D. p-ANCA
   E. Rheumatoid factor

6. A 77-year-old man is reviewed on the ward with an acutely painful swollen knee. He is on diuretic medication for heart failure.
   What do you expect the synovial fluid result to show?
   A. Rhomboid-shaped positively birefringent crystals
   B. Needle-shaped negatively birefringent crystals
   C. Rhomboid-shaped negatively birefringent crystals
   D. Needle-shaped positively birefringent crystals
   E. Rod-shaped positively birefringent crystals

7. A 50-year-old man is seen by his GP with bilateral knee pain. The pain has been worsening over the last 12 months and is associated with stiffness. He has some difficulty getting up out of bed and the pain gets worse towards the late afternoon/early evening. He thinks there has been some swelling. He also describes some pain at the base of his thumb. It is beginning to interfere with his work as a builder.

What type of arthritis is this?

A. Gout

B. Osteoarthritis

C. Pseudogout

D. Psoriatic arthritis

E. Rheumatoid arthritis

Chapter 4: Connective tissue disorders and vasculitis

1. A 70-year-old woman presents with pain and stiffness in her shoulders and hips. Her inflammatory markers are elevated and you diagnose polymyalgia rheumatica. You commence oral prednisolone.

What other investigation is recommended?

A. DEXA scan

B. Isotope bone scan

C. PET scan

D. Shoulder and pelvis X-rays

E. Temporal artery biopsy

2. A 25-year-old woman is referred with joint pain. She tells you that she has always been "bendy" and was able to do the splits as a child.

What feature in the history would make you consider a less benign condition?

A. Inguinal hernia

B. Knee pain

C. Prominent, sunken scars

D. Stretchy skin

E. Widespread musculoskeletal pain

3. A 33-year-old lady attends clinic for her routine follow-up appointment. She was diagnosed with SLE 2 years ago and has been stable on hydroxychloroquine. She tells you that she is planning a family.

What is the most important initial advice to give her?

A. Prescribe heparin for use during pregnancy

B. Re-check ANA

C. Refer for joint obstetric/rheum care

D. Stop anti-inflammatory medication

E. Stop taking hydroxychloroquine

4. A 64-year-old woman with Sjögren's syndrome attends her GP reporting sweats. She has had some weight loss.

Which condition are you most concerned about?

A. HIV

B. Hodgkin's lymphoma

C. Hyperthyroidism

D. Non-Hodgkin's lymphoma

E. Tuberculosis

5. A 45-year-old woman is referred with Raynaud's syndrome.

Which other feature of the history and examination is not a diagnostic criteria of limited cutaneous systemic scleroderma?

A. Calcinosis

B. Dysphagia (oesophageal dysmotility)

C. Malar rash

D. Sclerodactyly

E. Telangiectasia

6. A 22-year-old man presents to the Emergency Department with bilateral swollen ankles. He has been feeling generally unwell and reports feeling more short of breath on running.

What is the most likely diagnosis?

A. Crystal arthritis

B. Psoriatic arthritis

C. Rheumatoid arthritis

D. Sarcoidosis

E. Septic arthritis

7. A 57-year-old man has progressive muscle weakness. He struggles to get out of a chair but can still write and type without any problem. He doesn't describe much pain. His blood results show a raised CK.

Which autoantibody is most specific for his diagnosis?
A. ANA
B. Anti-CCP
C. Anti-Jo-1
D. Anti-La
E. Anti-Ro

8. A 33-year-old woman has had four miscarriages over two years. Antiphospholipid syndrome is suspected.
Which of the following laboratory tests supports the diagnosis?
A. Anti-cardiolipin antibody positive in last month
B. Anti-cardiolipin and lupus anticoagulant positive in last month
C. Anti-beta2-glycoprotein 1 positive in last month
D. Lupus anticoagulant positive in last month
E. Lupus anticoagulant and anti-cardiolipin antibody positive now and 3 months ago

9. A 43-year-old woman with SLE reports pain in the small joints of her hands.
What do you expect the X-rays to show?
A. Erosions of the MCP joints only
B. Erosions of the MCP and PIP joints
C. Erosions of the PIP joints only
D. No erosive change
E. Soft tissue swelling

10. A 47-year-old man presents with an intermittent fever, joint pain and a salmon-pink rash.
Which laboratory test do you expect to be significantly elevated?
A. Ferritin levels
B. Folate levels
C. Iron levels
D. Vitamin B12 levels
E. Zinc levels

Chapter 5: Metabolic bone disease

1. At what age is peak bone mass reached?
A. 12 years

B. 18 years
C. 25 years
D. 30 years
E. 50 years

2. A 76-year-old woman has a low impact fracture. Her DEXA scans confirm osteoporosis.
Which of the following may have put her at increased risk of osteoporosis?
A. Family history of osteoporosis
B. Hypothyroidism
C. Late menopause
D. Low alcohol intake
E. Obesity

3. An 80-year-old man presents with pain in his left thigh. He was recently referred to ENT with tinnitus.
What might his blood results show?
A. Low ALP
B. Low ALT
C. Raised ALP
D. Raised ALT
E. Raised GGT

4. A 34-year-old woman has a DEXA scan. She was diagnosed with coeliac disease 10 years ago. She has a 6-month-old baby whom she is breastfeeding. She wishes to have more children in the future. The DEXA scan confirms osteoporosis.
Which treatment is recommended?
A. Denosumab
B. Intravenous bisphosphonate
C. Oral bisphosphonate
D. Vitamin D and calcium supplements
E. Vitamin D and good dietary calcium intake

5. A 19-year-old male has been treated for anorexia nervosa for 3 years. He is osteoporotic.
What treatment is most recommended to increase his BMD?
A. Alendronic acid
B. Denosumab
C. Exercise and balanced diet
D. Vitamin D
E. Zoledronic acid

Chapter 6: Skeletal injuries and disorders

1. An 86-year-old woman has fallen and is taken to the Emergency Department. Her radiograph shows an extracapsular neck of femur fracture. She is admitted to the trauma ward for treatment.
   What is the single most appropriate definitive management of this injury?
   A. Hemiarthroplasty
   B. Hip fixation
   C. Physiotherapy
   D. Total hip replacement
   E. Traction immobilisation

2. A 4-month-old boy is brought to the Emergency Department by his mother. She says that he is not moving his right leg over the last week. She is told that there is a spiral fracture of the femur bone. He is given analgesia and is placed in traction.
   What is the single most likely mechanism of his injury?
   A. Birth injury
   B. Brother fell on him
   C. Leg caught in cot sides
   D. Non-accidental injury
   E. Simple fall

3. A 12-year-old boy presents to the Emergency Department with pain in his hip after running around in the playground at school. The pain came on suddenly and he is now limping and not wanting to walk on it. He is slightly overweight.
   What is the single most likely cause of his hip pain?
   A. Bone tumour
   B. Fracture
   C. Osteoarthritis
   D. Perthes' disease
   E. Slipped capital femoral epiphysis

4. A 40-year-old man is injured following a road traffic accident and is brought immediately to the resuscitation room. He is unconscious and bleeding profusely from his thigh. His BP is 70/35mmHg, his pulse is 140bpm and respiratory rate 40.
   What should be the first priority?
   A. Cervical spine immobilisation collar
   B. CT scan
   C. Intravenous fluids
   D. Intubation
   E. Leg tourniquet

5. A 30-year-old woman attends her GP six months after having hip fracture fixation surgery for a displaced intracapsular neck of femur fracture sustained in a road traffic accident. Her hip was initially doing well but has gradually become painful over the last 4 months. Her CRP is <5 and WCC is 10.2.
   What is the single most likely diagnosis?
   A. Avascular necrosis
   B. Bone metastasis
   C. Missed femoral fracture
   D. Osteoarthritis
   E. Septic arthritis

6. A 14-year-old girl is diagnosed with a slipped capital femoral epiphysis and is treated with surgery. The cause of her SCFE is unknown and is being investigated; she is not overweight and has had no history of trauma.
   What is the single most appropriate test?
   A. Bone scan
   B. Genetic testing
   C. MRI scan
   D. Serum electrophoresis
   E. Thyroid-stimulating hormone (TSH)

7. A 40-year-old male pedestrian is hit on his left side by a car at 30mph. He is brought immediately to the resuscitation room. He has C-spine collar and blocks placed and was complaining of pain around his hips and neck at the scene. His BP is 70/35mmHg, his pulse is 140bpm and respiratory rate 40.
   What single step should be the first priority?
   A. CT scan
   B. ECG
   C. Hip radiograph
   D. MRI neck
   E. Pelvic binder

Chapter 7: Exercise-related injuries and soft tissue disorders

1. A 25-year old man twists his knee whilst falling to the floor following a tackle in a football match. His knee swells up immediately but he is able to put some weight through his leg to hobble off the pitch. He is able to raise his leg straight from the bed.

What is the single most likely injury he has sustained?
  A. Tibial fracture
  B. Meniscal injury
  C. Anterior cruciate ligament tear
  D. Patellar tendon rupture
  E. Medial collateral ligament strain

2. A 23-year-old man has been taken to hospital following a severe seizure and on waking, he notices his shoulder is painful. His radiograph doesn't show a fracture but his shoulder is unable to externally rotate.

What is the single most likely diagnosis?
  A. Acromioclavicular joint dislocation
  B. Anterior shoulder dislocation
  C. Frozen shoulder
  D. Posterior shoulder dislocation
  E. Rotator cuff tear

3. A 46-year-old woman felt a pop in the back of her calf while putting out her rubbish bins. She is diagnosed with an Achilles tendon rupture and placed in a cast. She takes thyroxine for hypothyroidism and has had a recent chest infection requiring antibiotics. She takes NSAIDs for osteoarthritis.

What single risk factor is associated with this injury?
  A. Antibiotics
  B. Female gender
  C. Hypothyroidism
  D. NSAIDs
  E. Thyroxine

4. A 60-year-old woman complains of pain and weakness in her shoulder, especially when trying to brush her hair. She attends her GP as it is now been going on for 3 months and ibuprofen gel is not helping.

What is the single investigation that should be done first?
  A. CRP
  B. CT shoulder
  C. Diagnostic shoulder injection
  D. Shoulder radiograph
  E. Ultrasound

5. A 63-year-old man mildly twists his knee when walking. He feels a sudden pain and his knee becomes swollen over the next 24 hours. He has full range of movement and can raise his leg from the bed. He has a tender joint line and anterior and posterior drawer tests are negative.

What is the single most likely diagnosis?
  A. ACL tear
  B. Meniscal tear
  C. Patellar dislocation
  D. Patellar tendon rupture
  E. Pre-patellar bursitis

6. A 72-year-old woman has pain on the medial aspect of her knee after she slipped and twisted on a wet floor. Since then the knee is painful and can give way. On examination there is medial joint line tenderness and a small effusion.

What should be the single first-line investigation?
  A. MRI
  B. Radiograph
  C. CT
  D. Joint aspirate
  E. Ultrasound

7. A 43-year-old joiner attends his GP with elbow pain which is worse when he flexes his wrist. He has full range of movement of his elbow and no redness or swellings.

What is the single most likely diagnosis?
  A. De Quervain's tenosynovitis
  B. Golfer's elbow
  C. Olecranon bursitis
  D. Osteoarthritis
  E. Tennis elbow

8. A 55-year-old male computer software engineer presents with a painful little finger that he is unable to straighten. His little finger has been a bit sore for a while, especially after using his computer; however, his finger only became stuck like this yesterday.

What is the single most likely cause?

A. Dupuytren's contracture
B. Extensor tendon rupture
C. Flexor tendon rupture
D. Trigger finger
E. Osteoarthritis

Chapter 8: Infection

1. A 60-year-old man presents with a sudden onset swollen, red, hot and painful elbow. He is reluctant to move his arm due to pain. He has a temperature of 38.1°C, his heart rate is 90bpm and his blood pressure is 131/82mmHg. His blood tests reveal a raised WCC at 14.5, a CRP of 112 and a normal urate level of 141.

What is the single next appropriate step in his management?

A. Intravenous antibiotics
B. Joint aspiration
C. NSAIDs
D. Oral antibiotics
E. Surgical washout of joint

2. A 67-year-old has suffered with pain in his knee over the last week. Today his ankle has also started to swell, becoming hot and painful. He is unable to put weight through the affected leg. He is apyrexial and his pulse is 78bpm. His WCC is raised at 18.9, his CRP is 77 and his urate is normal. A radiograph of his knee and ankle shows chondrocalcinosis.

What is the single finding most likely to be seen on microscopic analysis of an ankle joint aspiration?

A. Calcium pyrophosphate crystals
B. Gram-negative bacilli
C. Gram-positive cocci
D. Monosodium urate crystals
E. Red cells

3. A 22-year-old woman has pain and swelling in her calf two months after an accident in which she sustained a contaminated open fracture of her tibia. The tibia was fixed with an intramedullary nail and the wounds closed primarily after a thorough debridement; recovery was uncomplicated. The anterior tibia is warm and tender to touch and she is getting pain all the time. She is otherwise well. WCC is 11.9 and CRP is 27.

What single investigation should be completed first?

A. D-dimer
B. Knee aspirate
C. MRI
D. Radiograph
E. Venous Doppler

4. A 25-year-old IV drug user presents unwell to the Emergency Department complaining of lower back pain. Her WCC is 27 and CRP is 189 and a radiograph shows osteomyelitis of the fourth lumbar vertebrae. An MRI confirms that the intervertebral disc is also involved. Her neurological exam is normal and she has normal heart sounds.

What is the single most likely cause of the discitis?

A. Contiguous spread
B. Direct inoculation
C. Haematogenous spread
D. Idiopathic
E. Immunocompromised patient

5. A 54-year-old type I diabetic stepped on a rusty nail in the garden. He didn't notice until later, as he has diabetic neuropathy. He suddenly becomes unwell and is rushed to hospital. He is unwell with a pulse of 140bpm, BP of 80/62mmHg and a respiratory rate of 35.

What is the single most likely pathogen?

A. *Clostridium perfringens*
B. Methicillin-resistant *Staphylococcus aureus*
C. *Mycobacterium tuberculosis*
D. *Pseudomonas aeruginosa*
E. *Staphylococcus aureus*

6. A 60-year-old woman with diabetes is being treated by her podiatrist for an ulcer over her medial malleolus. She becomes acutely unwell with increasing pain and red hot swelling of the ankle and surrounding region. She is taken by ambulance to the Emergency Department. Temperature is 38.3°C, pulse 150bpm, BP 74/56.

What is the single most appropriate immediate management?

A. Ankle joint aspirate

B. IV antibiotics

C. NSAIDs

D. Surgical debridement

E. Clean and dress wound

7. A 25-year-old IV drug user presents to the Emergency Department complaining of severe lower back pain and weakness in both her legs over the last two days. Sensation is lost at levels lower than L4. Her WCC is 27 and CRP is 189 and she is pyrexial at 38.9°C, but haemodynamically stable.

What single management step should be the next?

A. IV antibiotics

B. MRI

C. Strict bed rest and log-roll

D. Surgical stabilisation

E. Tissue sampling

8. A 43-year-old woman attends the Emergency Department with a swollen, hot, red left knee. Her temperature is 38.9°C. A joint aspiration is performed.

Which of the following organisms is most likely to grow on culture of the synovial fluid?

A. *Neisseria gonorrhoeae*

B. *Staphylococcus aureus*

C. *Staphylococcus epidermidis*

D. *Streptococcus pneumoniae*

E. *Streptococcus pyogenes*

Chapter 9: Spinal and peripheral nerve disorders

1. A 29-year-old woman is 38 weeks' pregnant and is suffering with pain and numbness in her index finger and thumb which is worse at night. This has only started in the last 2 weeks and she has not noticed any weakness in her hands. Two-point discrimination testing is normal.

What is the single most appropriate first-line treatment?

A. Carpal tunnel decompression

B. Night splint

C. Physiotherapy

D. Steroid injection

E. Ulnar tunnel decompression

2. A 47-year-old woman presents to the GP with sudden pain down the back of her leg and numbness on the top of the foot down to the big toe following taking some rubbish to the recycling centre. Her big toe is weak to extension and she has a weak ankle reflex.

What is the single most likely cause for her symptoms?

A. Common peroneal nerve compression

B. Compartment syndrome

C. Cord compression at L5

D. Extensor hallucis longus tendon rupture

E. L4/5 disc prolapse

3. A 78-year-old man is having difficulty doing up the buttons on his clothes and both his hands feel clumsy. He is diagnosed to have cord compression at C7.

What is the most likely examination finding in this patient?

A. Absent biceps reflexes

B. Absent supinator reflexes

C. Deltoid weakness

D. Loss of sensation on outer aspect of shoulder

E. Positive Hoffmann's sign

4. A 23-year-old man is stabbed in the back. He has a spastic paralysis and loss of vibration and proprioception on the same side as the injury and has lost pain and temperature sensation on the opposite side below the injury level. He has a flaccid paralysis on the same side and same level of the injury.

What single part of the spinal cord has been transected?

A. Central cord
B. Dorsal columns
C. Hemi transection
D. Lateral corticospinal tract
E. Spinothalamic tract

5. A 90-year-old man presents with weakness in his arms and legs following a fall. He is brought to the Emergency Department by ambulance. He is alert, his observations are stable and he takes warfarin for atrial fibrillation. He is normally fully independent and usually requires no walking aids.

What is the single next step that should be taken?

A. CT head and spine
B. MRI spine
C. Cervical spine immobilisation
D. IV vitamin K
E. Cervical traction

Chapter 10: Tumours and malignancy

1. A 55-year-old woman with known breast cancer presents to the Emergency Department with worsening back pain associated with numbness in her legs. An urgent scan is performed, which shows a tumour pressing on her spinal cord. Metastatic breast cancer is suspected.

What is the first treatment you should offer?

A. High dose steroid
B. IV bisphosphonate
C. Morphine
D. Urgent chemotherapy
E. Urgent radiotherapy

2. A 79-year-old man presents to his GP with pain in his spine. He is fatigued and admits to weight loss and constipation.

Which combination of blood tests are most likely to support your suspected diagnosis?

A. Bone profile, anti-CCP, CRP
B. Bone profile, FBC, U&Es, serum electrophoresis
C. Bone profile, LFTs, CRP, serum urate
D. HLA-B27, CRP, FBC
E. HLA-B27, CRP, U&Es

Chapter 11: Musculoskeletal emergencies

1. A 65-year-old woman has been suffering for the last month with pain while she is chewing. When she brushes her hair she gets a sharp electric shock-type pain on her forehead but is also suffering from quite debilitating headaches that can come on at any time.

What is the single gold standard test for diagnosing her condition?

A. CRP
B. ESR
C. Fundoscopy
D. MRI head
E. Temporal artery biopsy

2. A 55-year-old fisherman suddenly develops pain in his lower back while he is working. Over the next few hours his legs become weak and his feet become numb. He has an episode of faecal incontinence and on examination has a full bladder.

What single step should be the next in his management?

A. Colonoscopy
B. CT scan
C. MRI lumbar spine
D. Lumbar spine radiograph
E. Urine dip

3. A 62-year-old man has fallen over, sustaining a fracture to his distal radius. It is manipulated and put in a full plaster. He wakes up in the night with severe pain in his arm, prompting a return trip to the hospital. He unable to extend his fingers due to severe pain in his arm and he has numbness in all his fingers.

What single management step should be done first?

A. Analgesia
B. Ice
C. Nerve conduction studies
D. Split the cast and elevate
E. Urgent fasciotomy decompression

4. A 22-year-old man is in a serious road traffic accident in which he has an open femur fracture. His initial assessment reveals his leg is the only injury. A large wound is present on his anterior thigh and bone is exposed. His foot is pulseless and doesn't have any sensation.

What should be the first management priority?

A. Anti-tetanus immunoglobulin
B. IV antibiotics

C. Manipulation and splint
D. Radiograph of femur
E. Trauma CT

5. A 55-year-old woman was scratched on the finger by her cat's claws and teeth while playing. The next day her finger swells and is fusiform; she is unable to either passively or actively extend her finger due to pain. She is tender down her finger and into her palm.

What is the single definitive management plan?

A. Analgesia
B. Elevation
C. IV antibiotics
D. Open washout of flexor sheath
E. Physiotherapy

12.2 SBA answers

Chapter 3: Arthritis

1. Answer E
Symptoms of stiffness and swelling suggest an inflammatory process and the symmetrical polyarticular distribution strongly suggests rheumatoid arthritis as the most likely diagnosis.

2. Answer A
Ankylosing spondylitis is strongly associated with the HLA class I antigen HLA-B27, which is present in up to 90% of patients.

3. Answer B
Morning stiffness which improves with exercise and worsens with inactivity, and responsiveness to NSAIDs are all characteristic of inflammatory symptoms. Sudden onset is often more common in mechanical aetiology and response to analgesia is non-specific.

4. Answer C
The site and nature of the skin rash with involvement of the nails suggests psoriasis. Approximately 1 in 5 patients with psoriasis can develop an inflammatory arthritis. Symmetrical

involvement of the DIP finger joints is characteristic of one of the subtypes of psoriatic arthritis.

5. Answer B
Anti-CCP is the most specific autoantibody (rheumatoid factor is less specific), although a patient may be seronegative (i.e. not be positive for autoantibodies) but still have a clinical diagnosis of rheumatoid arthritis.

6. Answer B
Typical gout aspirates show needle-shaped negatively birefringent crystals.

7. Answer B
Osteoarthritis does tend to affect weight-bearing large joints but the carpometacarpal joint at the base of the thumb is also commonly affected. Patients with osteoarthritis do report joint stiffness but it is less prolonged. Activity makes the pain of osteoarthritis worse, hence the pain gets worse during the day.

Chapter 4: Connective tissue disorders and vasculitis

1. Answer A

A DEXA scan will give a baseline measurement of bone mineral density. This is useful as patients are potentially on steroids for 2 years. Isotope bone scans and PET scans may highlight areas of inflammation but this isn't necessary here. Shoulder and pelvis X-rays are likely to be normal or show background degenerative change. A temporal artery biopsy is only indicated if someone is reporting symptoms of temporal arteritis.

2. Answer C

Sunken or atrophic scars are a feature of classical Ehlers–Danlos syndrome. The other answers can be present in a diagnosis of joint hypermobility syndrome.

3. Answer D

All pregnant women should avoid non-steroidal anti-inflammatory medication, e.g. ibuprofen or naproxen. Patients with stable lupus do not need to be referred for specialist care when planning a family. Hydroxychloroquine is safe to continue during pregnancy. It would not be helpful to repeat an ANA screen.

4. Answer D

Patients with Sjögren's syndrome are at greater risk (5–9 times) of developing non-Hodgkin's lymphoma. Always suspect non-Hodgkin's lymphoma in a patient with Sjögren's who presents in this way. Check for lymphadenopathy during your physical examination.

5. Answer C

A malar rash is not a feature of scleroderma but would prompt you to consider a diagnosis of SLE.

6. Answer D

This is a presentation of sarcoidosis. Septic arthritis should be considered if a joint is swollen; although, with more than one joint affected, this is less likely.

7. Answer C

Anti-Jo-1 antibodies are often positive in cases of polymyositis. ANA may be positive but is less specific to polymyositis.

8. Answer E

For a diagnosis of antiphospholipid syndrome, one or more of the following antiphospholipid antibodies should be positive on two occasions at least 12 weeks apart:

- anti-cardiolipin antibodies
- lupus anticoagulant
- anti-beta2-glycoprotein 1

9. Answer D

SLE tends to cause a non-erosive arthropathy.

10. Answer A

Ferritin levels are markedly raised in patients with adult onset Still's disease.

Chapter 5: Metabolic bone disease

1. Answer D

Peak bone mass is usually reached in one's early 30s.

2. Answer A

Family history of osteoporosis. All other answers are protective factors.

3. Answer C

This is Paget's disease and ALP will be raised. Extra bone growth in Paget's can cause compression of peripheral nerves; in this instance the vestibulocochlear nerve is affected, causing tinnitus.

4. Answer E

It is preferable for a patient to take their calcium through their diet as it is well tolerated and reduces unnecessary medication. She is pre-menopausal so is still relatively protected by oestrogen effects on the bones. Bisphosphonates can affect foetal bone growth so are usually avoided if further pregnancies are planned. Other treatment should be reserved for when she has completed her family.

5. Answer C

There is little evidence for pharmaceutical intervention in osteoporosis due to eating disorders. He is yet to reach peak bone mass. The ideal treatment is therefore weight-bearing exercise and a balanced diet. It is worthwhile prescribing vitamin D if levels are low.

Chapter 6: Skeletal injuries and disorders

1. Answer B

The blood supply to the femoral head is likely to be intact following an extracapsular neck of femur fracture. Fixation rather than replacement of the femoral head preserves the patient's hip and has a low risk of avascular necrosis.

2. Answer D

A femoral fracture in a non-walking child is highly suspicious of NAI. Spiral fractures are more likely from a twisting mechanism rather than a direct impact. Birth injury is unlikely as the symptoms have been present for less than one week.

3. Answer E

Slipped capital femoral epiphysis (SCFE) is the most likely diagnosis. Fracture is unlikely from the mechanism of injury. Bone tumour, Perthes' and osteoarthritis are also unlikely as the pain had a sudden onset. Obesity is a risk factor for SCFE.

4. Answer E

Control of catastrophic bleeding is the first priority in the trauma patient. Applying a tourniquet will stem bleeding to preserve life. The next priority would be airway and C-spine protection.

5. Answer A

In a young patient intracapsular neck of femur fractures are often fixed to try to preserve the hip joint. There is a high risk of AVN due to blood supply disruption from the original intracapsular fracture. A missed fracture would have caused pain from the time of injury and

septic arthritis would have other systemic features. Although osteoarthritis and bone metastasis are possible, they are not the most likely cause.

6. Answer E

Risk factors for SCFE include being male, high BMI, growth spurts and hypothyroidism. A high TSH level would diagnose hypothyroidism. There is no genetic inheritance to test and serum electrophoresis is a test for bone marrow cancer and inflammatory diseases.

7. Answer E

The patient is haemodynamically unstable and due to the pain around his hip, has a suspected pelvic injury. The most appropriate step is to place a pelvic binder to reduce the pelvic volume. This could help stop bleeding in the pelvis. Stabilising the patient is the priority and other investigation can take place after this.

Chapter 7: Exercise-related injuries and soft tissue disorders

1. Answer C

A twisting injury with immediate swelling is pathognomonic of an ACL tear. Fracture is less likely, as he is able to weight-bear and the swelling associated with meniscal tears is not usually immediate. An MCL sprain is extra-articular and doesn't cause a significant effusion.

2. Answer D

Posterior shoulder dislocation is rare but more common after seizures. Radiographic findings are subtle and often missed. Frozen shoulder occurs over a period of weeks. Acromioclavicular joint dislocation does not affect external rotation. After anterior shoulder dislocation the arm is held in external rotation and internal rotation is inhibited.

3. Answer A

Fluoroquinolone antibiotics can precipitate tendon ruptures. Hypothyroidism, NSAIDs and thyroxine are not causes of tendon ruptures.

The mechanism of injury is not sufficient to solely cause a tendon rupture.

4. **Answer D**
A shoulder radiograph should be completed first, as this can diagnose common conditions such as OA and serious conditions such as bone metastases. An ultrasound and MRI would be useful to diagnose a rotator cuff tear; however, if the patient has OA it is unlikely you would perform a rotator cuff repair. You would not usually perform a shoulder injection without a recent radiograph, as in the unlikely event that there is primary bone cancer or osteomyelitis, you may inadvertently make the condition worse.

5. **Answer B**
Degenerative meniscal tears usually present after a minor knee twist. Swelling appears immediately in ACL tears and is uncommon in this age group, plus his drawer tests are stable. The patient is able to straight leg raise, confirming his patellar tendon is intact and his patella is not dislocated.

6. **Answer B**
The patient is likely to have a degenerative meniscal tear as a consequence of OA. A simple radiograph is likely to show OA and should be performed in the first instance. An MRI in this age group should not be a first-line investigation, as surgery for meniscal pathology is unlikely to be performed. There is no evidence to suggest septic arthritis and therefore a knee aspirate is not required. CT and USS are not first-line investigations.

7. **Answer B**
Golfer's elbow is tendinopathy of the flexor origin on the medial side of the elbow pain creases when the wrist is flexed. Tennis elbow and de Quervain's are tendinopathies of the extensor tendons. OA is likely to restrict movement and olecranon bursitis usually presents with swelling over the tip of the olecranon.

8. **Answer D**
A trigger digit is a fixed flexion of the finger which is sudden; it can often be straightened gently. Dupuytren's contracture and OA can cause fixed flexion but this comes on gradually over months to years and is permanent. Tendon ruptures would not cause a fixed deformity and the finger would have full passive range of movement.

Chapter 8: Infection

1. **Answer B**
This is clearly an infected joint due to the clinical symptoms and blood results, and should be proven on joint aspirate. Joint aspiration should be performed wherever possible before antibiotic therapy; this is to ensure that a sensitive narrow-spectrum antibiotic therapy is given. Antibiotics would be given first only if the patient was haemodynamically unstable.

2. **Answer A**
Calcium pyrophosphate is a crystal seen in pseudogout. Pseudogout can affect single or multiple joints. There may be a significantly raised WCC and CRP and systemic symptoms and confusion in the elderly. Chondrocalcinosis on the radiograph is pathognomonic of pseudogout.

3. **Answer D**
Osteomyelitis is the concern and therefore a simple radiograph could diagnose this. This would be the first step in the diagnostic pathway and it would also rule out other pathologies such as re-fracture. The blood results show an infected picture rather than one of deep vein thrombosis.

4. **Answer C**
Haematogenous spread from sharing of non-sterile contaminated needles or entry of bacteria through needle puncture through the skin into a vein is the most likely cause of the infection in her spine. Contiguous spread from other infections, such as endocarditis, is possible but heart sounds were normal with

no murmur. She has no direct history of being immunocompromised but sharing of needles should always prompt a thorough history of blood-borne viruses such as HIV.

5. **Answer A**
This infection is serious and occurred very fast and is likely to be a gas-forming organism. *Staphylococcus aureus* and MRSA do not normally cause such a severe deterioration. *Pseudomonas aeruginosa* is usually a colonising microbe on chronically infected wounds. *Mycobacterium tuberculosis* infections tend to cause "cold abscesses" and do not trigger acute inflammation.

6. **Answer B**
The patient is systemically unwell, and IV antibiotics should be given immediately without delay. This is likely to be a serious infection of the diabetic ulcer and surrounding soft tissues. Osteomyelitis should be considered.

7. **Answer C**
Strict log-roll and bed rest should be the first priority in order that no further damage is caused to the spinal cord. There is a potential for the spine to be unstable, as infection is present and neurological signs evident. All other steps can be undertaken once the patient is prevented from doing further damage.

8. **Answer B**
Staphylococcus aureus is the most common cause of septic arthritis.

Chapter 9: Spinal and peripheral nerve disorders

1. **Answer B**
The case presented is of carpal tunnel syndrome, which is likely to be caused by water retention in pregnancy. The symptoms are of short duration and not severe. She is due to deliver in the next couple of weeks, after which symptoms will hopefully then subside. First-line management should be night splints.

2. **Answer E**
The signs presented are of a L5 nerve root compression (lower motor neurone) which exits below the L4/5 disc. Cord compression would cause hyperreflexia (upper motor neurone). Although a common peroneal nerve compression and compartment syndrome would cause similar symptoms, you would expect a history of direct trauma to the nerve or calf.

3. **Answer E**
Hoffmann's positive sign is of an upper motor neurone lesion in the neck. C5 supplies the deltoid and outer aspect of the shoulder. Absent reflexes suggest a lower motor neurone lesion such as nerve root compression rather than cord compression.

4. **Answer C**
These are all the symptoms of a Brown-Séquard syndrome where half the cord is transection. As the spinothalamic tract crosses the midline at the level of the cord, pain and temperature are absent on the opposite side, whereas proprioception and vibration in the dorsal columns cross in the brainstem so are affected on the same side.

5. **Answer C**
Weakness in the arms and legs following trauma, no matter how trivial, should be suspected as a cervical spine injury. To prevent further damage to the cervical spine it should be immobilised. All other steps can be taken following this. Cervical traction is performed only in rare situations by experts and only following imaging to the C-spine.

Chapter 10: Tumours and malignancy

1. **Answer A**
High dose steroids are the most accessible treatment that will reduce swelling around the tumour site and reduce the compression on the spinal cord.

2. **Answer B**

In a patient with multiple myeloma, blood results will show anaemia, renal failure, hypercalcaemia and monoclonal gammopathy and paraproteinaemia on electrophoresis.

Chapter 11: Musculoskeletal emergencies

1. **Answer E**

This is temporal arteritis and a biopsy is the gold standard test, as the inflammatory cells can be seen in the vessel wall. ESR and CRP are almost certainly raised but not diagnostic. Fundoscopy is important to assess the effect on the optic disc but is not diagnostic.

2. **Answer C**

An urgent MRI scan is warranted, as clinical manifestations of cauda equina are present. This is to identify the cause of the compression and to plan urgent surgery. Radiographs will not show the spinal cord.

3. **Answer D**

The first management must be to release any pressure on the compartment and elevate to reduce swelling. This may be enough to prevent progression of compartment syndrome and avoid fasciotomy. Analgesia is important; however, there are already nerve symptoms, so action needs to be taken immediately.

4. **Answer C**

There is vascular compromise, so restoring the circulation is the first priority by manipulation and splinting. IV antibiotics, anti-tetanus, photographs and radiographs can be completed once circulation is restored.

5. **Answer D**

The patient has characteristic features of flexor sheath infection. Urgent surgical washout is the definitive management. Elevation, IV antibiotics and physiotherapy are important, but for the best outcome urgent surgical washout is needed to reduce the infection load.

Glossary

Actin	Smaller protein in muscle that binds to myosin in muscle contraction
Adaptive immunity	Specific, tailored immunity with memory
Angiogenesis	Formation of new blood vessels
Antigen	Something which is recognised by the immune system as foreign, leading to a response
Arthralgia	Painful joints
Arthritis mutilans	Severe inflammatory arthritis leading to collapsing of soft tissue and destruction of bone, resulting in telescoping of joints
Arthrocentesis	Removal of fluid from a joint, normally with a needle and syringe
Arthroscopy	Keyhole surgery in which a camera and instruments are put in the joint
Autonomic nervous system	Part of the peripheral nervous system that is controlled unconsciously, supplying the internal organs
Avascular necrosis	Abnormal bone resorption secondary to lack of blood supply to the bone, usually at the epiphysis
Axonotmesis	Nerve injury that results in damage to the myelin sheath; however, the neuron is intact
Bursitis	Inflammation of a bursa
Calcinosis	Calcium deposits in soft tissue
Carpal tunnel	A small tunnel in the wrist that is formed by the carpal bones and the transverse carpal ligament – it contains the median nerve which is compressed in carpal tunnel syndrome
Cauda equina	The terminal branches of the spinal cord from L1 to S5
Check rein	A restraint that prevents dislocation of a joint
Chondrocalcinosis	Calcium deposition in cartilage
Computerised tomography (CT)	Cross-sectional imaging using X-rays (ionising radiation)
Cortical bone	Thicker structural bone that surrounds the softer inner cancellous bone
Cubital tunnel	A tunnel at the medial elbow that contains the ulnar nerve
Dermatome	An area of skin that senses touch and is supplied by a single spinal nerve
Diaphysis	The central longitudinal part of the bone
Dorsal horn	Posterior part of the spinal cord that receives sensory information from the body
Dysphagia	Difficulty in swallowing

Dysphonia	Difficulty in speaking
Dysplasia	Abnormal cells
Effusion	Swelling within a joint
Endochondral ossification	Replacement of cartilage by bone during bone development
Endosteum	Inner vascular layer of a bone's diaphysis; supplies blood to the cortex from the inside (the main blood supply in adults)
Enthesitis	Inflammation where tendon or ligament inserts into bone
Epaxial	On the dorsum or the posterior part of the body
Epiphysis	Part of a long bone that is at either end of the bone and is within the joint
Epitope	The part of an antigen recognised by the immune system
Erythema nodosum	Raised red rash, usually on lower legs
Erythrocyte	Red blood cell that contains haemoglobin
Extracellular matrix	Non-cellular part of bone and cartilage that forms a 3D lattice structure – made from collagen and elastin fibres, as well as hyaluronic acid and proteoglycans such as keratin and chondroitin
Fibrocartilage	Strong and tough tissue that is made from elastin and collagen; usually holds together two joints very tightly
Fibrosis	Thickening of tissue in response to trauma/injury/inflammation
Gibbus	Kyphotic deformity of the spine (see Kyphosis)
Gram stain	Stain used to prepare microbiological specimens: Gram-positive organisms stain purple and Gram-negative organisms stain pink
Haematogenous	Carried by the blood
Haematopoiesis	Formation of blood cells from pluripotent cells
Haematoproteinuria	Blood and protein in the urine
Haplotype	A set of genetic variations that are inherited together
Haversian canal	Central part of an osteon that is occupied by longitudinal blood vessels that span the length of the bone
Human leucocyte antigen	Together with human major histocompatibility complex, HLA is an important protein for antigen presentation to the immune system
Hyaline cartilage	Smooth glass-like covering on synovial joints
Hypaxial	On the ventral or anterior part of the body
Iatrogenic	Injury or illness resulting from medical treatment
Immunoglobulin	Protein produced by plasma cells which bind to antigens and trigger an immune response
Innate immunity	Non-specific elements of the immune system (physical barriers and cells) which are the first line of defence
Intramembranous ossification	Bone that is formed directly without a cartilage precursor
Ischaemia	Loss of blood supply
Keratoconjunctivitis	Inflammation of the cornea and conjunctiva
Kyphosis	Excessive curvature of the spine which can result in a 'hunchback' appearance

Lamellar bone	Mature organised bone that has remodelled from woven bone, found in mature adult bone and remodelled fractures
Lower motor neurone lesion	A lesion in the peripheral nervous system characterised by weakness, hypotonia and reduced reflexes
Lymphocyte	A type of white blood cell
Magnetic resonance imaging (MRI)	Cross-sectional imaging formed using magnets
Malunion	A fracture that has healed with deformity
Metaphysis	Between the epiphysis and the diaphysis, this part of the bone is the most vascular and contains mostly cancellous bone
Metastatic	Distant spread of cancer
Microscopy	Microscopic assessment, usually of joint fluid, to determine presence of organisms, inflammatory cells or crystals
Mononeuritis multiplex	Isolated damage to different nerve sites
Myalgia	Muscle pain
Myelin	Insulation to peripheral neurons that is composed of fatty tissue
Myelocyte	A young granulocytic cell that can differentiate into a basophil, eosinophil or neutrophil
Myelopathy	Upper motor neurone syndrome secondary to spinal cord compression
Myosin	Large protein that gives muscle its red colour; binds to actin in muscle to initiate contraction
Myositis	Muscle inflammation
Myotome	The muscle group supplied by a single spinal nerve
Neurapraxia	A conduction block nerve injury; the nerve is structurally intact
Neurotmesis	Nerve injury in which the nerve has been cut and is not in continuity
Node of Ranvier	Part of the myelin sheath between two Schwann cells
Non-union	A fracture that has not healed
Normochromic	Normal amount of haemoglobin in each red blood cell
Normocytic	Normal-sized red blood cell
Osteoblast	A mononuclear cell that lays down bone matrix
Osteoclast	A multinuclear cell that resorbs bone
Osteocyte	A bone cell formed when an osteoblast becomes encased in the bone it secretes
Osteon	Longitudinal cylindrical channels within the bone that are formed by layers of lamellae and osteocytes
Pannus	An abnormal area of inflammatory tissue which covers the joint in rheumatoid arthritis
Paraneoplastic syndrome	A set of symptoms caused by a cancer releasing molecules which can affect distant sites
Parasympathetic	Unconscious control (see Autonomic) responsible for 'rest and digest'

Periosteum	Thick covering that surrounds the cortex of the bone in the diaphysis; it is the main blood supply to bone in children
Physis (growth plate)	Between the epiphysis and the metaphysis, it is where longitudinal growth occurs in children
Pott's paralysis	Spinal cord compression secondary to TB infection of the vertebrae
Radiculopathy	Lower motor neurone syndrome secondary to compression of a spinal nerve
Radiograph	A plane image formed by X-rays passing through the body; formed on a sensitive plate
Reiter's disease	A particular presentation of reactive arthritis with conjunctivitis and urethritis
Rigor	Uncontrolled shaking, usually of the arms secondary to a fever
Sacroiliitis	Inflammation of the sacroiliac joint
Saltatory conduction	Propagation of the action potential by jumping from node of Ranvier to node of Ranvier
Sarcomere	Subunit in striated muscle
Sarcoplasmic reticulum	A membrane that surrounds striated muscle; it stores calcium
Schwann cell	A nerve (glial) cell of the peripheral nervous system that wraps around the neuron to form the myelin sheath
Sequestrum	Dead bone secondary to infection
Sicca	Dry eyes and mouth
Spondyloarthritis	Inflammatory arthritis of the spine
Sympathetic nervous system	Unconscious control (see Autonomic) responsible for 'fight or flight' response
Syndesmosis	A fibrous joint held by a strong ligament between two bones
Synovium	The soft tissue inner lining of a synovial joint capsule
Tenosynovitis	Inflammation of the fluid-filled sheath around the tendon
Trabecular or cancellous bone	Soft non-structural central part of the bone found in the metaphysis
Upper motor neurone lesion	A lesion in the central nervous system characterised by weakness, spasticity and brisk reflexes
Uveitis	Inflammation of the middle layer of the eye
Valgus	Deformity in which the most distal part of the limb is deviated away from the midline
Varus	Deformity in which the most distal part of the limb is deviated towards the midline
Ventral horn	Anterior part of the spinal cord that delivers motor information to the muscles
Volkmann's canal	Transmits blood in a transverse direction between the periosteum and the Haversian blood channels, which transmit blood longitudinally
Woven bone	Immature disorganised bone that is quickly formed in children and the first part of fracture healing
Xerophthalmia	Dry eyes/reduced tears
Xerostomia	Dry mouth/reduced saliva

Index

Bold indicates main entries